Praise for Homeopath

"As a mom of two toddlers in daycare, they have experienced many illnesses. As soon as we recover from one cold, another is closely following. After my youngest had the flu, three cases of strep, and a recurring ear infection, unhealthy was our new "normal." I felt helpless, suppressing one of my daughter's symptoms after another. Finding homeopathy has helped restore the health of my family. I now have a toolbox that helps my daughter's body address her symptoms and work through them, strengthening her immune system instead of suppressing it. After learning about and using homeopathy, my family has significantly reduced our trips to the doctor and our use of pharmaceuticals."

—Meg S., Mom of Two

"I began using homeopathy when my children were babies. I sought out a homeopath at the time as I was very disillusioned with what mainstream medicine was offering, seeing it as not effective nor safe. That one choice alone changed my life and the life of my family. Not only did I have treatments I felt good about using (and that worked!), the experience taught me how to be a brave detective when it came to illness. It was deeply empowering to be able to look at symptoms as important clues about what was happening and what was needed. I never once ended up in the ER or having to take an emergency visit to a doctor because I was able to treat my family and myself through the use of homeopathy, and the other alternative treatments I was discovering. Beyond the resolution of any illness or condition, using homeopathy taught me how to look at the body in a different way. As opposed to fearing what it was doing, I learned of its brilliance and of the possibility for health when I was willing to learn from what it was doing. Homeopathy is truly the medicine of the people; being a direct route to gaining greater states of health as well as powerful agency over your life and the life of your family."

—Susan M., Founder of The Healer Within

"I love homeopathy and learning everything about it. I have used it successfully to support many acute conditions for my children, myself and my husband. We haven't taken an OTC (over-the-counter) medication in almost 10 years. At the top of my travel packing list is my remedy kit. It comes with me everywhere, so I'm never caught unprepared to help. I love my little remedies and so does my entire family!"

—Rania M., Mother of Three and lover of anything non-traditional

"Homeopathy has helped me in ways that conventional or herbal medicine has not. I started using homeopathic remedies 35 years ago when I was first introduced to them. Years ago, they helped eliminate a supposedly "incurable" viral infection, and since then have helped restore me to functioning in many ways, most recently in bladder and prostate health, when doctors offered me only surgery and herbal remedies stopped being effective."

—Jan K., Retired Land Surveyor

"After years of working on healing my chronic fatigue syndrome and fibromyalgia with herbs, vitamins, eating very clean, no more toxic chemicals, and still not feeling 100%, a friend had a nurse who turned her on to homeopathic cell salts, and that is what turned me into a huge learner, utilizer, seeker, and helping others know about homeopathy. It is becoming a passion for me. I have helped relatives and friends, and now through that enthusiasm, others have wanted to try it too. And now they are devoted as well. I can't possibly know enough, but by practice I am becoming familiar with the remedies."

—Ameena J., Licensed Massage Therapist, Reiki Master Teacher

"I often use homeopathic remedies if I feel a cold coming on. I'll buy remedies over the counter and they seem to help with congestion, sore throat and tiredness. It's an easy and safe way to take control of my health."

—Bonnie D., Acupuncturist

"Homeopathy came into my life after the birth of my 2nd child though it actually started with my firstborn in 1976 when I went to a study group on homeopathy. I began to use the remedies and have right up to now. I used them on all 5 of my children, on myself, on my foster children and now my adopted children. My grandchildren take homeopathy for common ailments. I took remedies when I fractured my whole leg and for teeth loosened from chemo and radiation. I believe every family needs to have a kit in their home."

—Michelle R., Foster Parent/Retired

"I first utilized homeopathy over 40 years ago when my son had chronic upper respiratory infections and allergies that continued to worsen from the overuse of prescription medicines. At that time the homeopath was able to gradually improve his overall health until these conditions diminished. After experiencing these results and understanding the safe effectiveness of this medicine I continue utilizing them for myself and family with evidence-based results."

—Susan K., Parent

"After my daughter had a major medical incident, in a fall she fractured a bone in her foot and had some massive bruising. Once we knew the bone was properly set, we used a remedy specific for healing the bones and the x-ray technicians could not even find where the bone was fractured. We used Arnica for the massive bruising and were amazed at how quickly the deep, deep bruising healed."

—Pat B., Grateful Mom

"Five years ago, during high pollen spring, I wanted to scratch my eyes out of my head. My eyes were so itchy, burning, and watery— I was so miserable and needed relief. Never had I had such bad eye allergies, even my eye doctor's recommendations weren't working. I ended up taking a remedy for my eye symptoms and a miracle happened quickly. I occasionally in the spring and fall have a minor flare up and generally one dose of the remedy does the trick."

— Patricia B., Small Business Owner

"We started homeopathy about 30 years ago when my pediatrician could not help with my breathing issues, homeopathy was the only thing to get me off my inhaler. We now choose homeopathy for our children because it works like magic when you use the correct remedy! Our Naturopathic Doctor has always helped us in finding the correct remedy for our children and when our 6-year-old was hospitalized for not being able to catch his breath the only thing that worked was the remedy we were prescribed by her. We did not have to use any "modern" medicine after he took the remedy, and he has not needed his inhaler ever since (it's been over a year)."

—Chrissie A., Mother of Three

"I am a registered nurse. About 30 years ago I turned to homeopathy for my young daughter who was struggling with asthma. Her pediatrician was unable to alleviate her severe symptoms without causing horrible side effects from the asthma medications. After dozens of trips to the ER in the middle of the night I knew I had to find something else to help her. I lived in the same town as my naturopath/homeopath and heard so many good things about her practice. I was skeptical at first because of my medical background but I immediately changed my mind when I witnessed how quickly homeopathy healed my daughter. I continue to see my naturopath for homeopathic treatment of my medical issues. My daughter and her entire family also enjoy their health care through her practice."

—Lorry B., Retired RN

"I chose homeopathy as a last resort when I found mainstream medical care was failing me. Medications and side effects were making my general health worse instead of better. I started with my naturopath and homeopathy 34 years ago. With homeopathy I felt my body was being supported and allowing itself to heal naturally. I find it balances me and keeps me healthy in body and mind. Allopathic medicine has its place in the medical world. However, I first turn to homeopathic remedies, and I find I very seldom have to resort to pharmaceutical medications. For me, homeopathy works amazingly!"

—Ann M.

"I have been benefiting from homeopathic treatment for over 30 years with a Naturopath. It has been a very beneficial journey. To have a good homeopathic doctor is like having a good treatment friend who understands my therapeutic needs and helps to meet them. It also helps me to understand my own body. Working as an attorney can be stressful on so many levels. Many times, over the years I have been able to describe my feelings and the treatment has been perfect to change my feelings for the better. There is just nothing else like it as far as I am concerned."

—Evans J., Attorney

"I began using homeopathy after suffering hot flashes (during menopause) once every five minutes, around the clock, for over 14 months. Someone introduced me to a homeopathic remedy and said, "at the start of the next hot flash, put two pellets under your tongue." About two minutes later, the hot flash started, I put the two pellets under my tongue, and within three seconds the hot flash had stopped. I had another one about three hours later, repeated the dose, and the hot flash stopped. Four days later, I had another one, took two tablets, it stopped. I haven't had once since - it's been 10 years. - (Note: a few months later I learned about a homeopathy school, went to it, and became a homeopath!)"

—Connie W., Massage Therapist

"I have had kidney stones due to a malformed kidney, which has sent me to the emergency room many times. It was recommended that I have surgery to remove my kidney. A friend suggested I try homeopathic treatment with a homeopath who was new in town. After visiting my homeopathic practitioner, I took the prescribed homeopathic treatment she recommended for me. This was on a Saturday. The very next day I painlessly passed a lot of small stones. I still get recurrences at times. I use the treatments, and the stones go away without any pain or medical intervention. I have been able to prevent hospital trips on several occasions."

—Twila, Registered Nurse

"I was in great discomfort with urinary infections and a urologist told me I had a "wrinkle" in my urethra. I looked into homeopathic solutions and finding a local homeopathic practitioner has been a tremendous asset to healing, not only complete physical healing of the "wrinkle", but mental and emotional healing as well. What I found in homeopathy was a very comprehensive, systematic inquiry into my past, present, and future - much more so than 'medical' information. I personally feel better using homeopathic treatments because they are much more attuned to what my body needs to function well. I plan to continue with homeopathic treatment as often as possible!"

—Lou, Retired Priest

"Using homeopathy taught me so much. I feel closer to my daughter and have learned to better understand her needs by being in tune with things like her moods, temperature, and discomforts. Whether it is a cold or the stomach flu, I am a more confident mom that I can use homeopathy effectively and alleviate her suffering."

—Kristine, Mom from Boulder, Colorado

"Homeopathy came into my life 4 years ago when I was seeking help for mental/emotional balance. I can attest that finding my homeopathic constitutional remedy was a key factor in supporting inner balance. It works with my pups too! One has a big ego, and his remedy calms him down. The other has a chronic back issue, homeopathic remedies give her relief."

—Marilyn M.

"I love the benefits of homeopathy because it's so individualized to one's lifestyle. It's natural healing and I love how simple remedies helped me heal from the flu and long-haul symptoms. The remedies I used helped me sleep better, relieve congestion and anxiety. Remedies can be tailored with different strengths and combinations to deliver healing benefits. I am so grateful to have found homeopathy."

—Renee B., RN, Holistic Esthetician

"Conventional health care has me feeling confused, frustrated and doubtful. My anxiety had been screaming at me and I needed something that could help ease this discomfort. I started to work with a Homeopath, and I am learning more about homeopathic remedies. I find homeopathy is not a cookie cutter medicine, rather highly individualized. Using these remedies are helping me find the balance and comfort my body needs."

—Nicole C., Busy Mom of 2 Boys

"I became interested in Homeopathy after I was referred to a homeopath as a way to improve my everyday health after being diagnosed with a chronic illness. I wanted to move away from traditional medications and the side effects that come with them. Since then I have joined a monthly homeopathy study group where I am learning to feel empowered by giving myself remedies for muscle aches, an occasional sore throat, stomach ailments, seasonal allergies, and cold symptoms. I'm looking forward to learning more in this book!"

—Paula M., Medical Coder

"Homeopathy has been used in my family since 1982, when my children were young, all 5 of them with wonderful results. Now my grandchildren take remedies instead of over the counter medicine, Gentle natural healing, I also used Homeopathy with teens where I was a house mom for teen shelter and with children in my care when I was a foster parent."

—Michelle R., Foster Mom of 5 + Teen Shelter House Mom

"Homeopathy has truly transformed my body health. I was feeling sluggish, tired and gaining weight while on several medications for health issues including high blood pressure and diabetes. Thanks to my homeopath's regime, I am off all medications, with very healthy numbers and I've even lost close to 20 pounds".

—Loriann J., Grandmother and Mother

HOMEOPATHY PRIMER

Getting Started with Homeopathy

A Study Guide, Learning Resource
and Reference Tool

Created by Abby Beale, CCH, RSHom (NA)
Compiled by Homeopathy Educator Press
Foreword by Shelley Keneipp, MH, DiHom (UK),
author of *The Parent's Guide to Homeopathy*

Published by
Homeopathy Educator Press
Wallingford, Connecticut
hello@homeopathyprimer.com

First Edition, 2024.

ISBN: 978-0-9745928-4-8

Cover and Interior Design: Karolina Wudniak, www.karolinawudniak.com

Images: iStock, Shutterstock, Pexels, Pixabay, Unsplash, Wikimedia Commons.
Icons: Rafiico Creative/CC BY 4.0, Font Awesome/CC BY 4.0, and Karolina Wudniak.

Contents

Foreword

It was 1986. My daughter was 12 years old and just entering puberty. Her emotions were all over the place and she was struggling. I walked into Santa Monica Drugstore in Santa Monica, California. Little did I know, this was a homeopathic pharmacy founded in 1944. It still exists to this day. It's "a small family business dedicated to serving the health needs of our community" as is stated on their website. The owner, a sweet elderly woman, asked if I needed help. I asked her to help me better understand what homeopathy was. I then explained what my daughter was going through. After asking me a ton of questions, she handed me a remedy called ***Pulsatilla***. The changes I saw my daughter go through were astounding. She became balanced, grounded, centered, and happy once again.

Years later, I had an opportunity to take a class from a homeopath who was teaching moms how to use homeopathy for their children. From then on, I used homeopathy for my two daughters and our family. I later decided to become a homeopath and did most of my training with two British Homeopaths, Colin Griffith and the late Martin Miles. After practicing for a while, I wanted to share what I knew and wrote a book, *The Parents Guide To Homeopathy: Safe, Natural Remedies For Children From Newborns Through Teens.*

Today, we are now living in an era where alternative healthcare modalities are growing by leaps and bounds. There are an increasing number of Americans who want to be more self-sufficient and to take back some of their responsibility for caring for themselves and their families. Parents are now wanting to learn how to deal with acute conditions and first aid situations that arise with their families.

As healthcare costs continue to rise out of control, Americans are realizing they don't need or want to run to the doctor for every little thing. We are seeing a return to the valuable heritage of knowing how to handle these acute situations at home, just like many of our grandmothers and great-grandmothers knew. Americans are turning to home remedies and finding that Aunt Gloria's natural remedies actually work quite well.

No one knows better than a mom what is needed for an ailing child. Homeopathy has proven itself as a practical, safe, and effective tool for ongoing good family health.

In Colonial American times, for the people traveling West on the wagon trains, homeopathy played a very big part in helping to stay healthy. Not every wagon train had a doctor, nor were there many doctors out west. In the 1860s, many wagon trains departed from Saint Louis, Missouri. There was a homeopathic pharmacy, Luyties, where people bought homeopathic kits and a book, *The Homeopathic Physician*, by Constantine Hering, MD (the father of United States homeopathy) to help guide them. In June of 1900, a statue was erected and still stands in Washington D.C. of Samuel Hahnemann, to commemorate the founder of Homeopathy (see photo on page 23).

For over 230 years, homeopathy has proven itself to be the most gentle, natural and safe medicine. People who use homeopathy are amazed at how quickly their symptoms can be resolved with a good remedy.

Homeopathy is a health care system using natural remedies made from plants, minerals, animals and elements from the periodic table. The remedies are prepared in high dilutions which make them safe, gentle, non-toxic, with no side effects. It is a healing system that is used throughout the majority of countries around the globe where homeopathic hospitals, pharmacies, and scores of homeopathic clinics exist.

This book is a vision of homeopath Abby Beale. Her vision has brought together over 35 experienced users including homeopaths, student homeopaths and home users to work together in a collaborative way to produce this guide. Her passion and devotion to homeopathy has produced a real masterpiece. And her great foresight has brought together some of the best in our homeopathic community to produce what will probably go down in history as a "homeopathic classic". This guide is a valuable option for American and other international consumers to use in their everyday life for year after year. It can be used by many including moms, dads, caregivers, nurses, physician assistants and doctors as well.

You hold in your hands a guide which will cover many acute conditions that might arise in an average household. It is comprehensive and well organized. You will learn how to deal with these conditions and get satisfactory results with no further outside interventions. This guide covers many common acute conditions that arise from birth through adulthood. It explains in a "user-friendly" way, just what you need to know in a clear and concise manner. You will find yourself becoming empowered and more confident in the use of homeopathy as you embrace its use. There are also clear, practical, and invaluable guidelines for how to care for a sick person, or when to seek care from your health care provider, or when to go to the emergency room. I am grateful this is getting out in the world.

Wishing you all the best of health and great success with your use of homeopathy!

Shelley Keneipp, MH, DiHom(UK)

About the Contributors

This book has been created by 35 volunteers who believe that homeopathy is the smartest medicine on the planet and want others to know about it! The list of contributors below consist of practicing homeopaths, naturopaths, nurses, student homeopaths, parents and other experienced homeopathic consumers who spent many hours either writing, editing or proofreading this manuscript. It has been a labor of love from every single one of them, to you!

A HEARTFELT THANK YOU TO ALL OF THESE WONDERFUL CONTRIBUTORS:

Shahin Afnan, Dip Hom, CCT

Barbara W. Baxter, M. Mus., M. Div.

Abby Beale, CCH, RSHom (NA)

Loretta Butehorn, PhD, RSHom (NA), FSHom

Sally E. Carlson, CA-All lines

Martha DeMarco, CCH, RSHom (NA)

Claire Dishman, CCH, RSHom (NA)

Jacquelynne R. Featherly, CCH, RSHom (NA), CN, MIFHI

Sefira Fialkoff, MS—International Development

Michelle S. Fielding, CCH

Tara Framer, CCH

Isabel Frankel, CCH

Faythe E. Goldman, BFCP, CCT

Irene Gomulka

Catherine (Casey) Hammond, RN

Robbin Howard

Zelda L. Johnson, DNMc, MAHAS, MSPH

Shelley Keneipp, MH, DiHom (UK)

Mr. Vijay Kumar

Julie Mann, CCH, RSHom (NA)

Dr. Nancy A. Mazur, ND

Holly Milton-Benoit

Dale C. Moss, MA

Carole Neary, DHom, MA, HMC, CHP, CEASE

Sujata Owens, CCH, RSHom (NA), DHMS (India), BSc (India)

Dor Remsen, BS, MEd

Tanya Renner, CCH, RSHom (NA), NBC-HWC

Frank Russo, RN, FNP, IACH (Diploma), CCH

Kausar Saiyed

Erika Simonian, CCH

Helen Tye Talkin, Ph.D

Vera Volfson, CCH, RSHom (NA)

Heather Welch-Smith, CCH

Connie J. Wehmeyer, LMT

Kristina M White, CCH

Cheryl Wood, CCH, RSHom (NA), C.HP

Glossary of credential abbreviations:

BFCT: Bach Flower Certified Practitioner

BS, MEd: Bachelor of Science, Master of Education

BSc: Bachelor of Science

CA-All Lines: Licensed Casualty Adjuster

CCH: Certified Classical Homeopath

CCT/CEASE: Certified CEASE Therapist, CEASE: Complete Elimination of Autism Spectrum Expression

CHP/C.HP: Certified Homeoprophylaxis Practitioner

CN: Certified Naturopath

DHMS/Dip Hom: Diploma in Homeopathic Medicine

DNMc: Doctorate Studies in Natural Medicine

DHom/DHom (UK): Degree in Homeopathy/Degree in Homeopathy from the United Kingdom

FNP: Family Nurse Practitioner

FSHome: Fellow of the Society of Homeopaths

HMC: Homeopath Master Clinician

IACH (Diploma): International Academy of Classial Homeopathy, Diploma

MA: Master of Arts

MAHAS: Masters in Health Arts and Science

M.Div: Masters in Divinity

MH: Master Homeopath

MIFHI: Masters of the Institute For Human Individuality

M.Mus: Master of Music

MS: Masters of Science Degree

MSPH: Master of Science in Public Health

NBC-HWC: National Board Certified Health and Wellness Coach

ND: Naturopathic Doctor

RSHom (NA): Registered member of the North American Society of Homeopaths

Some extra special THANK YOU's go out to:

- **Shelley Keneipp,** MH, DiHom (UK), the author of *The Parent's Guide to Homeopathy*, who shared ALL her work with us and allowed us to use pertinent material from her book. She also personally shared her expertise and contributed to MANY chapters of this book.

- **Faythe E. Goldman** who was our Project Administrator and was the important glue sticking the pieces together! She has been very generous with her time and sharing of her expertise.

- **Tanya Renner** for creating the **Introduction to Cell Salts** chapter.

- **Kristina White** of www.YourLifeandLand.com for creating the **Homeopathy for Pets and Plants** chapter.

- **Sally Carlson, Robbin Howard, Dale Moss, Connie Weymeyer,** and **Cheryl Wood** for sharing a lot of their time and expertise in either the writing, editing and/or reviewing.

- **Abby Beale,** the Managing Editor of this guide, who saw the need for this educational book and did what was needed to get it done.

ABOUT HOMEOPATHY EDUCATOR PRESS

Homeopathy Educator LLC managing member is **Abby Beale, CCH, RSH(om)NA**. She saw a need for this guide years ago and has worked hard and smart to get it out into the world. It is under this legal entity that this project has come to fruition with the talented help of many volunteer contributors.

Abby is offering an **affiliate opportunity** to anyone interested in sharing this book with others while earning a commission for their efforts. See www.HomeopathyPrimer.com for more information.

Though Homeopathy Educator LLC is a for-profit entity, Abby is planning to share excess revenues, after reasonable expenses, equally among the current existing homeopathic associations in the United States. See list in **Appendix 4—Additional Resources** on **page 350**.

About Abby Beale, CCH, RSHom (NA)

Abby Beale is a nationally certified classical homeopath and gifted homeopathic educator. She believes that homeopathy is the coolest medicine on the planet and thoroughly enjoys sharing it with others. She has formally been studying homeopathy since 2003 and enjoys the continuous learning the profession requires. Abby runs an informal introductory session called Tea with a Homeopath, offers educational webinars and study groups.

In her earlier life as a speed reading and learning expert, she has authored *10 Days to Faster Reading, The Complete Idiot's Guide to Speed Reading, Speed Reading: A Little-Known Time-Saving Superpower* and *Success Skills: Strategies for Study and Lifelong Learning.*

Why this book was created

Becoming an effective home prescriber of homeopathic medicine is a learned skill that combines knowing about homeopathy and how it works, honed observation skills for effective case-taking and personal experience using the remedies. This homeopathy primer was created to help its readers develop a practical understanding and experience of homeopathy, including how to use it for themselves and their families, and how to treat minor accidents and illnesses at home. We hope that this book will not only be used by an individual, but by groups of moms, dads, caretakers, etc. looking to incorporate homeopathic medicine into their healthcare toolbox. We also hope experienced homeopaths, interested medical professionals and other holistic health providers will use this to increase their knowledge about treating acute illnesses while teaching and spreading the word about homeopathy to others.

What to know about using this book

We want you to know there are many ways to use homeopathy and knowing what resources you have at your fingertips will make it even more useful. Here's what you need to know:

- The information presented in this book is meant as a study guide, learning reference and resource tool to be used alongside many of the more common remedies found in 30c homeopathic kits, sold by homeopathic pharmacies, manufacturers, and distributors in the United States as well as some others worldwide. With the ever-changing landscape of homeopathic remedy manufacturers, we have found - at the time of publication - that the **Blue Helios Basic 36 Remedy Kit in 30c potency** is a gold standard to start with. It's available directly from Helios in the UK or on Amazon and a few other purveyors. In addition to these kits' contents, there are more common remedies available through your local health food stores and online sellers like Amazon and Boiron. It's a good idea to connect with your local health food store to make sure they have a chosen remedy in stock before venturing out. For a list of homeopathic pharmacies, see **Appendix 4—Additional Resources** on **page 348**.

- Remedies can be known by different names or spellings. You will find the complete reference chart in **Appendix 2—Remedy Name Chart** on **page 327**.

- You will know easily if a mentioned remedy is in the **Helios Basic 36 Remedy Kit** in 30c potency or not:

  - If there is no marking next to a remedy name, this indicates it is found in the **Helios Basic 36 Remedy Kit** in 30c potency (see the list of 36 remedies in the kit in **Appendix 2—Remedy Name Chart** on **page 327**).
  - If you see an asterisk next to a remedy name such as *Cocculus or *Zingiber, it means it is NOT in the Helios kit but will most likely be found at a local store or online.

- You will see some kits available online in 200c potency or combination 30c and 200c. We discourage novice prescribers from using 200c potencies as they are meant for more experienced prescribers and professional homeopaths. The only exceptions are using a few doses of Arnica 200c after a serious injury or surgery, or taking Thuja 200c if you experience a strong reaction after a vaccine. No other dosing in 200c is advocated in this book until you are more experienced.

- Every discipline has its own vocabulary and homeopathy isn't any different. In the first few chapters, you'll read about **What Everyone Needs to Know About Homeopathy** and **Taking the Case and Giving the Remedy**. These will provide a solid basis for you to proceed with your homeopathic learning. Additionally we have compiled **A Glossary of Homeopathic and Clinical Terminology** found in **Appendix 3** starting on **page 331**. We encourage you to reference it as often as you need when you come across an unfamiliar word or concept.

- To help you learn the essence of the remedies, we suggest you have a blank notebook or create a computer file where you can create your own "materia medica", or list of remedies and their uses. This is a wonderful way of deepening your understanding. As you learn about a remedy, you can fill in the areas listed below or create any other categories that you come up with that are useful to remember from your experience of using the remedies, the keynotes, or most frequently seen symptoms.

  - The location(s) the symptoms are usually seen
  - The sensations or what the symptom feels like
  - The modalities or what makes the person better or worse
  - The causes or aetiology of the symptom
  - The affinities or what it could be used for
  - The concomitants or symptoms that occur at the same time as the main complaint
  - Your experience using this remedy - give the case notes and reactions

- Inside the chapters you will find many remedy suggestions, either compared in charts or in text, along with their unique characteristics needed for choosing a good remedy. Additionally, you will see these helpful sections:

  - **It's an Emergency When** will help you know when to call for help to get local emergency services. For the convenience of this North American published book, we suggest calling 911 but please use your own country's emergency service number. Sometimes in the book, you'll also see recommended remedies to give on the way to the hospital.
  - **Additional Support** which includes other non-homeopathic ways you can support the person with their symptoms.
  - **When to Contact Your Healthcare Professional** helps you know when you need to look for help from a healthcare provider or professional homeopath.

- At the end of every chapter, you will be challenged to respond to "What's the first remedy to think of when…". This will help reinforce some of the remedies learned in the chapter. Know that there are certainly other choices to be made but the answers to this activity provide a good starting point to manage the symptom. The answer key is located in **Appendix 1—What's the First Remedy Answer Key** starting on **page 323**.

- There are many wonderful **Additional Resources** shared in **Appendix 4** starting on **page 345**.

- **Appendix 5—Bibliographic Resources** lists all the resources used in creating this guide on **page 351**.

- For easy referencing, see **Index** starting on **page 353**.

Suggested Starter Books

Homeopathy: Beyond Flat Earth Medicine, Dr. Timothy Dooley, MD, ND, available online at no cost or in bound form through online booksellers.

Homeopathy: Start Here, Ann Jerome PhD, CCH, available through Amazon in both paperback and Kindle editions.

The Parent's Guide to Homeopathy, Shelley Keneipp, MH, DiHom (UK), available through the author's website www.LifelongHomeopathy.com.

Additionally, there is a list of more practical reference books located in **Appendix 4—Additional Resources** starting on **page 345**.

CHAPTER 1
What Everyone Needs to Know About Homeopathy

> **Quote from *The Organon*:**
>
> "In the state of health, the spirit-like vital force (dynamis) animating the material human organism reigns in supreme sovereignty. It maintains the sensations and activities of all the parts of the living organism in a harmony that obliges wonderment. The reasoning spirit who inhabits the organism can thus freely use this healthy living instrument to reach the lofty goal of human existence."
>
> —*Aphorism 9, by Samuel Hahnemann, Founder of Homeopathy*

Welcome to the amazing world of homeopathy! As in all disciplines, there is a specific language and vocabulary that describes homeopathy. Getting familiar with the terms is a key part of understanding this discipline. In this chapter, note that the bold terms are defined in more detail in Appendix 3—Glossary of Homeopathic and Clinical Terminology starting on page 331.

WHAT IS HOMEOPATHY?

Homeopathy is a safe, gentle, and natural system of healing that works with your body to relieve symptoms, restore function, and improve one's overall health. It is a science of healing which stimulates and strengthens the **vital force** using the energy of highly diluted substances found in nature. Homeopathic products are called **remedies**. These remedies can assist the body in restoring its healthy balance and stimulating the self-healing process into action. When a remedy is chosen and taken, it is absorbed into the body and permeates all body systems. The body receives the message from the similar energy pattern that exists in the homeopathic remedy. The person receives a little bit of the same energy but on a subtle level. It acts as a healing stimulus to the body allowing the **vital force** to find its **homeostasis** or balance.

The word **homeopathy** comes from the Greek words *homoios* and *patheia*, which translates into "similar suffering." In 1796, a German doctor, Samuel Hahnemann, based his approach to healing on the principle of the **Law of Similars** (also referred to as "like cures like" described in the following section) and thus, homeopathy was born. He wrote his philosophies about health and healing in a book that has become the basis for homeopathy, *The Organon*. *The Organon* itself is not a quick read but recommended for serious students looking to gain a better understanding of this amazing healing modality.

THE THREE BASIC TENETS OF HOMEOPATHY

These are the three basic tenets of homeopathy:

- **The Law of Similars**: "Similia Similibus Curentur," literally means, "likes are cured by likes." This means that a material substance that is capable of producing certain symptoms in a healthy person can also remove, ameliorate, or alleviate these symptoms in an ill person when the same substance is given as a homeopathic remedy.

- **The Minimum Dose/Potentization**: This theory is the idea that only the smallest amount of substance that will bring about healing should be used. To minimize side effects and create gentler medicines, Samuel Hahnemann developed a process known as "potentization," by which all homeopathic remedies are made. It is a series of **dilutions and successions** that require striking the bottle repeatedly against a hard surface (such as a leather bound book or the palm of the hand) which causes vigorous shaking.

- **The Single Remedy**: This theory is the idea that only one homeopathic remedy be given at a time, so the results can be assessed without any confusion. Even if you have several symptoms in different parts of your body such as a headache, diarrhea and a skin rash, a single remedy would be used to help you recover from all of these symptoms.

HERING'S "LAW OF CURE"

Constantine Hering, a German homeopath who emigrated to the U.S. in the 1830's, observed that healing occurs in a consistent pattern. He described this pattern in the form of three basic laws which homeopaths can use to evaluate and recognize that healing is occurring. This pattern has been recognized by acupuncturists for hundreds of years and is also used by practitioners of herbalism and other healing disciplines:

- Hering's First Law – Healing progresses from the deepest part of the organism (from the mental and emotional levels and the vital organs) to the external parts (skin and extremities).

- Hering's Second Law — As healing progresses, symptoms appear and disappear in the reverse order of their original appearance. Homeopaths have consistently observed that their patients re-experience symptoms from past conditions.

- Hering's Third Law — Healing progresses from the upper to the lower parts of the body. For instance, a person is considered to be on the mend if the arthritic pain in his neck has decreased, although he now has pain in his finger joints.

- Hering's Law is used more frequently to assess chronic symptoms. When trying to apply Hering's Law for an acute situation, the symptom's progress may sometimes be too rapid to notice.

WHAT ARE HOMEOPATHIC REMEDIES MADE FROM?

Homeopathic medicines, known as "remedies," are mostly made from natural sources (e.g., plants, minerals, and animals), and are environmentally friendly. The substances used to prepare homeopathic remedies include but are not limited to:

- plants (e.g., wolf's bane, deadly nightshade, dandelion, plantain)

- elements of the periodic table (e.g., gold, iron, phosphorus, hydrogen)

- minerals (e.g., iron phosphate, arsenic oxide, sodium chloride)

- microbes, bacteria, viruses (e.g., flu virus)

- animal products (e.g., insects such as honeybees, the venom from poisonous snakes, the ink of the cuttlefish)

- **sarcodes and nosodes** that are made from healthy and diseased tissues and hormones (e.g. **Thyroidinum** (thyroid tissue) and **Folliculinum** (estrogen))

There are even a few homeopathic remedies prepared from chemical drug substances such as penicillin or streptomycin. All remedies are substantially diluted, so that it is a healing substance rather than the poisonous or toxic substance it would be in its undiluted material state.

Many of the remedies being used today were the same ones used 200 years ago. New ones are being proven and added all the time to broaden the scope of possible treatment. You might be interested to know that remedies are tested on healthy adults, not animals.

Note: For the purposes of this book, the remedy suggestions will focus mainly on those remedies found in a basic remedy kit or available for order from a homeopathic pharmacy. **Sarcodes and nosodes** are not found over-the-counter and are used primarily by professional homeopathic practitioners.

HOW SAFE IS HOMEOPATHY?

Since most homeopathic remedies are devoid of chemical toxicity, homeopathy is one of the safest modalities of healing. It is an ideal system of healing for people of all ages, even the most sensitive such as an expectant mother or a newborn baby.

Homeopathic remedies in **potency scales** above 8X or 4c have an extremely low risk of side effects and no known medical or drug contraindications. The labeling of lower **potency** products that might cause concern provide appropriate warning. Some homeopathic products are restricted to homeopathic professional's use only and not for sale to the general public to ensure they are used properly.

Remedies can be safely taken alongside other conventional medications and are sometimes recommended to complement other treatments. If a remedy is given at 30c potency or lower and it's not the right choice of remedy, there generally is no reaction and another suitable remedy is sought.

If you have any concerns about the use of homeopathy, it's best to consult a trained professional homeopath. Refer to the homeopathic organization websites listed in **Appendix 4 — Additional Resources on page 346** to find a qualified homeopath. Conventional medical professionals with no formal training in homeopathy are unfamiliar with and uninformed about homeopathy and its long-standing history as a safe and effective treatment. As a result, understand they may tell you to avoid them. Ultimately, it's your choice about what you do to care for yourself and your family.

Important Note: Potencies over 30c should be given in consultation with a professional homeopath.

THE DIFFERENCE BETWEEN HOMEOPATHY AND ALLOPATHY

Hippocrates, the Father of Medicine (born in 460 B.C.), stated that there are two ways of treating ill health: the **Law of Similars** and the **Law of Opposites**.

The **Law of Similars** is also known as "like cures like" (see more detail on previous page). For example, why do people in hot climates eat hot food? They eat hot food because it is a Similar. It makes them hotter, they break into a sweat, and as a result they cool off. Another example is if a person has a sunburn and they can tolerate a warm application, the heat of the sunburn would dissipate.

Homeopathy is based on the philosophy of **homeostasis**, the body's ability to maintain internal stability while compensating for environmental changes. It addresses the root cause of the disease and sets out to eliminate the manifesting symptoms by bringing the body back into balance. All symptoms are considered and addressed by a remedy that encourages the body to heal them. This elimination process can appear as discharges such as the releasing of negative thoughts (mental discharge), sweating (a physical discharge), or an outburst of tears (an emotional release). These releases help rid the person of imbalances and thereby stimulates deeper healing.

The **Law of Opposite**s is the one followed by mainstream medicine, also referred to as "**allopathy**". The word "allopathy" was coined by homeopathic practitioners in the early 1800's to differentiate their practice from contemporary medicine providers. The word allopathy comes from the Greek words *állos* and *patheia* which translates into "other/different suffering." Examples of opposite practices include the use of antibiotics, antihistamines, antidepressants, antioxidants, etc.

Allopathy works by treating the symptoms of a disease, rather than its root cause. A conventional doctor, also referred to as an allopath, is trained to evaluate the symptoms a person is experiencing in order to identify a diagnosis or name for the condition. Only then can the doctor prescribe treatment which usually includes a chemical drug meant to reduce the symptoms. The chemical reaction, or effect (sometimes called the side effect), caused by the drug generally suppresses the condition. This **suppression** may reduce the symptoms temporarily, but it does not remove the cause. One example is an ear infection, when treated with antibiotics may make the person feel better for a while, but the infection often returns. Another example is with seasonal allergies. A person can take an allergy medicine and may feel somewhat better when the chemical is active in their body but once the substance is depleted in the body, the symptoms return, frequently stronger than before.

THE DIFFERENCE BETWEEN HOMEOPATHY AND NATUROPATHY

Homeopathy and **Naturopathy** are both considered branches of holistic medicine. They support and encourage a healthy immune system and aim to restore higher levels of health. Naturopathy is a natural medical system that takes a holistic approach to health and healing through many helpful modalities such as nutrition, lifestyle counseling, vitamins, and herbal tonics. In addition, some naturopaths who are

well-trained in homeopathy may also recommend homeopathic remedies as part of their treatment plan. Some naturopaths may also prescribe chemical (pharmaceutical) medicine when deemed necessary, but only if their state laws allow them to prescribe it.

Homeopathy also takes a holistic approach to health but focuses primarily on homeopathic remedies. These highly-diluted energetic substances are individually chosen to best match the totality of symptoms a person is experiencing in the way that they are uniquely experiencing them. As described earlier, it is based on the **Law of Similars**. It is used when a person is exhibiting active, uncomfortable and/or specific symptoms that need to be addressed.

To simplify, the main difference between the two practices is that naturopathy is a natural health system that utilizes many different treatments and modalities which can include homeopathy, while homeopathy is solely focused upon the use of homeopathic remedies to stimulate healing.

There are so many alternative, integrative and complementary approaches to health such as chiropractic, Reiki, acupuncture, vitamins, essential oils, and the list goes on. Like naturopathy, they should not be confused with homeopathy, which uses homeopathic remedies to provide symptom relief.

Professional homeopaths use a book called a **repertory** which is a compilation of symptoms and the remedies that can address those symptoms. They also use another book called a **materia medica** that

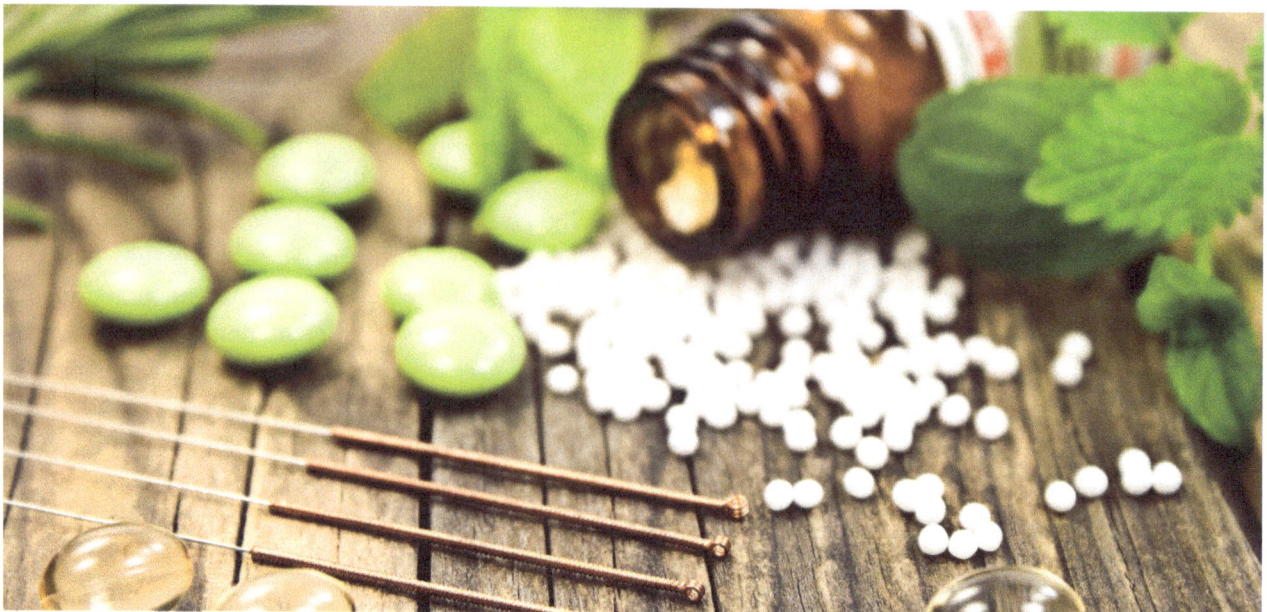

describes remedies and helps to compare remedy choices. In this book, we have identified and described some of the more common remedies used for acute conditions so you can more easily compare and make smarter remedy choices.

A BRIEF HISTORY OF HOMEOPATHY

Unfortunately, Hippocrates' idea of the Law of Similars as a cure for ailments was not further explored until the 15th century when a German doctor, named Paracelsus, decided to look deeper into this method. Paracelsus is known as the "Father of Chemistry," because he recognized the interaction of chemicals. He astutely observed the properties of plants, animals, and minerals. He gave careful attention to dosages. He noted a very small dose could be curative. He believed that disease affected the "vital spirit" and the body, and when given the proper medicinal preparations, the person could fully recuperate.

It wasn't until 300 years later, in the late 1700's, that Doctor Samuel Hahnemann took up the torch of the **Law of Similars** again. He believed the way medicine was being practiced at the time was inflicting injury to his patients. The treatments in vogue during his time included bloodletting, the use of leeches, and purgative therapy (a laxative effect) with poisonous drugs, for example excessive use of mercury. He turned his attention to the methods set forth by Hippocrates and Paracelsus. Hahnemann believed, as Paracelsus stated, "The art of healing comes from nature, not from the physician. Therefore, the physician must start from nature with an open mind." Hahnemann set forth the philosophy and principles of homeopathy in his book, *The Organon of the Medical Art*, which he updated six times.

THE DIFFERENCE BETWEEN ACUTE VERSUS CHRONIC[1] AILMENTS

An **acute illness** is one that has a gradual or abrupt onset, is self-limiting, and lasts for a short time—like a flu or stomach ache. A person with an acute illness will either recover and regain health, or continue with more chronic symptoms. A **chronic illness** is a set of symptoms that have not gone away after many months and limits the function of an individual. A common cold is considered an acute illness while recurrent seasonal allergies are considered a chronic condition. An ankle sprain is considered an acute problem while arthritis is considered chronic.

The body innately wants to heal. In chronic illness, the body tries to restore itself to health but seems to get stuck along the way. Chronic symptoms may accumulate and change but don't go away.

Using homeopathy for treating a chronic disease can be very complicated and requires a high level of competence in homeopathy, as well as some medical education. *This primer is designed to teach the use of homeopathy for home care in acute illnesses and injuries only.* To this end, we have included in this book some guidelines to help you decide when the condition you are addressing is or may be beyond the reasonable scope of home care, or when you may need the assistance of a skilled homeopath or other health care professional.

- **Acute Illness** produces symptoms that appear very quickly, are relatively short in duration, and go through a typical progression of changes. This covers injuries, fevers, flus, colds, cuts, bruising, teething, stomach upsets, etc. Ordinarily the vital force has its own self-healing resources and can find its own resolution. When the vital force isn't accomplishing this on its own, homeopathy can assist in encouraging the body to heal itself. Given the correct remedy, there will be less suffering and generally no suppression of symptoms.

- **Chronic Illness** is a long-term condition for which the body has no immediate internal solution. A chronic condition tends to get progressively worse over many months or years and remains as an ongoing health issue. The self-healing mechanism has somehow been compromised. Repetition of acute illness is not referred to as acute anymore. If someone suffers repeated colds over a long period of time, the real problem lies in the dysfunction of the immune system, nutritional deficiencies, and/or environmental or chemical toxins. These conditions require constitutional homeopathic

---

1 **Important note:** Chronic conditions should be treated by a clinically trained, experienced, and professional homeopath.

treatment which assesses every system of the body, including current symptoms, psychological make-up, family history, history since birth, and more. Through this treatment, lifestyle improvements are frequently identified and recommended.

NOTES ABOUT HOMEOPATHY IN THE UNITED STATES

In 1844, homeopathic practitioners created a national organization, The American Institute of Homeopathy (AIH), the first medical society formed in the United States. Partly in response, the orthodox physicians created their own medical society in 1846. One of the first actions of this rival medical group was to purge all members who were homeopathic practitioners, even though they had graduated from conventional medical schools. This new medical society named itself the "American Medical Association" (AMA).

In 1855, medical physicians would lose their membership for even consulting with a homeopathic practitioner or any other "irregular" practitioner. Losing membership in the AMA at that time also meant losing their license and the ability to practice medicine.

In 1862, Congress passed the first Homestead Act, which granted the head of a family 160 acres of land if they agreed to cultivate it for five years. In 1863, in Saint Louis, Missouri, people wanting to take advantage of the Homestead Act prepared their wagons for the adventure to the West. Most wagon trains did not have a doctor for the journey and the doctors in the West were few and far between, especially in the Plains states. There was a pharmacy by the name of Luyties where the pioneers could buy a homeopathic kit and a book, *The Domestic Physician* by Constantine Hering, MD (the Father of United States homeopathy). Thousands of pioneers used this book and remedy kit to treat illnesses that arose on their journey. Homeopathy was an invaluable modality for the pioneers who settled in the western part of the United States. It has since been used for generations to treat families in an effective and safe way with no toxic or harmful side effects.

Despite the political maneuvering within the medical communities, homeopathy continued to gain in popularity. In 1900, there were 22 homeopathic medical schools, more than 100 homeopathic hospitals, over 60 orphan asylums and senior living facilities, and over 1,000 homeopathic pharmacies in the United States.[2] A statue of Dr. Hahnemann was also erected in Washington, D.C. at that time and proudly stands to this day. The location is 1300 Corregidor St NW, Washington, DC.

In 1910, The Flexner Report was published which profoundly impacted medical education in the United States. The report, ironically funded by the Carnegie and Rockefeller families who were staunch supporters of homeopathy, gave poor marks to homeopathic and other "irregular" medical colleges. Of the 22 homeopathic schools in 1900, only two remained by 1923.

In 1928, penicillin (the first antibiotic) was discovered by Alexander Fleming. By 1944, it was undergoing large-scale pharmaceutical production and was being used to treat patients on a global scale during World War II. Interestingly, homeopathy's renaissance was launched when antibiotics efficacy began to falter due to many bacteria developing resistance to this new drug.

The resurgence of homeopathy in the 1970's was fueled primarily by the lay public. In the 1970's, fewer than 100 homeopathic practitioners were still practicing in the United States. By the 1980's, there were over 1,000. By the early 1990's, homeopathy became a major component of naturopathic medical education. Some conventional physicians also began to embrace homeopathic medicine and several training programs developed around the United States.

Every year, more and more medical doctors, physician assistants, and nurses are studying homeopathy and incorporating it into their practices. And more and more families are learning about its efficacy, ease of home use and safety record.

RESEARCH INTO HOMEOPATHY

Over 200 years of clinical experience, along with modern research published in The Lancet, Pediatrics, Pediatric Infectious Disease Journal, The British Medical Journal, The British Journal of Clinical Pharmacology, The Journal of Head Trauma

---

2   *A Condensed History of Homeopathy* by Dana Ullman: https://homeopathic.com/a-condensed-history-of-homeopathy.

Rehabilitation, and The Clinical Journal of Pain have all confirmed homeopathy's effectiveness. Included in some of the research are double-blind clinical trials, especially from the British and German homeopathic communities.

The use of homeopathy is advocated by the World Health Organization. Its use is commonplace in many parts of Europe including Switzerland, Germany, the United Kingdom, and France as well as in India, Israel, Brazil, Mexico, Canada, the Netherlands, Greece, Australia, New Zealand, and Russia. There are homeopathic hospitals, not to mention scores of homeopathic clinics, in Moscow, France, India, Denmark, Shanghai, and the United Kingdom. The Royal Family of the United Kingdom has been using homeopathy as its main healthcare modality since the 1840s and has its own homeopathic physician for consultations.

To learn more about current research into homeopathy, go to Homeopathy Research Institute located at https://www.hri-research.org.

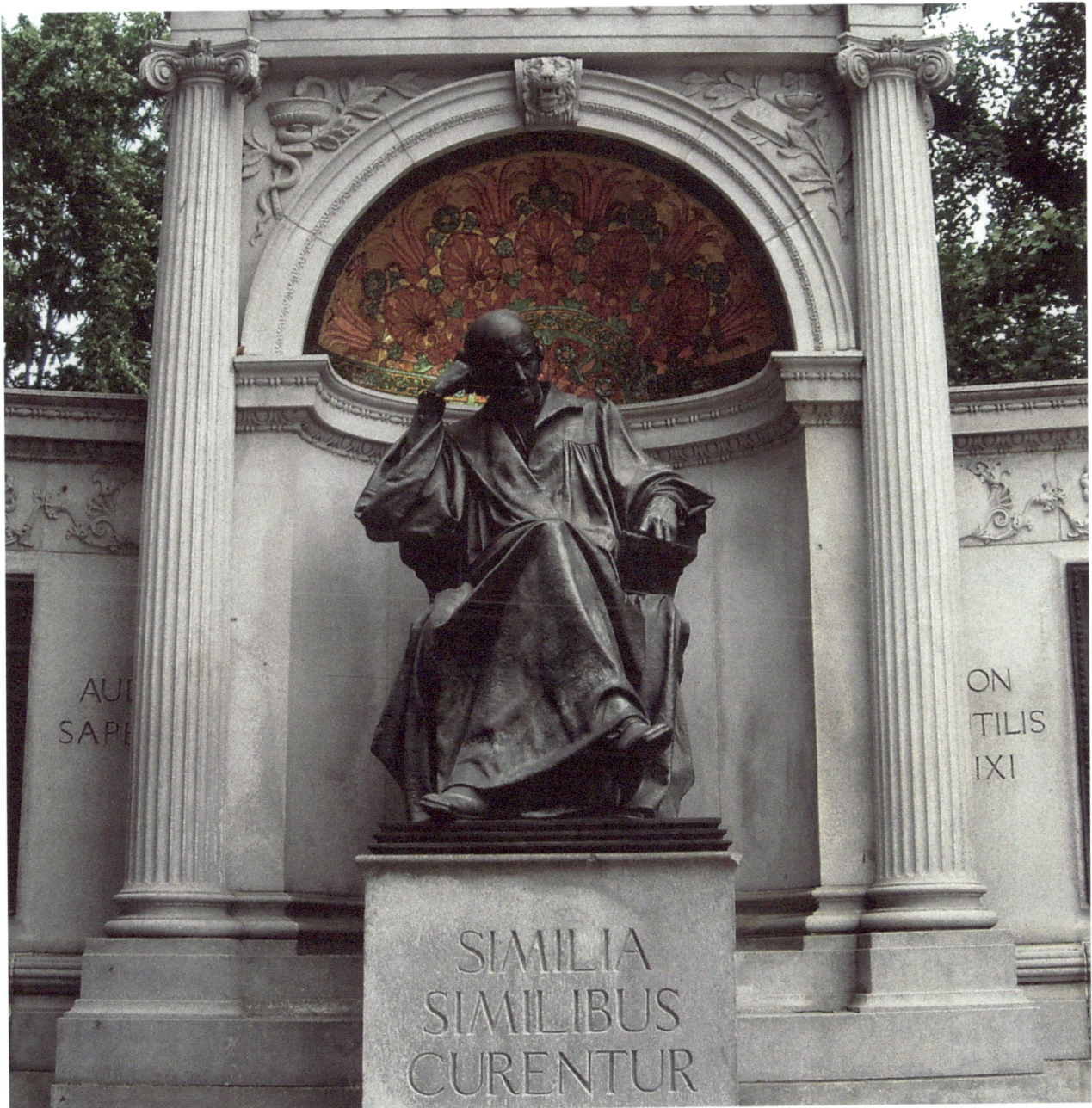

Samuel Hahnemann Monument was created in 1900 and was last restored in 2011. It is located at 1300 Corregidor St NW, Washington, DC. [© AgnosticPreachersKid/Wikimedia Commons/CC BY-SA 3.0.]

CHAPTER 2
Taking the Case and Giving the Remedy

The most repeated theme in this book is "Observe and Evaluate"! These two words are what can help anyone be successful with homeopathic prescribing. In this chapter, you will begin to learn how to become good observers and things to consider when you evaluate each situation.

TAKING A CASE—GATHERING THE SYMPTOMS

Homeopathy is powerful in that it evaluates the whole person, considering ALL of the physical, emotional, and mental symptoms. Homeopathic case taking looks at each person as a unique individual. Each person suffers from their health conditions in their own unique way. Observing four different people suffering from the same cold virus, we see that one person will develop a horrible sore throat, another a deep cough, another with a frontal headache or yet another with an ear infection.

When taking a case it is important to allow the person to describe in their own words what is happening to them at the present moment. This is the first step of what is called, "taking a case". It is important to listen to and make note of what their own description is. It's important to not second guess what the person is feeling by saying something like "you seem upset." If you observe that they are upset, when you are later asking questions about their emotional state, you can ask how they are feeling about what is happening. This allows the person to get in touch with and express how they are "feeling" about what is going on. For instance, they might say "I am fine" even though they are feeling hurt. This statement could be very helpful for choosing the correct remedy. Ask all the questions you want, but allow them the time to tune in to what is happening.

THE ART OF OBSERVATION

Gathering the symptoms for any homeopathic case takes good observational skills on your part. Since homeopathy focuses on each person's unique symptoms, it's important to have a comprehensive method for gathering them. Learning to observe symptoms is a little like learning a foreign language. Symptoms are the language that the mind, body, and emotions use to express when the vital force is not in balance. While taking the case, it's important to look at the person to see if there are any obvious symptoms such as mood, skin coloring, expression, or energy. Additionally, it is of great use to find out what was going on in the person's life when the symptoms started manifesting. There may have been a trauma or a stressful event which is part of the whole picture to be considered in the analysis.

- Skin coloring can be useful; for instance, observing if a boil is very red or purple.

- Energy is important: a person whose energy is lively will need a different remedy from a person who is laying on the sofa, or from another who is weak but restless. Have their sleep patterns changed in any way?

- Sensitivity to the environment is important because it can give us a clue as to how the person reacts to drafts, heat, cold, weather changes, sunlight, moon phases, or noise.

- Pain and other sensations are good guides as well. Pains can be achy, sharp, shooting, burning, crampy, pinching, erratic, steady, throbbing, etc. Sensations can be numbness, trembling, weakness, heat, cold, heaviness, pressure, spasms, etc.

- Timing can be important. If the person is always waking at 4:00 AM, this can point to a specific remedy.

- Thirst and appetite can also be helpful in guiding you to the correct remedy, especially if there's a change from the person's normal state.

- The most valuable of all are known as strange, rare and peculiar (SRP) symptoms. The more strange, rare or peculiar they are, the more likely you will be led to the correct remedy. See SRP description on the bottom of page 25.

How To Select An Indicated Remedy

The main goal in choosing a remedy is to match the symptoms the person is experiencing with the symptoms the remedy would stimulate if given to a healthy person. In homeopathy, we call this "finding the simillimum." We look at the totality of the symptoms, not just the main symptom(s). The key to remedy selection is careful observation of the small differences that distinguish one person's experience of a problem from what someone else might experience. For example: Janet and Joe were both exposed to a virus on the same day. Within two days, Janet was burning with heat, had a red face, wide pupils, burning throat, and a headache that pounded with each heartbeat. She felt worse whenever she moved and was very irritated by noise. Joe slowly became ill over the span of a week and had a

pale face, scratchy throat, low fever, dull headache, felt chilly, and his eyelids drooped. He felt better when he jiggled his foot and worse when he thought about how sick he felt. Janet needed **Belladonna**, and Joe needed **Gelsemium**. They both reacted to the same virus by developing a headache and a sore throat, but their responses were not the same. By observing all their symptoms and getting specific information about their headaches and sore throats, you have the information needed to select the correct remedies.

Learning CLAMS Case-Taking

Asking targeted questions and observing the person are the predominant ways to help you gather the most helpful information for finding a good remedy in an acute situation. Using the **CLAMS acronym**[1]—**Cause, Location, Additional Symptoms, Modalities and Sensations**—will help guide you with your acute case-taking. Not all areas have to be responded to but the more information you can gather, the better. You can go in any order as long as all areas are at least asked about. **See page 30** for a CLAMS Template you can copy and use for your case taking.

The first thing to note is what is/are the current complaints/symptoms. These are the areas you will need to focus on.

C—CAUSE is finding out what caused the complaint/symptoms and when did they start. This is a very important piece, if known, that will help you find an appropriate remedy for the situation. What was happening in their life or where was the person around that time? Was it a sudden symptom or did it come on slowly? Some examples are symptoms that started after a beloved pet died, after getting chilled or wet, when a child left home/got married, after watching a scary movie, after eating out, etc. The question to ask is "What was going on in your life or where were you when this started?"

In the previous example of Janet and Joe, their etiology was they were both exposed to a virus.

---

1   Another version you may see of the CLAMS acronym accomplishes the same thing but the C and A of the words are written differently. C is Concomitants (same as Additional Symptoms) and A is Aetiology (same as Cause).

L—LOCATION is where exactly the site(s) of the discomfort(s) or pain are e.g., left or right side, top, side, back, inside, outside, above or below. This includes where on the body the symptom is. If the symptom extends to another part of the body such as a sore throat that extends to the right or left ear would be important to note. Sidedness is always important when doing homeopathic case-taking. The question to ask is "Where exactly is the discomfort/pain?"

In the previous example of Janet and Joe, both felt the pain in their throats, so the location was the same. You can always ask a follow up question that helps you know if the pain is more on one-side or another. Another question for both would be to ask exactly where the headache is located.

A—ADDITIONAL SYMPTOMS are symptoms that are present at the same time with the current problem(s) but may not be directly connected to it. Examples of an additional symptom include red eyes that can develop when the person has a headache, a sore throat with frequent sneezing, a headache when coughing, diarrhea with nausea, and so on. It is a symptom that only appears in relation to something else and does not have its own sensation, location, or modalities. The question to ask is "Is there another symptom present at the same time as your current complaint?"

In the previous example of Janet and Joe, Janet had a headache with a burning throat while Joe had a dull headache with a scratchy throat.

M—MODALITIES are actions or circumstances that make a person or their symptoms feel better or worse. It doesn't include the use of aspirin or other commonly used medications but does include the application of heat or cold. An example is when a person feels worse from being in a hot, stuffy room and better from being in the fresh air. Or they may feel better from sitting than lying down. Some conditions are better from motion and worse from rest. Others are better from hard pressure and worse from rubbing. There are also times of day and night that a person may feel better or worse. The question to ask is "What makes your symptoms better or worse?"

Modalities are also helpful for the comfort of the person who is sick. e.g., a person who needs **Pulsatilla** will feel worse in a warm stuffy room, so fresh air will make them feel better.

Modalities also act as a significant clue in deciding a remedy. For example, worse on initial motion, but better from continuous motion is a good indicative modality for **Rhus tox**.

In the previous example of Janet and Joe, the modalities for Janet were worse from motion and noise, and Joe's were better from motion and worse from thinking of his ailments.

S—SENSATIONS mean what does each symptom feel like such as burning, throbbing, stabbing, radiating, bursting, constricting, bloating, etc. Is the pain achy, sharp, shooting, burning, crampy, pinching, intermittent, steady, throbbing, etc? And is there numbness, trembling, weakness, heaviness, pressure, spasms, etc? Anything that the person can describe around the sensation of the symptom(s), the more helpful the information will be. The question to ask is "What does your discomfort/pain/symptom feel like?"

In the previous example of Janet and Joe, Janet's sensation about her sore throat was that it was burning. Joe's sensation was that it was scratchy.

As you engage in using CLAMS case-taking, here are some other things to look for that may be an acute presentation of their symptom:

MOOD/FEELINGS/ATTITUDE: Is the person feeling sad, angry, irritable, depressed, clingy, weepy, demanding, indignant, etc.

SLEEP: What's their sleep like since being sick? Is there a change in sleep quality? Any nightmares?

APPETITE: Is their appetite increased or lacking? Any new cravings since feeling unwell?

THIRST: Is their thirst increased, taking only small sips, or none? Is there a preference for cold, iced or warm drinks?

ENERGY LEVELS: Has the energy level gone up or down?

STRANGE RARE AND PECULIAR SYMPTOMS: Knowing these can be especially helpful—particularly if the symptom has lots of clarity and/or volume. For instance, a person with burning abdominal pains who feels better when hot water is placed on the abdomen is exhibiting a symptom that is different than you might expect. Other examples are the person has a dry mouth, but no thirst; thus, indicating the remedy, **Pulsatilla**. Or the person who has burning pain in the stomach but still wants a heating pad; thus, indicating the remedy, **Arsenicum**. Or a person who gets a cold after having her/his hair cut, indicating the remedy, **Belladonna**.

Often these symptoms are described under only one remedy, which makes finding the simillimum easy. Be careful though about selecting a remedy based on only one symptom. It's important to look at the totality of symptoms when making remedy choices.

Other things to consider inquiring about depending on the symptoms:

DISCHARGES: Where are discharges coming from? What's the color, texture, or smell? Any blood present?

URINE/STOOL: Any changes in frequency, color, consistency, smell, or any blood present?

PERSPIRATION: Is it different now when unwell? Does it have a different odor than when well or are there particular places it is occuring other than when well?

TEMPERATURE: Is there a fever present? Does it increase or decrease during the day or night?

SENSITIVITY TO ENVIRONMENT: Is the person sensitive to drafts, heat, cold, weather changes, sunlight, moon phases, or noise?

ADDITIONAL CONSIDERATIONS FOR CASE TAKING

- To avoid missing important information, it is very helpful to mentally use an image of the entire body and ask questions from top to bottom and inside out. For example, ask first about symptoms starting from the top of the body (head, eyes, nose, mouth, ears, face), then throat, then chest, abdomen, back, etc. After questions from top to bottom, then ask about bones, muscles, skin, etc. Remember to include questions about how the person feels in general, such as "I feel achy all over" or "I feel chilly."

- When questioning someone about their symptoms, be careful to avoid leading them to specific answers, especially if you suspect that a particular remedy may be needed. It is quite possible to unwittingly lead someone to answer in a way that will confirm what you want to hear and end up with the wrong remedy. For example, in questioning Janet it would be wiser to ask, "How does your throat feel?" instead of "Does your throat burn?". You will get much more accurate information with a more open question. If you must ask a specific question, you can provide several alternatives for the person to choose from. For example, you might ask Janet "Does your throat ache, burn, or tickle or other sensation?" This question will encourage her to provide you with more information than you can receive with a "yes" or "no" answer, and you will avoid leading her to a specific answer and possibly the wrong remedy. Be sure to let the person talk freely. Often, they will tell you exactly what is wrong if you simply let them tell you. In addition, be sure to observe with your own eyes and note what you see. The person doesn't need to tell you that they have a red face or one cheek red and the other not—you will be able to see it.

- After noting the information about all the person's symptoms, you correlate the symptoms of the person with the remedy descriptions to find the closest match. In doing this, we use a hierarchy of symptoms, giving more consideration to the symptoms with the most clarity and volume. For instance, if a person emphatically says, "It's a burning pain right here!" That symptom has more clarity than other symptoms the person might have. If the person describes a symptom more than once, it has more volume than other symptoms. It is more important that these symptoms with the most clarity and an amplified volume be in the remedy description than other symptoms of less importance.

- Systemic symptoms are also given more weight than other symptoms. Systemic symptoms are symptoms that involve the whole person, i.e., "I feel chilly and weepy." These symptoms can be physical, emotional, and/or mental.

- In some cases a remedy may be needed initially, but then the person moves on to a different remedy. An example would be that a person got chilled in a north wind and the condition came on fast.

In this case **Aconite** would be the remedy. Later the person may develop a cough and need a cough remedy to feel completely well.

- Finding the simillimum is achieved through careful observation, open questioning, and systematic thinking. By using these techniques every time you choose a remedy, you will find remedy selection becomes easier and easier. The adage "practice makes better" applies here.

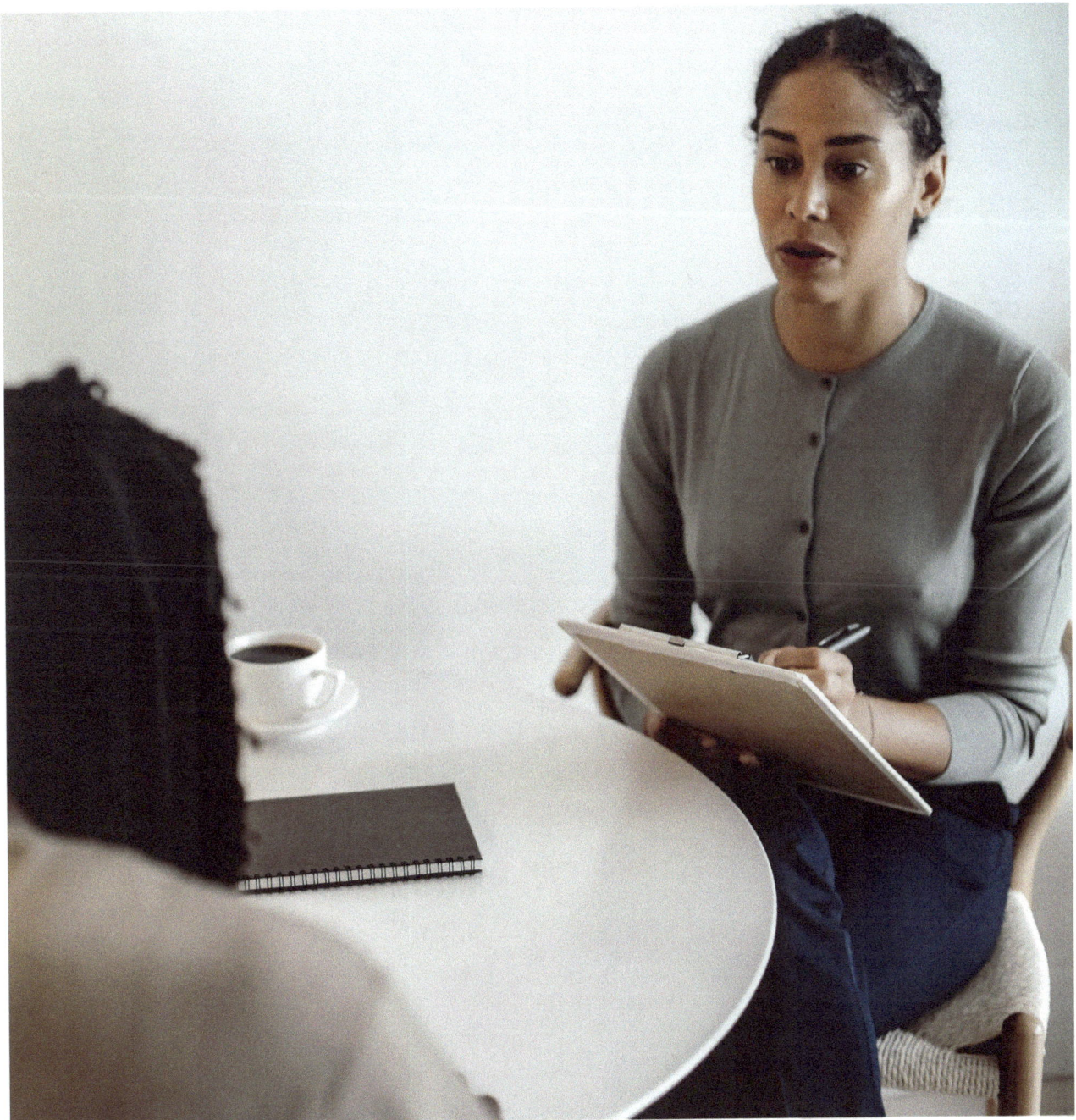

CLAMS for Homeopathic Case-Taking Template

Asking targeted questions and observing the person are the predominant ways to help you gather the most helpful information for finding a good remedy. Using the CLAMS acronym will help guide you with your acute case-taking. Not all areas have to be responded to but the more information you can gather, the better. You can go in any order as long as all areas are at least asked about.

What is/are the current complaint(s)? e.g., sore throat, headache, diarrhea, etc.

C—CAUSE?

L – LOCATION?

A – ADDITIONAL SYMPTOMS?

M – MODALITIES?

S – SENSATIONS?

Other things to ask about...

MOOD/FEELINGS/ATTITUDE:

SLEEP:

APPETITE:

THIRST:

ENERGY LEVELS:

STRANGE RARE AND PECULIAR SYMPTOMS:

DISCHARGES:

URINE/STOOL:

PERSPIRATION:

TEMPERATURE:

SENSITIVITY TO ENVIRONMENT:

HOW TO READ THE REMEDY CHARTS

To help you learn what remedies are most common for the symptoms discussed, you will find either a text description of the remedies OR typically if there are more than three remedies, you will see a remedy comparison chart like the one below. For most sections, each chart will have a minimum of four remedies and a maximum of seven to choose from listed in alphabetical order. Note that some charts may not need one of the themes from the far left column so it's been eliminated for easier readability. Also, a few charts have different themes. Understand that you don't have to match every section of a column but the more symptoms in common compared to the others will help you make a smarter choice.

COMMON REMEDIES FOR XYZ CONDITION							
	Remedy 1	Remedy 2	Remedy 3	Remedy 4	Remedy 5	Remedy 6	Remedy 7
ONSET							
SYMPTOMS							
MOOD							
INDICATIONS							
WORSE							
BETTER							

WHAT YOU'RE SPECIFICALLY LOOKING FOR:

Onset = Was there something that started the symptom such as sitting on a cold stoop or experiencing grief? Was it gradual or sudden?

Symptoms = What are the physical, mental or emotional clues the person is expressing that seem most helpful?

Mood = Is the person cheerful or irritable? Restless or quiet? Attentive or delirious?

Indications = Why would this remedy be given – temper tantrum, a condition that came on fast, thirstless, throbbing pain, etc?

Worse = What things make the person's symptoms feel worse?

Better = What things make the person's symptoms feel better?

What potency to give

Once you decide on the best remedy match, the next step is to determine what potency to use. Know that you cannot take (or give) a potency that you do not have on hand! Thankfully, a well selected remedy will greatly assist the body/mind to restore a healthful balance regardless of which potency is used. The most commonly used potencies for home care, and those being advocated for those new to homeopathy are 6c, 12c, and 30c.

How Often To Give A Dose

Frequency of the dose is actually the most important thing. Each dose, separated by a period of time, is a fresh input of the energy of the remedy for the vital force. Sometimes it is necessary to repeat a dose because the vital force has used up the energy of a previous dose. So a person who has begun to respond to **Belladonna** for a fever, or *Podophyllum** for diarrhea, might need a repeat dose after two hours if the symptoms begin to return. It is not unusual for remedies to be repeated quite a few times. This is where the observe and evaluate concept comes into play when deciding on how frequent a dose is needed.

The general guidelines are as follows:

- Give the potency you have on hand. This book is advocating for having a 30c kit on hand but if you only have 6c or 12c, use that.

- If the condition is life-threatening, give the remedy every 5–15 minutes. (see **RED** dosing method on **page 34**).

- If a condition comes on fast and furious, give the remedy every 15 minutes. (see **ORANGE** dosing method on **page 34**).

- There are two situations that use the **BLUE** dosing method on **page 34**.

  - If the onset is slower and less intense, give the remedy every 2–4 hours.
  - If the onset is mild, give the remedy every 4–6 hours.

- If the condition is quite slow to heal, as with a muscle strain, give the remedy 2–3 times per day for a few days. (see **BROWN** dosing method on **page 34**).

- Stop repeating the remedy as soon as there is a strong improvement of the symptoms.

- Repeat only if there is a return of symptoms.

Sometimes you are getting good results from a remedy, but then it fails to hold. At this point, you will need to administer the same remedy with more frequency. If there is still no holding power, you need to reassess the case and look to another remedy. It might be that your choice was not quite similar enough to match the manifesting symptoms. Or the first remedy was needed but now the person's symptoms have moved on, and requires another remedy to compliment the first remedy you gave. In this case, the second remedy will then finish the healing. This can be common, as previously mentioned, if a person was chilled in a north wind and feels unwell fast, indicating **Aconite**. Twenty-four hours later, they are coughing and have different symptoms. At that point you need to reassess, and look for a cough remedy.

Note: A common mistake that new prescribers make is not giving enough doses of the remedy. If you follow the instructions in the Suggested Dosage section that follows under each remedy, you do not need to worry about giving a person too much of a remedy. You do, however, need to make sure that enough of the selected remedy has been given before ever moving on to another remedy. One dose is rarely enough.

With homeopathy, less is more. As your condition improves you should decrease the number of doses and spread out the time between each dose. When you are well again, you stop taking the remedy altogether. Taking a remedy longer than needed can result in a **proving** of that remedy, meaning you get more of the symptoms the remedy is intended to alleviate. If this happens, it is best to immediately stop the remedy to let the symptoms subside.

Good rules of thumb for dosing:

- Observe and evaluate!

- If the remedy has given no relief whatsoever after 4 doses, retake the case and choose a different remedy. In this time frame, *care*ful observation of the person will help determine if you made the right choice or what other remedies you might consider. For example, you originally thought the person didn't want to move because they were lying on the couch, but after further observation, you notice that, yes, they are lying on the couch BUT are also moving around a lot and can't seem to get comfortable. This is restlessness, not stillness, which may warrant a different remedy.

- Repeat the same remedy ONLY if there is a return of the same symptoms. If the symptoms change, consider another remedy.

- Repeat only as necessary, and only when needed.

- If there is no improvement after several remedies, consult with your healthcare provider or a professional homeopath.

SUGGESTED DOSING METHODS

To help identify the best dosing practices, we have created different color levels to reflect the intensity and/or urgency of the symptoms and the suggested dosing schedule.

1. **RED** is for emergencies—quite serious or life threatening (e.g., anaphylaxis (serious allergic reaction), broken bones, fainting, etc.). The indicated remedy can be taken **every 10 minutes ON THE WAY TO THE HOSPITAL. DO NOT attempt to manage these at home.** If the remedy is helping, dosing can become less frequent and then only given as needed.

2. **ORANGE** is when a symptom comes on <u>quickly</u> (e.g., a sudden high fever, menstrual cramps, earache, etc.) and/or it's important to get quick relief (e.g., profuse vomiting and/or diarrhea, shooting pain after a tooth extraction, throbbing pain after slamming a finger in a car door, etc.). The indicated remedy can be given once every 15 minutes for up to an hour. If the remedy has an effect and the person is starting to feel better, dosing can then be hourly or even less frequent depending on the person's symptoms. If the intensity of the symptoms stops, then stop giving the remedy. Only give another dose IF the symptom returns. If the chosen remedy doesn't seem to have any effect on the person after an hour, re-evaluate and choose another remedy.

3. **BLUE** is for when a symptom comes on <u>slowly</u> and/or there are acute uncomfortable symptoms (e.g., colds, flus, coughs, headaches, back pain, etc.). The indicated remedy can be given every two to three hours for up to 4 doses when the onset is slower than the **ORANGE** method. OR if the symptoms are mild, the remedy can be given every four to six hours for up to 4 doses. It will be clear within a few doses whether the remedy is a good match, or if it needs to be continued a little longer, or stopped because the person is feeling better, or needs to be re-evaluated to choose a different remedy. You may need to repeat the remedy two to three times per day for a few days to help guide the symptoms to slowly improve. If you see no result within 24 hours, reassess the symptoms. You may not have been wrong with your initial choice; the condition may simply have moved on to require a related remedy. Change the remedy if you have followed the above guidelines with no results, or if the symptoms have clearly changed.

4. **BROWN** is for unpleasant conditions but not urgent situations (e.g., constipation, hemorrhoids, ingrown nail, etc.). The indicated remedy can be given 1-2x a day for up to 3 days and make sure to observe before continuing. If the remedy is having a positive effect, give for one day more and again observe. Stop when the condition has been ameliorated. However, if there are no positive results after the three days, then reevaluate and choose a different remedy.

5. **GREEN** is the support level (e.g., building up bone, repairing a bone break, iron deficiency, etc.). To provide support, there is usually a more frequent dosing of a 6c or 12c remedy or a cell salt potency which is a 6x or 12x. These can be taken once or twice a day (*see Chapter 3—Introduction to Cell Salts on page 39*).

HOW MANY IS A DOSE?

Most homeopathic remedies that are sold for internal use are provided in one of these forms:

A. **Sucrose globule/pellet**

B. **Lactose globule/pellet**

C. **Pressed lactose tablet**

Unlike chemical medicine, the effectiveness of homeopathic remedies does NOT depend on the size of the dose. It depends on the remedy and the potency. The proper dose is one that is large enough to ensure sufficient contact with the mucous membranes of the mouth to enable the remedy to be absorbed. Generally, the following doses will suffice though reading the label will provide guidance as well:

- **Tablets** (all sizes): 3 for adults, 2 for children, 1 for infants

- **#40 Pellets** (size of a BB): 3 pellets

- **#25 Pellets** (size of cupcake sprinkles): 5 pellets

- **#15 Pellets** (size of a granule or poppy seed): 10 pellets

#40	●	**4mm**
About the size of a BB		
#25	●	**2.5mm**
#15	⁝	**1.5mm**
About the size of a poppy seed		

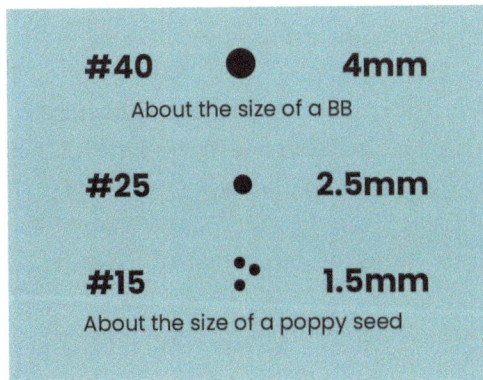

How to Administer a Remedy

Homeopathic remedies affect the body directly through the mucous membranes. This works best if the mouth is in its natural clean state, unaltered by food, beverages, brushing teeth, etc. We recommend:

1. homeopathic remedies be taken at least 10 minutes before OR after eating, brushing teeth, etc., and

2. holding them under the tongue as long as possible and letting them dissolve.

Since homeopathic doses are very small, care should be taken that they reach the mouth in as pure a state as possible. Measure the required number of tablets, pellets, or globules into the inside of the bottle cap or a small paper cup or spoon and gently pour them under the tongue to dissolve.

It is best not to let the remedies touch your hands as the medicinal substance is on the outside of the pellets. If it needs to be poured in your hand, lick the remedy off your hand as you guide the remedy under the tongue to dissolve.

Special Dosing Instructions for Infants, Young Children or Pets

When giving a remedy to an infant or pet, know that the infant could choke on the pellets while pets have a tendency to spit them out. To avoid these issues and to ensure they receive the remedy, you can choose from these possible actions:

1. Add one dose of the remedy to a half cup of water and let the remedy dissolve. Stir the water gently. Then using a medicine dropper, draw up water to fill the pipette and gently squirt into the infant or pet's mouth between the cheek and gums. That is one dose. Hold onto remaining water remedy for next dosing if needed.

2. Take one dose of pellets and crush them between two spoons creating a powder. Then dump the powder onto the infant, young child's or pet's tongue and let it dissolve.

3. For young children (not infants), take one dose of the remedy and place it between the gums and the bottom lip to dissolve.

4. A dose of a remedy can always be added to drinking water for pets but make sure after they get a drink from the remedy water (can be a lot or a little at one time—that will be a dose), you remove that water bowl until you are ready to give another dose. Provide clean water after.

5. A dose of a remedy can be added to a shot glass size of water, let it dissolve, stir gently, then ask the child to drink the water for the dose. Clean the glass, or any dropper or spoon used, with warm soapy water. Let them dry before dosing another remedy.

6. **WHEN YOU ARE RUNNING OUT OF A NEEDED REMEDY**

If you find yourself needing more remedy than you have, and don't have time to get more, you can add the pellets to 4-6 ounces (or about half cup) of clean water and let them dissolve. Stir the water with a clean spoon and take a teaspoon or good sip as one dose. Cover the glass to preserve the remaining liquid for your next dose. This will help extend the number of doses you will have until getting more pellets. This water solution can be used for a week if it's left in a cool, dark, dry place between doses; no need for refrigeration. It is ideal to make a new remedy mixture once a week though if still needed.

If you find you do need a remedy to last even longer, then refrigeration would be suggested OR add just a few drops of clear alcohol (e.g., vodka) to the water instead as it acts as a preservative.

WHEN YOU MIGHT WANT TO "PLUS" A REMEDY

Plussing is a way to make your remedy just a little stronger. Many times, during an acute illness, giving the same potency repeatedly will work. However, after several doses of the same remedy potency, some people find it helpful to "plus" the dose. Simply, place your dosing pellets into a bottle or jar of clean water with a top—can be as much as 16-20 ounces or as little as 6 ounces—and let them dissolve. Then vigorously shake the jar or bottle up and down (which can include pounding the bottom of the bottle or jar on your palm or a hardbound book) 10 times to energize the water. Then take a teaspoon or a good sip for a dose. This successive action makes the remedy just a little stronger. The next dose you need, if you need one, would require an additional 10 vigorous shakes before taking a teaspoon or sip.

WHAT MIGHT INTERFERE WITH A REMEDY?

A remedy's action can be interfered with by certain substances or circumstances, and it seems to be a variable phenomenon. If the person is generally sensitive to other medications or has allergies to their environment or foods, consider the interfering agents more seriously. However, if you are taking a remedy repeatedly over a short period of time, the chances of these factors interfering are greatly reduced.

The following have been known or are suspected of counteracting or interfering with the effects of homeopathic remedies for some <u>sensitive</u> people:

1. Coffee — caffeinated and, rarely, decaffeinated. All other forms of caffeine are fine.

2. Anything made with strong peppermint including tea, mints, mouthwash, or toothpaste.

3. Strong odors – including camphor, menthol, eucalyptus, tea tree oil, chemicals, perfumes, liniments.

4. Pharmaceutical drugs.

5. Electric blankets and waterbed heaters. Anything that emits a strong electrical current, like a microwave, X-Rays, or a router.

6. Marijuana, cocaine, and other illicit drugs.

7. Stress, trauma, major illness, high fever.

8. Dental drilling, sometimes cleanings.

9. Other energy healing modalities e.g., Polarity, Reiki, Acupuncture.

10. Anything to which you are particularly sensitive.

Interestingly, there are many stories about remedies being interfered with by coffee, yet there are others who suggest giving remedies in coffee. After all, the Brazilians who take two or three shots of espresso still receive benefits of homeopathy just fine. Some homeopathic practitioners feel that high potencies are interfered with more easily than lower potencies. But it's not consistent and each person's reaction will be different. Since the issue of interference is not straightforward, it's wise to be aware of those things that might hinder a remedy's action.

CARE OF REMEDIES

- Remedies should be stored in a cool, dry place away from excessive heat, moisture, strong sunlight, strong odors, and any electrical equipment.

- Keep your remedies at least 10 feet away from a cell phone, cordless digital phones, microwave ovens, computers, or stereo equipment. The further away, the better.

- It's best to store your remedies away from aromatic substances such as strong perfumes, oil-based paints, mints, camphor, liniments, etc., which have been known to counteract their effectiveness.

- If you are traveling, do what you can to protect your remedies from the x-ray machines at the airport although some homeopaths who travel say it's not an issue for them. Carry-on and checked bags are x-rayed. Some suggest wrapping all remedies, or your whole kit, in aluminum foil.

- Some people place their remedies in a lead-lined photographer's bag, especially if they have invested in a kit with many remedies. Avoid carrying remedies on your body if you go through the full-body scanner at the airport.

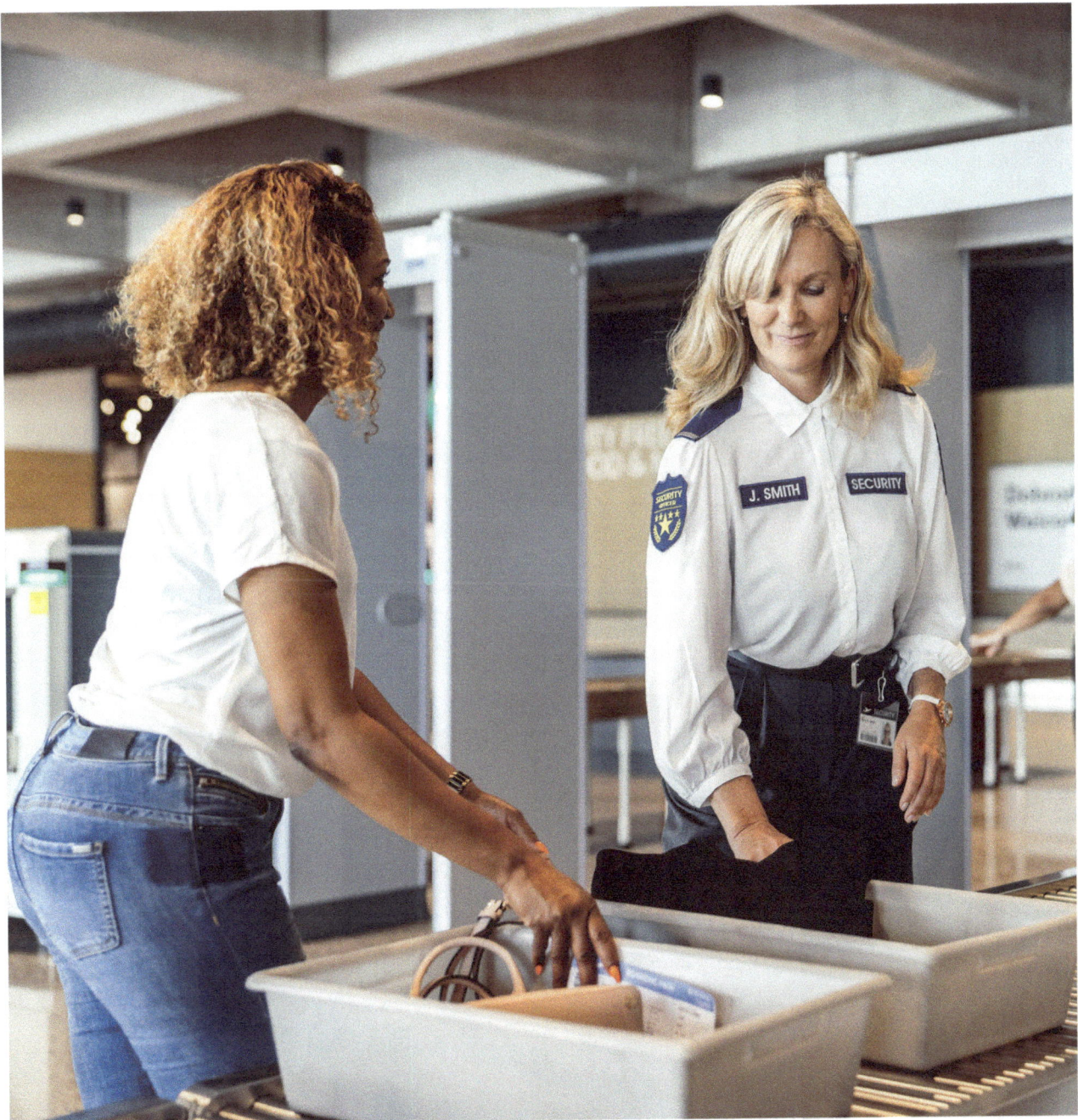

CHAPTER 3
Introduction to Cell Salts

Schüssler cell salts, also known as Schüssler tissue salts or biochemic cell salts, are a system of medicine developed by Dr. Wilhelm Heinrich Schüssler, a 19th-century German physician. This system is based on the belief that deficiencies in essential mineral salts can lead to health issues and that restoring these minerals can promote overall health and well-being.

Cell salts help restore mineral balance at the cellular level, promoting the body's natural ability to heal. Each mineral salt is associated with specific functions or symptoms and is recommended based on the individual's constitution or health complaint. For example, **Natrum muriaticum** (Sodium Chloride) is often suggested for conditions involving water balance and digestive issues, while **Ferrum phosphoricum** (Iron Phosphate) is recommended for addressing symptoms related to inflammation and fever.

WHY USE CELL SALTS

Today, our bodies are asked to manage increasing exposures to environmental insults while we experience declining availability of previously nutritious foods. Weakened digestive systems and poor nutritional status, alongside increasing toxicity, cause health disturbances and a decline in overall well-being. This book opens with a discussion on boosting essential nutrients because it is well-known that nutritional status is vital to well-being. If you are new to homeopathy, you will likely succeed quickly with these twelve remedies.

Let's review how our bodies are nourished.

Metabolism Basics:

1. Nutrients need to be provided in a bioavailable form.

2. The body needs to digest and absorb the nutrients efficiently.

3. The body must assimilate the nutrients into the appropriate cells and tissues.

We can't say precisely how the homeopathic cell salts assist in this process, but they likely help in each step of metabolism. As you become more experienced with these unique 12 cell salt remedies and homeopathy, you will form your opinions about how the cell salts work.

DISCOVERY OF 12 MACRO-MINERALS

Wilhelm H. Schüssler was a homeopathic physician and medical researcher in the late 1800s in the village of Oldenburg, Germany. Schüssler investigated the chemical makeup of human cells by analyzing ashes from human tissue. His early research led him to believe all cells can be reduced to 12 essential inorganic mineral salts. Schüssler believed that without these mineral salts, cells cease to function properly, and disease develops. Today, we recognize these 12 minerals as essential macrominerals.

Schüssler declared the following, "The inorganic substances in the blood and tissues are sufficient to heal all diseases which are curable by supplying to cells the cell salts needed for a normal condition to exist, thereby destroying the breeding place for the fungi, germs, or bacilli."

SCHÜSSLER'S HEALING SYSTEM IS BORN

With the discovery of the 12 essential salts, Schüssler concluded that the active ingredients in homeopathic remedies are the inorganic minerals that affect cellular metabolism. He believed homeopathy could be greatly simplified, and perhaps the only remedies the body needs are the 12 homeopathically prepared mineral salts. He named his new healing system the "Biochemic System of Healing." This healing system employs the 12 essential mineral salts in low potency prepared by the homeopathic process of trituration —repetitive dilution and grinding of a tiny amount of a substance in lactose powder. Unlike classical homeopathy, the cell salt remedies are usually selected following the "Law of Deficiency." In other words, careful observation of the body's signs and symptoms will point to mineral deficiencies. Tissues strengthen and heal when the appropriately chosen cell salt remedies are taken to restore the deficient minerals.

FOOD FOR THOUGHT

Schüssler's cell salts are used worldwide by professionals and home prescribers. The remedies are fast-acting and easy to use for simple ailments, making them well-suited to home care. Professionals use cell salts in a variety of ways. Sometimes, they are used between **constitutional remedies,** and other times as targeted support for a physical condition.

Homeopaths who favor their use find cell salts very helpful in addressing simple ailments and notice that

they can also provide deep-acting support. Occasionally, a well-selected cell salt for a physical complaint may act on another level, such as the emotional level. The release of emotions is noticed more frequently with **Natrum mur** and **Silicea** cell salts.

OTHER NAMES FOR CELL SALTS

- Cell Salt Remedies
- Biochemic Salts
- Biochemic Cell Salts
- Tissue Salts
- Tissue Remedies
- Biochemic Gems
- Biochemic Therapy

SCHÜSSLER'S 12 CELL SALTS AND THEIR COMMONLY USED ABBREVIATED NAMES:

1. **Calcarea fluorica (Calc fluor)**

2. **Calcarea phosphorica (Calc phos)**

3. **Calcarea sulphurica (Calc sulph)**

4. **Ferrum phosphoricum (Ferrum phos)**

5. **Kali muriaticum (Kali mur)**

6. **Kali phosphoricum (Kali phos)**

7. **Kali sulphuricum (Kali sulph)**

8. **Magnesia phosphoricum (Mag Phos)**

9. **Natrum muriaticum (Nat mur)**

10. **Natrum phosphoricum (Nat phos)**

11. **Natrum sulphuricum (Nat sulph)**

12. **Silicea (Sil)**—same as **Silica**

Cell salt potencies most commonly used: 6X or 12X.

SELECTING A CELL SALT REMEDY

If you are dairy or sugar intolerant, it's wise to check the cell salt ingredients you purchase. **Saccharum lactose** is a pharmaceutical grade of sugar from cow's milk that does not contain any casein, whey, or other milk proteins. According to cell salt makers, individuals sensitive to dairy can take these tablets safely. However, some lactose-intolerant people may do better with sucrose cell salt tablets. Cell salts can be ordered in a liquid form with an alcohol or glycerin preservative, avoiding the lactose and sucrose issue.

People who need to monitor dietary salt intake do not need to be concerned with the concentration of mineral salts in homeopathic cell salt remedies. All of the homeopathic mineral salts are nearly undetectable.

Homeopathic cell salts can be selected using traditional homeopathic materia medica and repertories, or common knowledge about mineral deficiencies. Ideally, you want to choose a cell salt based on multiple symptoms. Select one to four cell salts that address your most troubling symptoms.

EXAMPLE CASE #1: Nat mur for a dry rash

One hot summer day, a young boy complained about burning pain from a dry, raw, red rash under his nose. One pellet of **Nat mur 6X** taken three times daily cleared up the painful rash. Shortly after the rash cleared, he broke down in tears, which cleared up lingering emotions.

The **Nat mur 6X** cleared up the painful rash, restoring moisture to his skin, and helped him release emotions, which his parents were unaware he was holding. This case example illustrates how a remedy selected for the physical complaints acted on both the physical and the emotional levels, even though the remedy was chosen only for the rash.

EXAMPLE CASE #2: Mag phos for menstrual pains

A fifteen-year-old complained of menstrual pains. She spends the first day of her menses on the couch, curled into a ball with a heating pad on her abdomen. When the pain is intense, she makes a fist with her hands and kneads her lower belly with firm pressure. She says the pain comes and goes in waves. She is also notably averse to disagreements – more than usual.

For this case of menses pain, either the "Law of Similars" or the "Law of Deficiencies" can be used to select the cell salt **Mag phos 6X**. **Mag phos** covers the physical symptoms and the emotional sensitivity.

The cell salt **Mag phos** covers many types of spasmodic and neuralgic pains, which are better from heat and firm pressure. Abdominal colic, muscle cramps, neuralgia headaches, spasmodic bladders, and heart palpitations are a few symptoms. **Mag phos** can help resolve pain, mainly when the pain is better with heat and pressure.

Interesting side note: the homeopathic remedy *Colocynthis (bitter apple) covers this case of menstrual cramps, too, and this plant contains high magnesium levels.

You can start selecting remedies using the Cell Salt Reference Key on **page 44**.

*Also, see some suggested cell salt books in the **Appendix 4—Additional Resources** starting on **page 346**.*

CELL SALT POTENCY

Homeopathic cell salts are prepared by the homeopathic pharmaceutical process of **trituration**—repetitive dilution and grinding with a mortar and pestle of a small amount of mineral salt in lactose. The resulting low-potency remedy (typically 3X, 6X, or 12X) is pressed into quick-dissolving tablets or dissolved in water. These low-potency cell salts contain a tiny amount of the original mineral salt.

> **Note:** For our purposes, mineral remedies in potencies greater than 12X are not considered cell salts, even when the remedies are made from the same material. For example, **Nat mur 30X, 6C, 12C**, or **30C** are not cell salts because they do not fall in the **3X-12X** potency range. However, you may reference the **Nat mur** materia medica to deepen your understanding of the characteristics of **Nat mur 6X**.

CELL SALT DOSING

Follow the label instructions for quantity per dose on the bottle or tube.

Dry Dosing

- Tablets can be dispensed into the bottle top and then tipped into the mouth or hand for self-administering.

- Tablets can be crushed between two spoons, and the powder can be tipped into the mouth.

Water Dosing

- Mixed with a bit of water and sipped.

Special Note for Mag phos: The cell salt **Mag phos** works best when taken in warm water.

Dosing For Babies

- Single tablets can be held against the inside of a young child's cheek. The tablet will dissolve quickly.

- A tablet can be dissolved in a small amount of water in a teaspoon, and the liquid is given straight from the spoon or a medicine dropper.

- Nursing mothers can take the remedies themselves as they will transfer via breastmilk.

Frequency of Dosing

Dosing frequency depends on the condition. If you are working with an acute condition that appears suddenly and lasts only a short period, for example, menstrual cramps, or a cold or flu, decide on the best-indicated cell salts, taking a few of each remedy every 10-30 minutes for a few doses until the person starts to feel better. Then, continue to take, but lengthen the time between doses until symptoms are much improved.

Cold example: Combine **Ferrum phos 6X**, **Nat mur 6X**, and **Kali mur 6X** if the symptoms fit, taking a dose of each remedy every 10-15 minutes at the first sign of a cold or sore throat for about three doses. As you notice the symptoms subsiding, you can reduce the frequency, taking them every 2-3 hours and then once or twice a day for a day or two until all symptoms are resolved.

When to Stop

- Stop as soon as the person's symptoms start to improve. Re-start if the same symptom(s) returns. When the symptom picture changes, you may need to change the remedy(s).

- Stop if the person experiences any worsening of the symptoms.

- If there is no improvement after 4-6 doses in an acute situation, such as a cold or menstrual pain, stop and try a different cell salt(s).

- If there is no improvement after trying three different cell salts, stop and consider contacting a professional homeopath or a healthcare provider.

- Sensitive people are more likely to do better with fewer doses of the remedy, while more rugged folks tolerate more frequent dosing.

For chronic conditions, such as arthritis or bone conditions, such as osteopenia or recurring cavities, where the person has had the condition for some time, the condition is often more complex. Hence, it takes time to resolve. In this case, take a dose of the indicated cell salt or a combination of salts two times a day for two to three months. It often takes three months to see a change in a chronic condition. It is important to be consistent and have patience. If you are new to homeopathy, consider consulting a homeopath for chronic conditions.

Important Note: Taking breaks from dosing cell salts is important so the body does not develop a tolerance. It can be done using either of these two ways: 1) The salts can be taken Monday through Friday, with the weekends off, OR 2) the cell salts can be taken for three consecutive weeks and the fourth week off.

COMBINING CELL SALT REMEDIES

In most classical homeopathic practices, only one homeopathic remedy is taken at a time. However, practitioners who use the cell salts often combine one to three cell salts at a time and may change the remedy selection quickly as the symptom picture changes. The cell salt remedies lie between a mineral supplement and a higher potency homeopathic remedy, which contains no physical substance.

Several popular cell salt combinations are on the market, for example, **Bioplasma** and **Biochemic phosphates**. **Bioplasma** contains all 12 cell salts, while **Biochemic Phosphates** contain just the five phosphates: **Calc phos, Ferrum phos, Kali phos, Mag phos**, and **Nat phos.**

Generally speaking, the best healing work is done when the remedy(s) are individualized to the case rather than choosing the five or twelve cell salts combinations. In an acute case, avoid using **Bioplasma** as some of the remedies work against each other, and management of the case is easily confused.

Some people report a lift from **Bioplasma** after a physical workout or when recovering from a recent illness and a calming effect from **Biochemic phosphates**. **Bioplasma** should not be taken as a daily mineral nutritional supplement.

Suggested Dosing When Combining Cell Salts for CHRONIC Complaints:

If taking TWO Salts:

Cell Salt 1: Waking + late morning
Cell Salt 2: Mid-day + Bedtime

Two remedies can be taken on the same day but preferably not at the same time unless they are already combined in a ready-made formulation.

If taking THREE Salts:

Cell Salt 1: Waking

Cell Salt 2: Mid-day

Cell Salt 3: Bedtime

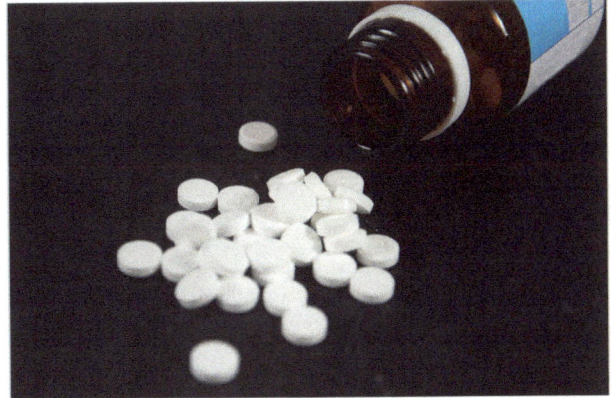

Another option is to rotate the selected cell salts weekly. For example, take Cell Salt 1 the first week, Cell Salt 2 the second week, and Cell Salt 3 the third week.

It's helpful for a person to create a relationship with their cell salts and use their symptoms and intuition about when to repeat them.

CASE EXAMPLE FOR COMBINING CELL SALT REMEDIES FOR AN ACUTE:

After traveling on an airplane, Jamal feels he is coming down with an acute illness. He is sneezing, his eyes are tired, his throat is dry, and he feels a dull ache in his ears. He selects the following cell salt remedies:

- **Ferrum phos 6X** for inflammation and enhanced circulation

- **Nat mur 6X** for sneezing and water balance

- **Kali mur 6X** for mucous membrane support

Dosing: Ferrum phos 6X, Nat mur 6X, and **Kali mur 6X**, one dose of each remedy, alternating them every few hours or Jamal can take all three remedies at the same time, every few hours. By the next day, he is feeling fine, and the cold symptoms have resolved, but he is a little tired, so he plans to take **Calc phos 6X**, one dose, four times during the next 12 hours as a restorative remedy and has discontinued the other cell salts. This plan is an example of how several well-selected remedies are combined.

To find where to purchase cell salts, see **Appendix 4—Additional Resources** *on* **page 349.**

REFERENCE KEY TO HOMEOPATHIC CELL SALT REMEDIES 3X-12X

	Action	Tissue Affinity	Worse/Better From	Symptoms
Calc fluor **Calcium fluoride**	Suppleness, elasticity.	Blood vessel walls, connective tissue, tendons and ligaments, bones and teeth.	Worse dampness and rest.	Bone tonic. Weak or strained joints/back pain. Hemorrhoids. Constipation with difficulty expelling stool due to tissue weakness.
Calc phos **Calcium phosphate**	Nutritive, restorative, convalescence.	Blood, bones and teeth. Digestion.	General aggravation from cold or drafts.	Bone tonic. Weak or strained joints/back pain. Digestion. Colic. Diarrhea. Heavy menses with fatigue.
Calc sulph **Calcium sulphate**	Blood cleanser	Liver, blood, skin.	Desires fresh air. Worse stuffy rooms.	Yellow discharges with skin conditions or cold/allergy symptoms.
Ferrum phos **Iron phosphate**	Inflammation. Heat, redness, swelling and pain. Oxygen carrier.	Blood. Circulation.	Pain improves with motion or constriction.	Congestive conditions and inflammation such as sore throats, colds, earaches, fever, sprains and strains.
Kali mur **Potassium chloride**	Cleanser. White discharges and mucus.	Skin, mucous membranes, digestive tract.	Worse rich foods.	White discharges from mucous membranes or skin. Cough, runny nose, sore throats, burns. Earache with swollen glands and white tongue. Also supports slowed digestion accompanied by white-coated tongue. Heartburn, gas, diarrhea or light-colored firm stool. Digestive headache.
Kali phos **Potassium phosphate**	Nerve and brain nutrient.	Nerve tissues.	Symptoms worse from mental/physical exertion and cold.	Soothes jangled nerves. Nervous conditions with fatigue, impatience, restlessness, irritability. Headache or tension from tight muscles or nervous tension. Tension pain may extend down the back.
Kali sulph **Potassium sulphate**	Oxygen carrier. Lubricant for sticky "stuff."	Blood, lungs, mucous membranes, skin.	May be better with fresh air and worse in a stuffy room.	Yellow sticky discharges such as yellow/sticky sinus and ear congestion. Yellow diarrhea, yellow nasal discharge. Earache with yellow tongue and ear discharge.
Mag phos **Magnesium phosphate**	Antispasmodic. Nerve tonic.	Muscles and nerves.	Generally better with heat and pressure.	Well indicated for spasmodic/nerve pain such as abdominal or menstrual cramps, leg cramps, spasmodic coughs. Earaches w/ sharp pain. Neuralgic head pain.
Nat mur **Sodium chloride**	Water distributor	Mucous membranes, digestive track, bodily fluids.	Many food/beverage sensitivities.	Conditions too dry/too wet. Both states coexist. Discharge is clear, watery or whitish like raw egg white. Sore throats. Heartburn. Postnasal drip. Hay fever. Colds. Stools with mucus or dry and hard with ineffectual urging.
Nat phos **Sodium phosphate**	Acid/Alkaline balancer.	Digestive tract, tissues, joints.	Worse cold foods/beverages, fat and sweets.	Acid indigestion. Infant colic. Lactic or uric acid buildup. Sleeplessness from indigestion/heartburn. Achy, swelling joints.
Nat sulph **Sodium sulphate**	Liver mover.	Liver, digestive tract, respiratory tract.	Worse rich foods. Better fresh, warm and dry air.	Digestive complaints. Sick headache, heartburn, yellow diarrhea, esp. with flatulence. Respiratory complaints. Cold and congestion with yellow mucus, wheezing and chest tightness.
Silicea	Cleanser. Helps to expel small foreign objects.	Connective tissue, skin, hair, nails, teeth and bones.	Worse chill. Better warmth.	Poor metabolism, especially of minerals. Pus-infection. Congestion. Skin eruptions and weakness. Sweaty parts, especially hands and feet.

For a basic guide to cell salts, look at *Schussler's Biochemic Pocket Guide With Repertory* available for sale online.

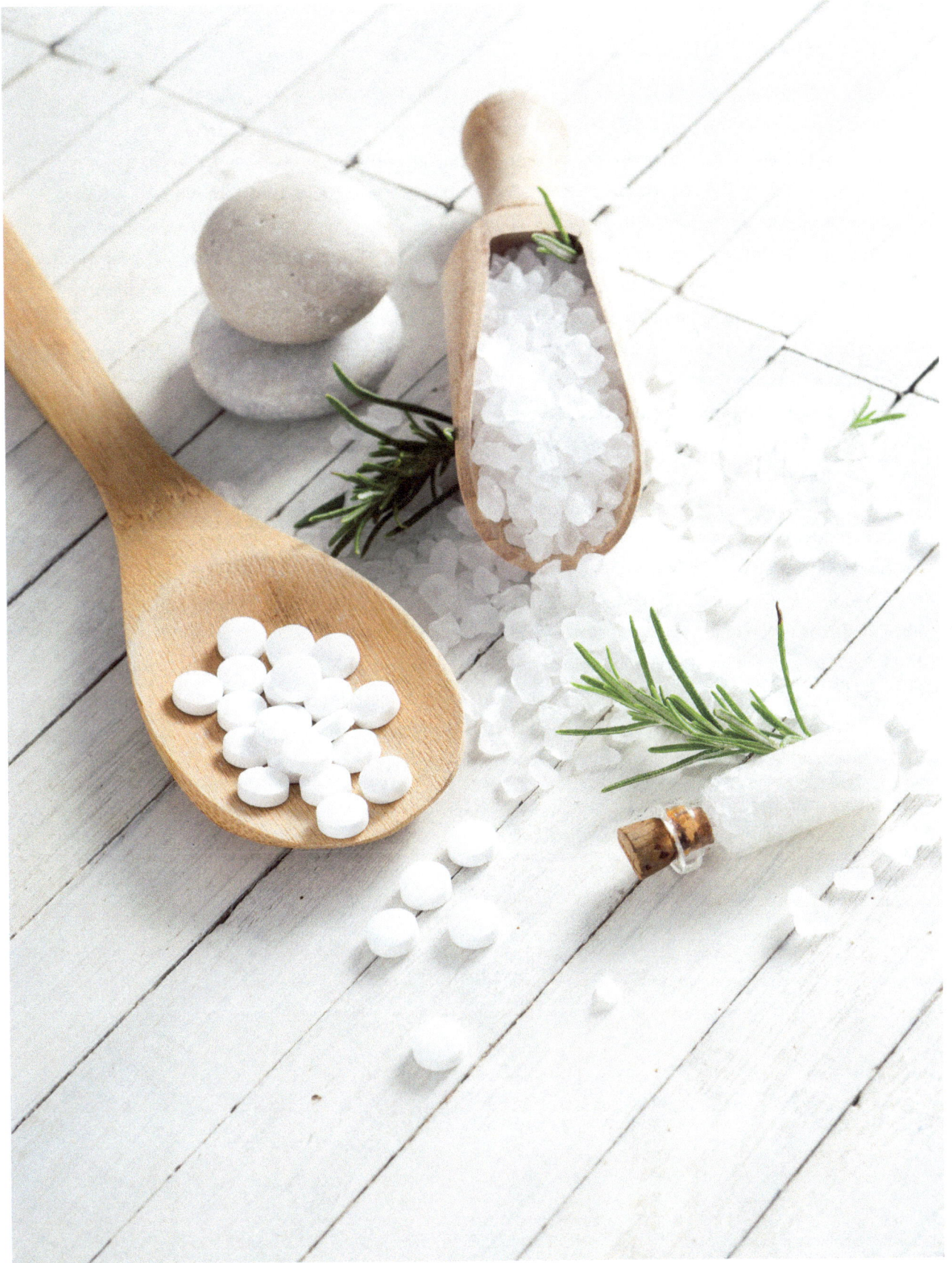

? CELL SALT QUIZ

Using the Cell Salt Key, see if you can match a different cell salt to each symptom condition:

1. Congested, throbbing pains are in the temples or over the eyes, with a red face.
2. Nervous conditions cause irritability, restlessness, and impatience.
3. Dull, heavy headache accompanies a watery nose or increased saliva, and sometimes firm stools.
4. Earache and sinus congestion have yellow sticky mucus.
5. Neuralgic headaches cause darting pain. Heat and pressure relieve the pain. Cold aggravates the pain.
6. Back pain from strain or produce a sensation of weakness in the back. May have constipation.
7. Constipation causes difficulty expelling stool, which may be due to hemorrhoids.
8. The muscles cramp and produce spasmodic pains, or nerve pains, as in menstrual cramps or from overused muscles during exercise.
9. Headache accompanies white-coated tongue or hawking white mucus.
10. A raw sore throat is from post nasal drip with clear water mucus from nasal passages.
11. Skin eruptions are ones that are pus-filled.
12. First signs of illness are experienced as a sore throat with pain, redness, or swelling.
13. Acid reflux or indigestion is from overindulgence of fats or sweets.
14. Colds with chest tightness, wheezing, are accompanied by yellow expectoration or nasal mucus.
15. A headache is on the crown of the head, with acid, sour regurgitation, and creamy-coated tongue.
16. A fever comes on quickly with throat or sinus inflammation.
17. A cold produces sticky yellow mucus in sinuses or ears accompanied by a yellow-coated tongue.
18. Allergy symptoms appear with yellowish discharge and a desire for fresh air.
19. A sick headache produces dullness and a bitter taste in the mouth.
20. A headache is from too much mental work and worry.

Answer key on page 323.

CHAPTER 4
First-Aid for Injuries

Immediate use of homeopathy to aid in recovery from trauma to the body or mind can prevent an emergency from becoming more serious and complicated. What remedies are needed to bring the psyche or body back into balance will depend on the nature of the trauma and the symptoms produced by it.

YOUR FIRST TASK — ASSESSING SHOCK

Any trauma, whether minor or major, is always accompanied by some degree of shock. That's why your first action should be the assessment of shock. Then homeopathy can be applied to do what it does best: provide gentle healing, in a short amount of time and with little need for any further intervention.

SHOCK

Shock is a potentially critical condition brought on by the sudden reduction in blood flow through the body. Shock may result from trauma, heatstroke, blood loss or an allergic reaction. It also may result from severe infection, poisoning, serious burns or other causes. When a person is in shock, their organs don't get enough blood or oxygen. Untreated, shock can damage organs or even cause death.

Before determining the severity of any injury, it's important to evaluate for shock. The remedies that will be needed depend on the symptoms and the cause of the shock, but for most trauma-induced shock you should please evaluate if the person is in shock and give either **Aconite** or **Arnica**:

- **Aconite:** The person needing **Aconite** is very fearful, anxious, extremely reactive to pain, and inconsolable. The eyes can have a glassy appearance, and/or with dilated pupils. The person is likely to be screaming, crying out, and trembling with terror and pain. **Aconite** definitely presents as a hyped-up state!

- **Arnica:** The person is stunned, irritable when offered help, exhausted, and uncooperative. The person says "I'm fine" and doesn't want to be touched, even withdrawing if you approach them. They may complain of pain, feeling as if they've been beaten up, but will steadfastly maintain that they are fine. The stronger their denial, especially if visibly injured, the more likely they are to need **Arnica**. They feel like they have been beaten up. In contrast to **Aconite**, someone needing **Arnica** will seem dull and even a little out-of-body.

Dosing: Use ORANGE method.
Observe and evaluate.

For shock induced by allergic reactions, see **Anaphylactic Shock** *later in this chapter* **page 52**.

For shock from blood loss, heatstroke, burns, etc., see **Clinical Shock** *later in this chapter on* **page 52**.

For guidance on emotional shock and/or fright, see **Chapter 19—Mind and Emotions** *starting on* **page 219.**

GENERAL INJURIES

Even the healthiest bodies react when they encounter a strong intrusion from the outside world. Common allergens, bites, stings, and poisonings force the body to mount a defense that may result in uncomfortable and sometimes life-threatening symptoms. To help manage these, this chapter provides some common-sense advice and homeopathic remedy ideas.

If you are facing an extreme reaction and are unsure how to handle it, you should always be prepared to dial 911 (or the appropriate emergency number in your area) to call for an ambulance.

IT'S AN EMERGENCY WHEN

- The person is drowsy, sleepy, and/or vomiting.
- The person loses consciousness; has a seizure; is unable to move or feel any part of the body; cannot recognize familiar people or surroundings; has balance, speech, or vision problems; or has clear fluid draining from the nose or mouth. Get them to the emergency room or urgent care center immediately.
- One pupil of the eyes seems more dilated than the other or both pupils are dilated. This symptom alone is reason enough to go to the emergency room immediately.
- If the person has fallen and has a severe headache or they fall asleep right after hitting their head – or if you suspect a skull fracture – do NOT move them: call 911. Then while awaiting help, keep the person warm. You can still give the appropriate remedies while waiting.
- The person just does not seem right or they are quite out of it for more than six hours. Take them to the emergency room or urgent care facility. Never worry about overreacting or wasting someone's time; you are being responsible by making sure the person is all right. In dealing with a head injury or the possibility of internal bleeding, everything must be checked out by medical professionals.

BLEEDING/HEMORRHAGES

We need blood to survive, so losing too much of it is a danger that needs quick medical intervention.

IT'S AN EMERGENCY WHEN

- There is visible bleeding from an injured artery, in which case the flow is bright red and comes in spurts, or from a vein, which produces a steady flow of darker red blood. Blood flow must be stopped or at least reduced as soon as possible to avoid having the person go into shock.

While waiting for emergency help and if the 911 operator doesn't offer guidance:

1. Consider removing any foreign objects (when applicable) and apply pressure directly over the site with a clean gauze pad, or by squeezing the edges of the wound together. Cover the wound with a clean and sterile dressing. If the bleeding continues through the dressing, don't remove it but apply more dressings and more pressure.

2. If the bleeding comes from a limb, elevate that limb above the heart if possible. Keep the person calm and still, checking their pulse every five minutes. If the pulse rate is increasing, it may mean that there is internal bleeding. Signs of internal bleeding are dizziness or faintness, rapid but weak pulses, shallow breathing, and cold, clammy skin.

While waiting for help, consider the following remedies:

- **Aconite**—Acute for hemorrhages accompanied by a lot of anxiety, fear, and panic. The blood flows bright red, and the person is thirsty, feverish, and restless.

- **Arnica**—The first remedy for bleeding from any physical trauma. It helps stabilize the bleeding and prevents infection and shock.

- **Belladonna**—For arterial injuries with sudden hemorrhaging: the blood is bright red, gushing out; it feels hot and coagulates easily. The person's face is red and hot, but their limbs may be cold. Useful in uterine hemorrhages with bearing-down pains.

- **Carbo veg**—Continuous passive venous hemorrhage in someone who has cold, bluish skin, is in a state of shock and collapse, and desperately wants to be fanned.

- **China**—Intermittent hemorrhages, profuse and exhausting, that nearly drain the person dry. Dark, clotted blood flows from any orifice. Substantial loss of blood is likely to be accompanied by ringing in the ears. Useful in removing severe anemia and weakness after major blood loss.

- ***Hamamelis**—Passive venous hemorrhages of usually dark blood. There is no anxiety, but there is exhaustion, a hammering headache, and feelings of soreness and bruising. Also used for hemorrhoids.

- **Ipecac**—Bright red, gushing blood, accompanied by nausea, labored breathing, and fainting. The tongue is clean, the skin cold and covered with cold sweat. Thirstless and irritable. Worse lying down, but better in the open air.

BLOWS AND CONTUSIONS/BRUISES

A hard blow to any part of the body will cause blood vessels under the skin to burst and release blood into the surrounding soft tissue. The affected area then turns deep purple and/or blue. Later it will turn yellow, before eventually disappearing. Homeopathic remedies not only help to reduce swelling, bruising, and pain, they will also speed up the healing process.

For any injury likely to result in bruising, give **Arnica** immediately. **Arnica** is the first remedy for bruising and hematomas (a bump of clotted blood).

If a blow may have injured a vital organ, such as the kidneys, spleen, stomach, liver, or lungs, the person must be evaluated by a healthcare professional to ensure that there is no internal bleeding.

Note: Pain is a necessary communication from the body that there is something wrong. Although you may give a remedy to make someone more comfortable, it is very important to also give an injured person rest and proper support measures to ensure complete healing. For instance, **Ruta** can reduce the pain of a sprained ankle, however it is still imperative to rest the ankle and not let the person run or play sports until it is fully healed. Pain is a warning to stop. If it is not heeded, further damage can result.

BLOWS TO THE ORGANS/SOFT TISSUE

The most common remedy for blows to organs and soft tissues is ***Bellis per**. This is a remedy for damage to the breast, the abdominal area (housing the stomach, liver, and spleen), the kidneys (located on either side of the spine just below the rib cage), or the pelvic area (housing the intestines, bladder, and reproductive organs).

Give ***Bellis per** every two hours for at least three doses. Because this remedy can disrupt sleep, it's best to give it at least six hours before bed. However, if needed, it is better to give the remedy rather than worry about impaired sleep.

For a blow to the breast, if ***Bellis per** does not help, consider ***Conium**.

For blows to the penis or testicles **Calendula**, **Arnica**, or **Hypericum** are helpful. If inflammation develops after a contusion, consider **Arnica**, ***Conium**, ***Hamamelis**, or **Pulsatilla**.

WHEN TO CONTACT YOUR HEALTHCARE PROFESSIONAL

- If someone has received a blow to a vital organ or the body cavity containing it. The injury must be checked out to ensure that there is no internal bleeding or hidden damage.

CUTS AND ABRASIONS

See **Chapter 18—Skin** on **page 200.**

INFECTED WOUNDS

See **Chapter 18—Skin** on **page 201**.

NERVE INJURIES

Nerves are made up of fiber bundles which are wrapped around layers of tissue and fat that can be damaged by overstretching, trauma, long sustained pressure, or slicing. If a nerve is damaged or cut, the signals to and from the brain weaken or cease altogether, causing muscles not to work properly. It can also cause pain, especially burning and shooting sensations, or a loss of feeling in the injured area.

IT'S AN EMERGENCY WHEN

- There is an extremely severe deep cut, raising the possibility that some nerves may have been severed.
- You suspect nerve damage anywhere along the spinal column.

WHEN TO CONTACT YOUR HEALTHCARE PROFESSIONAL

- Any sensations of numbness, pain, or burning that are not resolving.
- You suspect nerve damage is happening due to repetitive use, i.e., as in carpal tunnel syndrome.

Remedies to consider:

- **Arsenicum:** For pains that burn like fire, with a sensation of hot needles, although paradoxically the injured area feels better with warm applications. The skin is sensitive to the touch and the person is restless, anxious, and demanding, especially at night.

- ***Coffea cruda:** This remedy is useful for a nerve injury with pain triggered by the least motion or noise and so intolerably intense that it keeps one awake at night and in a heightened state of awareness. The remedy can help induce sleep. Those needing this remedy can be hysterical, hypersensitive to everything, weeping or screaming.

- **Hypericum:** A tonic for injured nerves, especially in such nerve-rich areas as the fingertips, toes, knees, coccyx, elbows, and parts of the face, lips, and mouth. It is particularly useful if the tissue has been crushed, like a finger caught in a slammed door. There is a feeling of pressure, with pains that are intense and violent, appearing suddenly but disappearing gradually. They tend to shoot upwards, and the surrounding area is very tender and sore, sometimes with tingling, twitching, trembling, or numbness.

Dosing: Use ORANGE method. Observe and evaluate.

HEAD INJURIES

See **Chapter 5—Head** on **page 78**.

ALLERGIC REACTIONS

Allergic reactions can be mild (the person may sneeze for a few minutes) to severe (anaphylactic shock and potentially fatal respiratory arrest). An allergic reaction is the body's response to an allergen—any substance that the body is trying to defend itself against. This defensive response typically triggers a release of histamine into tissues, causing inflammation and other symptoms.

Common allergic responses to an allergen include: sneezing; runny nose; eyes that are swollen, puffy, red, watering, or excessively dry; swelling and itching in other parts of the body; inflammation; rashes; vomiting and/or diarrhea, and hives (itchy, stinging welts on the skin). Hives can also be produced by an emotional upset and other causes (for more about hives, see **Chapter 18—Skin** on **page 205**). Extreme allergic responses can include: paleness; swelling of lymph glands; swelling of the tongue, blocked air passages and constricted breathing; extreme itching or sweating; rapid pulse; shallow and/or irregular breathing; confusion, collapse, or unconsciousness.

Asthmatic responses to an allergen include: mild to severe wheezing; shortness of breath; coughing; chest tightness; rattling; increased mucus in the bronchi (tubes that carry air from the windpipe into the lungs); and sometimes sneezing. Coughing may lead to retching (gagging) and sometimes vomiting.

Asthma can become a chronic allergic reaction and is often a hereditary condition. The remedies listed below are helpful in an acute episode; however, the underlying cause of the asthma should be addressed by a professional homeopath through constitutional treatment. It is advisable to use prescribed medications, including inhalers, as needed during constitutional homeopathic care until the breathing difficulties are under control.

IT'S AN EMERGENCY WHEN

- The person is experiencing an **extreme allergic response** such as anaphylactic shock (read more in the next section) and obstructed breathing. Blood pressure can drop dramatically, causing faintness and irregular heart palpitations that can set off extreme panic in a person. In the case of a severe allergic response, call 911. The person should be taken to an emergency room immediately.

Apis can save a life on the way to the hospital in this situation if there is an extreme allergic reaction. Give a few pellets every 15 minutes, even while waiting at the hospital. If the person is unconscious, dissolve some pellets in a glass of water and apply some of the solution to their wrist or on their lips.
*See the next section on **Anaphylactic Shock** for other remedies to consider.*

COMMON ALLERGENS AND ASSOCIATED REMEDY(S)

Allergen	Remedy(s)
Animal Dander	**Arsenicum**: watery and burning discharge, sneezing without relief, dry nasal cavity, anxiety, restlessness, difficulty breathing. **Allium cepa**: eyes burning, biting, smarting, itching. Need to rub eyes. Redness and tearing.
Car Fumes Pollution	**Carbo veg**: head feels heavy and hot, intense pain at the base of skull, weakness, exhaustion, external body cold, but feels hot inside, thirst, nausea. Close to collapse from not enough fresh oxygen, quick respiration, spasms of cough with weakness. ***Petroleum**: nausea with or without vomiting, profuse salivation, dizziness, heavy feeling, stomach painful with cold empty sensation, can have heavy pulsing pain in head.
After Exposure to Cold	**Rhus tox**: water-filled blisters or hives that itch intensely after exposure to cold.
Dust	**Arsenicum**: watery and burning discharge, sneezing without relief, dry nasal cavity, anxiety, restlessness, difficulty breathing.
Pesticides	**Arsenicum**: breathlessness, weakness, diarrhea, anxiety.
Poisonous Plants	**Arsenicum**: burning, itching, sensitivity to touch, swelling, scratching makes itching worse, very chilly, but better with warmth. **Rhus tox**: intense itchiness and redness with fluid-filled blisters, heat, inflammation, burning, swelling, sensitivity to cold air.
Shellfish	**Arsenicum**: burning, itching, sensitivity to touch, swelling, scratching of hives makes itching worse, very chilly and better with warmth. ***Urtica**: hives from shellfish, burning, stinging, intense itching, possible pains in the joints (especially if reaction is to shellfish).

Dosing: Use ORANGE method. Observe and evaluate.

HAY FEVER/SEASONAL ALLERGIES

*See **Chapter 8—Nose** on **page 97**.*

SHOCK

*For general shock, see the beginning of this chapter on **page 47**.*

ANAPHYLACTIC SHOCK

In anaphylactic shock, the body releases large amounts of histamine (a chemical compound involved in immune reactions and neurotransmission) into the bloodstream, causing blood vessels to dilate and airways to narrow. This type of shock can come on quickly. You might suddenly feel too warm, have the sensation of a lump in your throat or difficulty swallowing, break out in hives or localized redness, experience tingling or itching, or feel your tongue and lips swelling. Blood pressure can drop dramatically, resulting in faintness; the pulse may become weak and rapid, with heart palpitations that can set off panic and agitation.

🏥 IT'S AN EMERGENCY WHEN

- The person is experiencing anaphylactic shock. **DO NOT DELAY**, as time is of the essence, especially if hives have come on very quickly and/or the throat is swelling. Give **Apis** on the way to the hospital (see below).

Remedies to consider while you wait for care, or on the way to the hospital using the RED dosing method:

- **Apis**: This remedy can save a life in an extreme allergic reaction. Swelling is rapid, and there is no thirst. There may be panting and a feeling of not being able to get enough air or take another breath. Someone who needs **Apis** may be whiny, weepy, restless, anxious, irritable, and fidgety. On the other hand, they may be tired and want to lie down.

- ***Carbolic acid***: This remedy is for anaphylactic shock following a bee or wasp sting, with respiratory problems, fainting, swelling, and hives. The part affected will be weak, with intense itching and severe burning and pricking pains that come and go. There may be cold hands and feet, trembling, and profuse cold, clammy sweats. The person rapidly loses vitality and strength, even to the point of collapse.

People needing ***Carbolic acid*** are likely to have strong chemical and environmental sensitivities, and a very acute sense of smell can be a strong indicator for this remedy. If you or someone close to you has a known allergy that can cause anaphylactic shock, you might want to purchase this remedy to have on hand in an emergency.

CLINICAL SHOCK

Clinical shock is typically caused by losing substantial body fluids through bleeding, vomiting, diarrhea, or sweating to the point of total dehydration, as might happen with heatstroke or sunstroke. It can also result from surgery, a head injury, poisoning, or systemic infection. Clinical shock manifests with skin that is cold and clammy, either pale or of a bluish color; a rapid and weak pulse; hyperventilating or difficulty breathing; disorientation, sleepiness, and/or restlessness; and weakness.

🏥 IT'S AN EMERGENCY WHEN

- The person is not responding to remedies for shock.
- The person becomes unresponsive.

💚 ADDITIONAL SUPPORT FOR SHOCK

- Do not move the person if you suspect a broken bone or they seem to be in severe pain. Keep them warm and comfortable. If nothing is broken, raise their feet above the level of the heart. Don't give them anything to eat or drink in case they require surgery.

Remedies to consider:

- **Arnica**: Heavy internal bleeding may also bring on clinical shock. This is a remedy to consider for someone who's been hit by a car – or any large, heavy object – particularly if they are denying they need help even while shrinking from being touched.

- **Carbo veg**: For acute shock with breathing difficulties. Shock responding to this remedy is usually due to a loss of body fluids from bleeding, vomiting, or diarrhea. The face is pale with a bluish tint. While gasping for breath, the person asks to be fanned, the faster the better, as there is an overwhelming need for fresh air. They are likely to be markedly indifferent to everything, weak, exhausted, and confused; if they have enough vitality left, they may be irritable. Though cold externally, they do not want to be covered because inside they are burning up. You can help by keeping their feet elevated, keeping the air around them cool, and letting them rest and regain their energy.

- **China**: For shock from loss of blood or depletion of other bodily fluids through vomiting, diarrhea, or excessive perspiration – anything that causes severe dehydration. Someone needing **China** is completely drained and weak, to the point of trembling and being shaky on their feet. Sensitive, irritable, and unable to think straight, the person may complain of ringing in the ears or blurred vision. Similar to **Carbo veg**, they like being fanned, but not too hard, because that takes their breath away – and they're already having enough trouble trying to breathe.

- ***Veratrum**: Also for shock from loss of bodily fluids, especially from vomiting and diarrhea. Shock manifests as cold sweats, beads of clammy perspiration on the forehead, and chills so intense that they flee to the shower or a hot bath to warm themselves up. Even their skin has a bluish tint. Given how much sweat they're producing, it's no surprise that they have a huge thirst; but paradoxically, despite their chilliness, it's cold water they crave. The pulse is feeble, but they are restless, and their condition worsens quickly.

Dosing: Use the ORANGE method. Observe and evaluate.

ELECTRICAL SHOCK

Electrical shock is caused by contact with a live electrical wire or being struck by lightning. The shock may be a mild jolt or so severe as to cause powerful muscle contractions, heart palpitations, and difficulty breathing. The person may even lose consciousness and stop breathing.

IT'S AN EMERGENCY WHEN

- There is a loss of consciousness or a persistent state of shock with confusion.
- The person is nonreactive, having convulsions or trouble breathing, or is listless or limp.
- The person has stopped breathing — start CPR (cardiopulmonary resuscitation) and have someone call 911 immediately.

Check for electrical burns on the skin. After assessing for shock and giving **Aconite** or **Arnica**, give one dose of **Phosphorus** immediately. Repeat only if symptoms return.
*See also **Burns** on the bottom of **page 54**.*

SEPTIC AND TOXIC SHOCK

Septic shock is caused by an overwhelming bacterial infection. The symptoms include diarrhea, headaches, high fever (with or without chills), low blood pressure, muscle aches, nausea, vomiting, seizures, redness of the eyes, mouth, or throat, and/or a widespread rash that is red like a sunburn.

Septic shock is a serious condition that typically occurs from a wound infection going systemic. Look for red streaks traveling outwards from the wound toward the heart. These are a precursor to septic shock, not a sign of it, and they may be treated homeopathically to prevent septic shock from developing. At the first sign of red streaks, ***Pyrogenium** may be given using the ORANGE dosing method. If you do not have ***Pyrogenium** or if the red streaks continue to spread despite using the remedy, call 911 immediately.

Toxic shock syndrome is a serious condition caused by bacterial toxins; it can result from something as simple as leaving a tampon inserted for longer than 8 hours.

IT'S AN EMERGENCY WHEN

- You suspect septic or toxic shock. Do NOT give a remedy - dial 911 or your local emergency number.
- There is loss of consciousness or a persistent state of shock with confusion.
- The person has had a fever for more than three days.
- The person is nonreactive, having trouble breathing, having convulsions, and/or is listless or limp.
- The person has stopped breathing — start CPR (cardiopulmonary resuscitation) and have someone call 911 immediately.
- You suspect a woman has toxic shock syndrome from the use of tampons.

ADDITIONAL SUPPORT FOR SEPTIC SHOCK OR TOXIC SHOCK WHILE YOU WAIT FOR HELP

- Place the sufferer on their back, unless trauma to the spine or neck is suspected. Loosen any tight clothing. Make sure the airway is clear and that they are breathing.
- Keep the person warm (not hot, to avoid sweating and further loss of fluids).
- Raise their legs slightly above their head, unless they have a head injury. In case of a head injury, the head should be raised slightly above the feet.
- If vomiting seems likely, turn their head to the side to prevent choking and aspiration of the vomit. If they ask for a drink, avoid cold liquids.
- If there is a wound, pressure should be applied to stop the bleeding.

EMOTIONAL SHOCK

See **Chapter 19—Mind and Emotions** on **page 219**.

BURNS

Burns on the skin are injuries caused by exposure to heat such as a hot stove pan or exhaust pipe, to chemicals, electricity, the sun or radiation. They can vary in severity, ranging from mild redness and blistering to deep tissue damage. Burns are quite painful and can lead to complications like infection and scarring. The depth of the burn and its source will determine how best to handle it.

IT'S AN EMERGENCY WHEN

- The burn is more than three inches, it covers the hands, joints or face and there is little to no pain.
- The burn may appear dry, leathery and be white, black, brown, or yellow in color.
- There is a third degree burn - see description in following section.

DEGREES OF BURNS

First Degree

In a first-degree burn, i.e., most sunburns or a minor scald, the upper layer of the skin is intensely hot, with swelling, pain, and redness. For minor burns, immediately applying WARM water, not cold, nor hot, to the spot is a trick that will quickly reduce pain. The idea of cold water may appeal intuitively, but it is not homeopathic to the injury. Consider these two remedies first:

Cantharis is a remedy known for helping with heat burns from touching something hot on a stove or sunburns. The sensation is burning and smarting and can avoid blistering when given immediately after the burn occurs.

*Urtica is the most common remedy for first-degree or minor burns with no blistering. It exhibits pronounced stinging pains and also makes it the preferred remedy for scalds.

Second Degree

In a second-degree burn, the first and second layers of the skin are damaged, causing a lot of pain, redness, swelling, and creating blisters that may ooze a watery fluid. ***Causticum**, **Cantharis** or ***Urtica**, when given immediately, can prevent blistering.

Third Degree

In a third-degree burn, the first and second layers of the skin are blackened, charred, or deathly white, with damage to the nerves and underlying tissue. There is usually no pain at the immediate site of the burn, as nerve endings there have been destroyed. However, the surrounding skin does burn and is very painful. ***Causticum** is the most common remedy for third-degree burns and, if given immediately, can prevent blistering.

Persons with a third-degree burn should seek emergency care. Apart from the searing pain of the initial burn, the most agonizing aspect of a third-degree burn is debridement, or the removal of dead tissue. Dressing a third-degree burn is a task for professionals in burn management.

For chemical burns, flush the area with clean water for at least five minutes, then treat with ***Causticum** or **Cantharis** if the burn is fairly severe.

For electrical burns, the remedy of choice is **Phosphorus**. Note that electrical burns are often more extensive than they may look because damage beneath the skin is apt to be greater than surface damage. Treat this as a severe burn, but do NOT give ***Causticum** if you've already given **Phosphorus** or if you have given **Phosphorus**, don't give ***Causticum**: the two remedies are close in so many respects as to be incompatible. **Kali bich** may be used if the burn leaves a sharp-edged hole.

For ailments during convalescence from extensive burns on much of the body, ***Carbolic acid** is helpful. Burns needing this remedy heal very slowly and tend to ulcerate.

ADDITIONAL SUPPORT FOR BURNS

- Do not put any conventional creams, oils, butter, or ointments on a newly burned area. These can hold in the heat and cause more burning. If the oils or creams have to be removed later, it will cause additional pain and trauma to the skin. After any blisters have healed and the burning pain is gone, **Calendula ointment** may be used to promote healing.
- Never puncture burn blisters, as doing so risks them becoming infected. For burns that do become infected, **Hepar sulph** should be given, particularly if the person is very chilly, extraordinarily sensitive to pain and cold air, and irritable to the point of being abusive.
- Water from the tap can be scalding hot. If you have young children in the house, the hot water heater should be set no higher than 125 °F (51.6 °C). Never leave a child unattended in a tub, because a scald can happen in less than five seconds if a child inadvertently opens the tap. Keep hot liquids well back from the edges of counters, especially coffee or teapots. Turn the handles of pans on the stove inward to prevent a child from reaching up and pulling a pan of hot liquid onto himself.

*See the **Common Remedies for Burns** chart on the next page.*

COMMON REMEDIES FOR BURNS

	Apis	Arsenicum	Belladonna	Cantharis	*Causticum	Phosphorus	*Urtica
Type of Burn	Chemical burns to the eyes, sunburns, tongue burns.	Grease or oil burns, tongue burns.	Sunburns.	Chemical burns (body and/or eyes), electrical burns, grease or oil burns, scalds, tailpipe burns, tongue burns.	Chemical burn, scalds, tailpipe burns, tongue burns.	Electrical burns, radiation burns.	Scalds, sunburns, tongue burns.
Symptoms	Skin is sensitive, very swollen, puffy, either reddened or pale. Pains are intense, burning, prickling or stinging. No thirst. Tired.	Skin burns like fire, but they do not want anything cool on the burn. Burns that have formed blisters that may ooze a foul discharge or become bloody.	Skin is bright red, painful, burning, and may throb. Much heat. Very sensitive to noise, light, touch, motion.	Pains sharp, needle-like, burning. Skin feels raw, itchy, smarting, stinging, inflamed. Blisters are sensitive to touch. Extreme thirst, but do not give them iced drinks.	Pains are burning with intense soreness. Skin feels raw, stiff, tight. Burns that are slow to heal, old painful burn scars. Burns with painful, tender blisters.	Most intense pain of all burns; violent burning with much heat. Feels as though there is something crawling under the skin.	Skin feels sore, raw, intensely itching, stinging, burning. May swell. Skin may be raised in red blotches, or have tiny, clear fluid-filled blisters.
Mood	Whiny, weepy, restless, anxious, irritable, fidgety.	Anxious, agitated, restless, chilly, and weak.	Delirious, changeable temperament, inclined to anger.	Anxious, restless, crying, full of rage.	Sad, sense of hopelessness, easily tearful.	Easily vexed, fearful, overly sensitive.	Restless.
Indications	May become scared of being alone or become dull. Wants to lie down.	Skin turns bluish or black.	If severe burn, eyes can be glassy, sparkling with wild look, dilated pupils. May have throbbing headache. Craves cold water or lemonade.	Burns tend to ooze fluid, start out bright red, later may turn black. Adverse to cool applications and removing gauze for even a few seconds.	Blisters that keep breaking open and bleeding. Never been well since a burn.	Will take care of shock and help the burn. Strong craving for ice cold water. Very sensitive to light, sound, odors, touch, and electrical changes, like a thunderstorm.	Useful as a tincture and an internal remedy. For old burns that itch and sting. Sunburns with much itching. Usually want to rub affected area. Look tired and pale.
Worse	Heat, touch, sleeping, late afternoon, lying down, pressure, right side.	Cold applications, cold drinks, and night.	3 PM, getting overheated or chilled, touch, noise, jarring, light, heat of the sun.	Touch, scratching, coffee, and iced drinks.	3-4 AM and 6-8 PM, cold drafts, stooping, motion, and darkness.	Change of weather, cold air, cold wind, thunderstorms, evening, exertion, lying on left side.	Cold water, after sleeping, cool moist air, cool baths, touch, night, and strenuous exercise.
Better	Cool applications, cool air, cool bathing, sitting up, cold drinks, and being uncovered.	Warm (not hot) applications, and warm (not hot) baths.	Rest, light covers, sitting semi-erect, low lights, and quiet.	Cool applications, lying down, rest, and quiet.	Sipping cold water, warmth, damp wet weather, and gentle motion.	Sleep, warmth, sympathy, eating, company, no or low lights, slow intake of cold things, cool applications, and sitting.	Lying down (but not on the affected parts), and gentle movement.

Dosing: Use the RED or ORANGE method. Observe and evaluate.

FAINTING AND COLLAPSE

Fainting, or syncope, is a temporary loss of consciousness from a lack of blood flow to the brain. The most common type, vasovagal syncope, can result from an extreme emotional upset, shock, poor ventilation, overheating, severe pain, loss of bodily fluids, exhaustion, hyperventilation, and/or dehydration. A sudden drop in blood pressure on standing up may lead to postural syncope (also known as postural hypotension). Plummeting blood sugar from going too long without food can cause one to faint, although paradoxically it's also possible to pass out right after eating, or after exercising.

Fainting is nature's way of quickly making a body horizontal— a favorable position for restoring blood flow and oxygen to the brain. Any of the fainting remedies below may be placed on the inside of the cheek to bring the person back to consciousness. Put the remedy between the gum and cheek and let it dissolve. Alternatively, you may dissolve a few pellets of remedy in a small amount of water and rub that onto the person's wrist.

Never put your fingers inside a person's mouth if they are experiencing a seizure and do not attempt to give any remedies until the seizure has passed.

Be aware that while there are benign causes for a sudden loss of consciousness, such as stimulation of the vagus nerve through the simple act of urinating copiously (loss of fluids), fainting can signal other problems, such as heart block or other cardiac or neurological issues, especially if it occurs repeatedly or episodes of unconsciousness are protracted.

IT'S AN EMERGENCY WHEN

- The person is having a seizure or convulsions.
- The person has not regained consciousness after a few minutes—keep them warm while you wait for emergency care.
- The person has fainted after falling and hitting their head or receiving a serious blow. Do not move the person—keep them warm while you wait for emergency care.
- You suspect there is internal bleeding.
- The person is having trouble breathing.
- The person is diabetic and has fainted.
- Fainting occurs repeatedly.

ADDITIONAL SUPPORT FOR FAINTING AND COLLAPSE

- Place the person on their back and loosen any tight clothing, especially around the neck.
- Keep onlookers at a distance, for optimum ventilation.
- Put a cool compress on the forehead.
- If possible, keep the person lying where they have fallen or sitting for at least a few minutes after consciousness has returned. When they try to stand up, make sure they are supported in case they are dizzy.
- If the person is dehydrated, give liquids slowly but steadily.
- If they have fainted from lack of food, give them a nutritious, high-carbohydrate snack.
- Observe the person closely for the next 24 hours.

COMMON REMEDIES FOR FAINTING AND COLLAPSE

	Aconite	Arnica	Carbo veg	China	Gelsemium	Ignatia	Pulsatilla
Onset	Rapid.	Shock.	Loss of body fluids from bleeding, vomiting, or diarrhea.	Loss of body fluids.	Prior to an event.	An emotional upset.	Dehydration
Symptoms	Heavy perspiration, rapid pulse, heart palpitations, heavy hot head.	Stunned, feels sore, beat up, and bruised.	Exhausted, weak, gasping for breath. Face is pale, with a bluish tint. Needs fresh air. May ask to be fanned.	Gasping for breath. May complain of ringing in ears, or blurred vision. Very weak, with much sweating.	Trembles, diarrhea, headache at the forehead or back of head. Droopy eyelids. Dizzy.	Very sensitive to pain. May have stomachache, sore throat, tight chest, cramps in muscles, numbness, tingling.	Mouth feels dry, but they are not thirsty. If chilly, wants window open for fresh air.
Mood	Anxious, restless, and fearful that they are going to die.	Irritable when offered help, exhausted, uncooperative saying they are fine. Does not want to be touched.	Indifferent to everything, a bit confused, irritable, and very sluggish.	Irritable, oversensitive, nervous, and may have problems sleeping.	Anxious, afraid, confused, dull, and weak.	Nervous excitable, introspective, easily frustrated, moody, weepy, lots of sighing or yawning.	Wants attention and gentleness. Usually weepy or feeling sorry for themselves.
Indications	Fainting from fright, severe anxiety, shock, or fear.	Fainting from shock, physical trauma, or blood loss.	Fainting from exhaustion, or weakness, with breathing difficulties.	Fainting from loss of fluids, as in hemorrhage or diarrhea.	From stage fright, fear of exams or public speaking, performance anxiety.	Fainting from grief, sudden bad news, loss, or a major disappointment.	Fainting from being in a hot, stuffy crowded room, or from dehydration.
Worse	Being alone.	In a crowd.	Stuffy room, stale stagnant airflow.	Activity, sitting up, cold.	Damp weather, emotion, thinking of his ailment.	Excitement.	Heat, stuffy room, lack of hydration.
Better	Rest, fresh air, and cool drinks after regaining consciousness.	Rest, lying down with head lowered, not being touched, quiet, and being away from people.	Vigorous fanning with fresh air, feet elevated, cool air, rest, and belching.	Quiet rest, firm pressure, bending double, warmth, and fresh air.	Bending forward, fresh air, and lying down with head slightly elevated.	Keeping calm and being encouraged to take deep breaths.	Cool fresh air, rehydration, and motion if faintness or dizziness is gone.

Dosing: After the person has regained consciousness, use the ORANGE method.

HEAT EXHAUSTION

Heat exhaustion comes from excessive exposure to the sun or exertion in an overly hot environment. It can come on quite quickly if the humidity is high. Loss of the body's salts through sweating results in an electrolyte imbalance that then affects brain function. The person becomes weak, nauseated, fatigued, and usually has a headache. Their skin grows pale, cool, and clammy from profuse sweating. With a weak pulse and falling blood pressure, they may be anxious and irritable, feel dizzy, have blurry vision, and even faint.

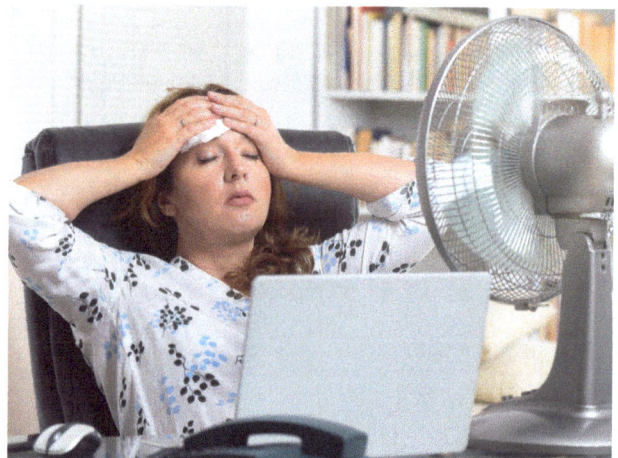

SIGNS OF HEAT EXHAUSTION

- dizziness and confusion
- headache
- excessive sweating and pale, clammy skin
- cramps in the legs, arms and stomach
- loss of appetite and feeling ill
- fast breathing or pulse
- cool, moist skin with goosebumps when in the heat
- thirsty

IT'S AN EMERGENCY WHEN

- You suspect sunstroke (see Sunstroke section that follows).
- The body temperature is rapidly rising.
- The person has had a seizure.
- The person is delirious for longer than 30 minutes.
- They do not respond to any of the remedies within an hour.

ADDITIONAL SUPPORT FOR HEAT EXHAUSTION

- Keep babies and small children out of the strong sun.
- Get an overheated person to a shaded or cool area. Keep them out of the sun.
- Be sure to keep well hydrated. Avoid caffeinated or very sugary drinks. A good rehydration drink for someone suffering from heat exhaustion would be: 16 pellets of **Bioplasma** (a combination of different tissue salts in homeopathic form); ¼ cup fresh lemon or lime juice; 1/16 - 1/4 tsp. sea salt (or potassium-based salt substitute); 16 oz. of water (you can add coconut water, if it's available); and a tiny bit of raw honey, organic sugar, or maple syrup to taste.
- Take **Natrum mur 6x cell salts** OR **Bioplasma cell salts** placed in water and sipped as a stopgap measure until a more appropriate remedy is found.

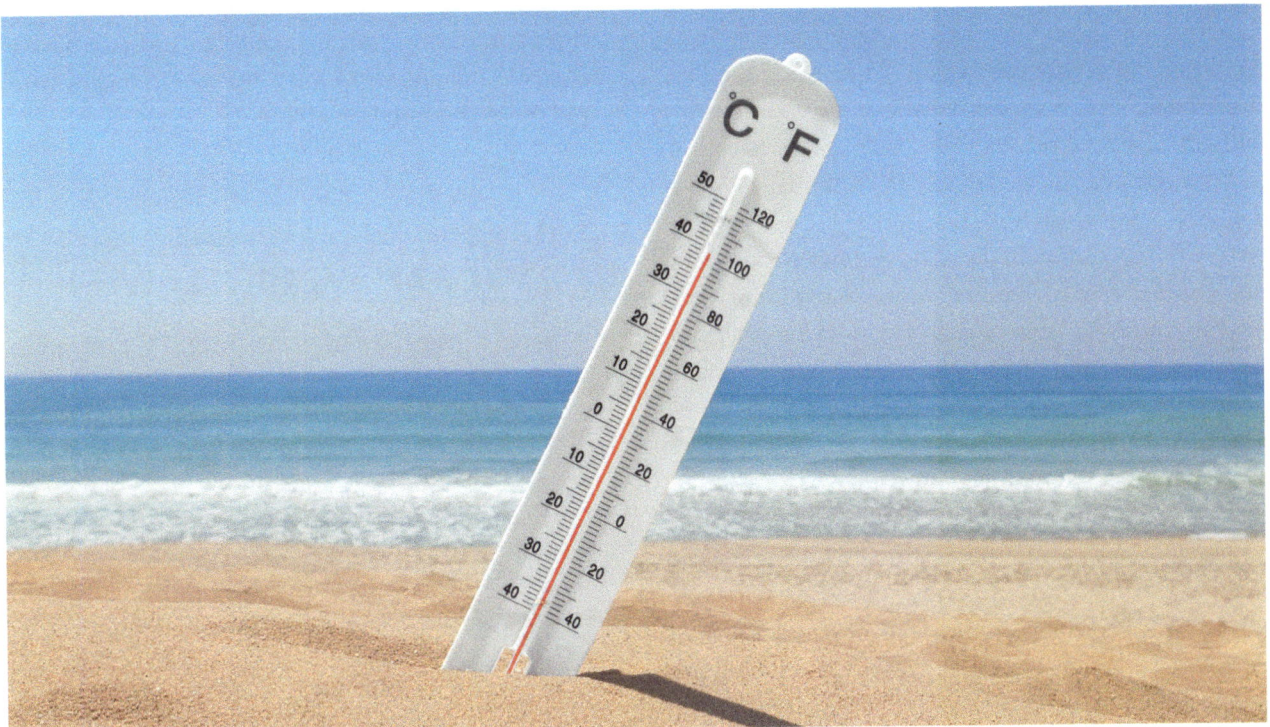

COMMON REMEDIES FOR HEAT EXHAUSTION

	Bryonia	China	Gelsemium	Natrum mur	Pulsatilla
Symptoms	Severe, splitting headache with bursting heavy sensation. Hurts to even move the eyes. Likely nauseous. Very thirsty for cold drinks. Dry mouth and throat.	Drained, very weak, trembling, and gasping for breath. May complain of ringing in the ears, or blurred vision. Much sweating.	Heavy eyes. Face flushed, but not bright red. Skin dry and hot, but hands and feet cold. May complain of chills going up and down spine. If there is a headache, it is at the nape of the neck.	Heat in the head with red face, nausea, and vomiting.	Air hunger, always taking deep breaths. Weak and can feel faint.
Mood	Grumpy, like a bear, and wants to be left alone.	Irritable, sensitive, and cannot think straight.	Drowsy and cannot think straight.	Weepy, dull, prefers to be alone.	May feel sorry for themselves, weepy, wants company or assurance.
Indications	Does not want to move.	Helpful for severe dehydration.	Looks as though they are drunk.	Head pain feels bursting like tiny hammers banging. Zigzag aura before eyes. Strong desire or aversion for salty food.	Very sensitive to heat and sun.
Worse	Hot weather, sun, exertion, touch.	Slightest touch, loss of vital fluids, at night.	Damp weather, emotions, thinking of his ailment.	Heat of the sun, moving the eyes, talking, reading, noise.	Heat, warm room, after eating, towards evening.
Better	Cold drinks and lying in a dark room.	Fluids and electrolytes.	Fluids and rest.	Open air, cool bathing, sweating, lying down.	Usually thirstless. Needs to drink fluids to get rehydrated.

Dosing: Use the ORANGE method.

SUNSTROKE AND HEAT STROKE

Sunstroke and heat stroke are much more serious conditions than heat exhaustion. As its name implies, sunstroke comes from excessive exposure to hot sun, while heat stroke results from prolonged subjection to high temperatures—usually in combination with dehydration—which leads to failure of the body's temperature control system. Heat stroke may happen as a progression from such milder heat-related illnesses as heat cramps, heat syncope (fainting), and heat exhaustion. But it can strike even if there are no previous signs of heat injury.

Whereas perspiration is profuse with heat exhaustion, someone suffering from sunstroke or heat stroke has become so overheated that their body can no longer cool itself through sweating. Any perspiration is sparse. More characteristically the skin is dry and hot, and the person may have a fever of 104 °F (40 °C). A fever that can rise even higher as homeostasis, the body's automatic rebalancing mechanism, is no longer working. This can happen very quickly, especially if the humidity is high. Dizzy, weak, fatigued, and nauseous, the person may vomit, become delirious, or have a seizure. Watch also for a very intense headache, with rapid pulse and rapid breathing.

IT'S AN EMERGENCY WHEN

If any of these symptoms are present, consider the situation an emergency:
- a body temperature of 104°F (40°C) or higher
- sweating stops
- rapid heartbeat
- rapid and shallow breathing
- fainting, (often the first sign in the elderly)
- lowered or elevated blood pressure
- confusion and/or disorientation
- seizure

ADDITIONAL SUPPORT FOR SUNSTROKE AND HEAT STROKE

- Reducing the body temperature of a person experiencing sunstroke or heat stroke is the most important thing you can do for them. They should be given emergency medical care immediately, but if no one is nearby, don't wait for help: do the following steps BEFORE and/or RIGHT AFTER calling 911.
- Get the person to a cool, shaded or air-conditioned area. Keep them out of the sun. Remove their clothing – or as much of it as you can – to allow faster dissipation of the heat from their body.
- Cool them off as quickly as possible by pouring or sponging liberal amounts of TEPID or COOL (not ice-cold) water over their body, or wrapping them in a sheet moistened with water. Put a cool compress on their head. Be aware that if the humidity is high, these cooling measures are less effective. Fanning will be needed to aid in evaporation and cooling.
- Alternatively, a cool shower or even an ice-bath (provided the person is young, healthy, and suffered heat stroke while exercising) can bring down the body temperature. So, too, can ice-packs be strategically placed at the person's armpits, groin, neck, and back, areas rich with blood vessels close to the skin's surface. Do not use ice on older people or those with chronic illness, young children, or anyone whose heat stroke was not brought on by vigorous exercise.
- Have the person slowly sip a few glasses of cool saltwater (½ teaspoon of salt in 16 ounces of spring water). Be careful not to give too much salt, as it may cause vomiting and further dehydration. You may also use the rehydration drink recommended for heat exhaustion in the previous section.
- Have them lie down and rest.

Important note: Anyone who has suffered from sunstroke or heat stroke will be susceptible to rapid overheating in the future. The person needs to reduce their exposure to both heat and sun.

Remedies to consider while you wait for care or on the way to the hospital:

- **Belladonna**: For symptoms that come on fast and furiously. There is intense heat radiating from the body, with a face that is bright red and hot, and skin is burning hot to the touch and dry. The person has a throbbing headache that is worse on the right side and better from bending the head backward. The eyes may be glassy and sparkling, with a wild look and dilated pupils. Someone needing **Belladonna** has great sensitivity to noise, light, touch, and motion; usually they crave very cold water or lemonade. If they have a high fever, they may be confused and delirious. Children can become agitated to the point of biting, screaming, and hitting. They will feel better with rest, light gauze coverings, sitting semi-erect, having the lights kept low or turned off, and absolute quiet.

- ***Glonoinum**: When sunstroke symptoms come on rapidly and violently. The person has a throbbing headache, the pain coming in waves so strong they feel their pulse in their head – and see the temporal veins pulsing – sense heat and blood rushing in, and fear the head may explode from too much pressure. They may even feel that their eyes are too large and about to burst from their head. They cannot bear anything hot near their head, whether a heated stove, a hat, or even a pillow. They are confused, very irritable, weepy, and possibly bathed in sweat. Anyone needing ***Glonoinum** must stay still, with their head elevated, given access to fresh air, and kept cool with cool applications and drinks. Once the crisis has passed, a long sleep will be beneficial. Give this remedy until the throbbing stops and repeat only if it begins again.

- **Belladonna** and ***Glonoinum** look very similar, although the latter appears to be in a more precarious state: the **Belladonna** face may be red, but ***Glonoinum** is close to purple; **Belladonna** skin is dry, whereas ***Glonoinum** is moist; **Belladonna** is worse from having the head uncovered, whereas ***Glonoinum** cannot tolerate any head covering.

Dosing: Use the RED or ORANGE method depending on urgency. Observe and evaluate.

POISONINGS

A high percentage of accidental poisonings happen to children under five years old. Keep all medicines, household cleaning products, industrial chemicals, and poisonous plants out of reach of little hands. Any corrosive chemicals should be locked up and inaccessible to children, for these can severely damage a child's esophagus if swallowed. Parents should make sure any plants in the home are not poisonous and that all medications are kept well secured. Never refer to any medicine or homeopathic remedy as "candy" or treat remedies as "rewards."

Post the phone number of your local poison control center on your refrigerator or near the phone, so it is readily accessible. Identify the source of the poison: some poisons cause internal symptoms, and others cause skin reactions. The more you can tell the physician, the 911 operator, or poison control center about the poison, the better they will be able to help you. If a child has ingested a poison and is fearful, give two doses of **Aconite**, 15 minutes apart.

If your child does get into your remedies and even ingests a whole tube, know that they may have a stomachache from the sugar but there is no poisoning from that. Remember it's energy medicine. Regardless, it is best to keep remedies away from children's reach.

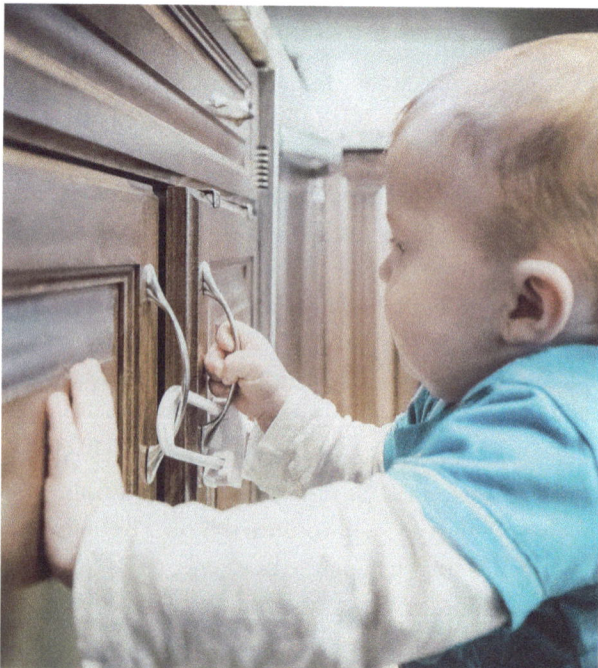

If the person is unconscious, try to keep their airway open and keep them breathing, with CPR or artificial respiration if necessary.

Note: To administer a remedy to anyone who is unconscious or whose breathing is compromised, dissolve the remedy in half a glass of water and dab it, either with a Q-tip or your finger, onto the lips or wrist (on the pulse point just above the thumb).

Remedies for the types of poisonings listed below will not interfere with any emergency treatment and can be given afterwards to ease symptoms and speed recovery.

ALCOHOL POISONING

Underage and inexperienced drinkers are particularly vulnerable to alcohol poisoning. When someone consumes excessive amounts of alcohol in a short period, their breathing slows and the brain and other organs are deprived of oxygen. Drinking too much too quickly can also affect heart rate, body temperature, and gag reflex. Symptoms of alcohol intoxication – which can include confusion, sleepiness, aggression, incoherence, irrationality, trembling, excessive laughing or crying, nausea, and vomiting – are heightened in alcohol poisoning. They may also include seizures, irregular or greatly slowed breathing (fewer than eight breaths a minute), pale or grayish skin, low body temperature (hypothermia), a severe headache, and blacking out. The staggering, speech-slurring drunk may be the butt of jokes in the movies, but someone suffering from alcohol poisoning is in grave danger and needs immediate help.

IT'S AN EMERGENCY WHEN

- The person is hard to awaken, is unconscious, or has had a seizure.
- The person cannot stop vomiting or is vomiting blood.
- The person is experiencing slow or irregular breathing, i.e., gaps of more than eight seconds between breaths.
- The person has a low body temperature (less than 98.6 °F or 37 °C).

ADDITIONAL SUPPORT FOR ALCOHOL POISONING

If alcohol poisoning is suspected, it is NOT a good idea to let the person sleep it off: not only can the blood alcohol level continue to rise, but they risk choking to death on their own vomit. The person needs fresh air and should drink lots of water to flush toxins out of their liver and to rehydrate. If they can walk, it is good for them to do so, preferably with someone supporting them. If someone has repeatedly been vomiting, they should be encouraged to drink small frequent sips of any of these suggestions to slowly replenish their electrolytes:

- A homemade fluid replacement can be made with apple (or any clear, pulp-free) juice and water (50/50 mix).
- Fresh, pulp-free watermelon juice with water is a quick way to replenish lost electrolytes.
- Liquid-IV.com sells a rehydrating powder to add to fresh water that boosts one's electrolytes.

Remedies to consider:

- **Nux vomica**: This is an all-purpose remedy for consuming too much alcohol, whether to the point of mild intoxication or to the more dangerous stage of actual poisoning. It will help expel toxins from the blood and liver, relieve or even prevent a hangover. In someone needing **Nux vomica**, the stomach and intestines may feel bruised and sore, with cramping, gas, and sour or bitter belching. The person is chilly and has a bone-dry mouth.

- **Pulsatilla**: If the person has ingested cheap wine, give **Pulsatilla** to help purge the body of chemicals in these wines. People needing **Pulsatilla** tend to be overheated, want fresh air, are usually thirstless, and may be weepy.

Dosing: Use the RED method. Observe and evaluate.

ADDITIONAL SUPPORT AFTER ALCOHOL POISONING

- **Bach Flower Rescue Remedy®** can be given to restore a sense of balance, calm, and harmony. It reduces the effects of a shock to the system from the alcohol. The person may feel faint and may tremble. **Bach Flower Rescue Remedy®** can also be given if a person is becoming hysterical or exhibiting wild or irrational behavior from the alcohol. It is a very gentle yet effective remedy in this kind of situation.
- **Rescue Remedy®** comes in different forms (tincture, pastilles, gum, etc.) and the tincture is the one to have around for general use. There is also a children's tincture that is preserved with vegetable glycerin instead of brandy in case there is concern about the alcohol.

Rescue Remedy® Dosing: Add two drops to a glass of spring water and have the person sip it frequently until they calm down OR dose directly under the tongue. Repeat as often as needed, but stop when emotional stability has returned. It would be a good idea to have them sip three glasses of water with **Bach Flower Rescue Remedy®** the day after the poisoning.

CARBON MONOXIDE POISONING

After sitting in a traffic jam for a long period of time on a sultry, windless day, you may react to vehicle exhaust fumes. Or in wintertime, a blocked tailpipe or leaky exhaust can allow a car to fill with carbon monoxide (CO) fairly quickly. A gas stove is also a possible source of CO poisoning, as well as burning charcoal in a closed environment.

ITS AN EMERGENCY WHEN

- The person has inhaled carbon monoxide in a closed space.

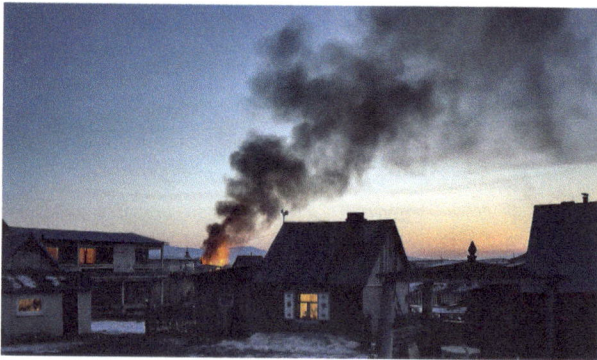

The stand-by remedy for carbon monoxide poisoning is **Carbo veg**. The head becomes hot and heavy, with an intense pain at the base of the skull. You are likely to feel weak, sick, and too exhausted to react to anything or make even the slightest exertion. Your vitality is so low that you may be at the point of collapse. Breathing may become quickened, and the face becomes red. Despite the body and breath being cold, you'll want to be fanned—a tell-tale sign of inadequate oxygenation—and will crave fresh air because of feeling hot internally. The picture of someone who needs **Carbo veg** is one of confusion, indifference, and sluggishness paired with irritability. Give this remedy every 15 minutes; but if symptoms are severe and persist after four doses, immediately contact a healthcare provider or dial 911.

Another choice for carbon monoxide poisoning is *Ammonium carb, a remedy that's invaluable for people with emphysema or those who become extremely short of breath – even choking – on going up stairs. People needing this remedy may be obese and have congestive heart failure. Their personality tends to be as acrid as their discharges. Disappointed in and with life, they cope by rejecting the world and leading the life of an outcast.

CHEMICAL POISONING

Toxic chemicals frequently seen in household items include ammonia, bleach, detergents, drain cleaners, glue, solvents, and pesticides, insecticides, or herbicides. Ingested poisons, however, can also include medications, whether prescription or over-the-counter, and poisonous plants (especially mushrooms and berries). Toxins may also be absorbed through the skin in the case of many chemical preparations.

IT'S AN EMERGENCY WHEN

- The person has swallowed any toxic chemical, corrosive or petrochemical product such as oven cleaner, lye, drain opener, kerosene, paint thinner, or gasoline.
- DO NOT INDUCE VOMITING or attempt to neutralize the poison with anything by mouth. Corrosives or petrochemicals are likely to do only more damage if vomited: strong acids or alkalis will injure the esophagus, while petroleum products (gasoline, kerosene, paint thinner, furniture polish, etc.) may be aspirated into the lungs.
- Check with your local Poison Control (check out www.poison.org) if you know the substance ingested to see if vomiting is advised, and follow their directions for inducing it. The same holds true for administering activated charcoal. Neither of these should be attempted on an unconscious person.

If the poison has been taken by mouth, symptoms may include convulsions, retching or vomiting, abdominal pain, and unconsciousness. Try to find out what caused the poisoning, but if the victim is unconscious, check pulse and breathing. Do artificial respiration and/or cardiac resuscitation, if necessary.

If you can, place the person in "recovery position" by gently tilting his head back and turning the victim onto his side, leaving the topmost arm stretched out in front and the other behind but parallel to his body. The uppermost leg should be bent at the knee and pulled forward to support the lower body. The purpose of the recovery position is to keep the tongue from blocking the airway and to prevent accidental aspiration of any vomit. Dial 911.

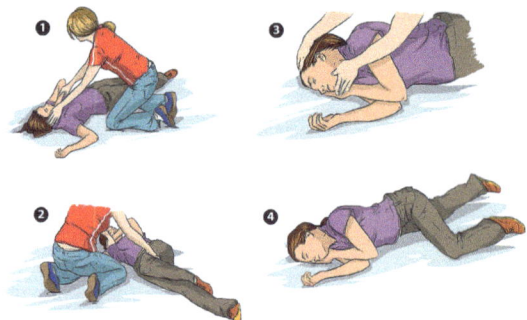

Recovery position

If the person is cold, cover them with a blanket.

If lips or mouth are burned, as is likely with any caustic chemicals, you may give sips of cool water or milk. *For more see the **Burns** section previously in this chapter on **page 54**.*

While waiting for emergency care, consider these remedies for minor chemical poisonings:

- **Arsenicum**: Burning pain in the throat, esophagus, or abdominal area. The mouth and throat may be dry, and there is thirst for small sips of cold water. Vomiting and retching may be severe. If a toxic chemical has come in contact with the skin, there is likely to be itching, burning, swelling, and even blisters. Although absolutely exhausted, the victim is extremely anxious with great restlessness. Despite strong burning sensations, they like warm applications to counter their innate chilliness.

- **Phosphorus**: This remedy is useful when there is an oversensitivity to chemicals or food containing monosodium glutamate. There may be palpitations or an elevated heartbeat and labored breathing from the least exertion. The lungs are tight, congested, and feel as though there is a heavy weight pressing on the chest. A sensation of rawness and burning from the throat to the bottom of the rib cage creates a thirst for ice-cold drinks. Skin reactions are mild itching, burning, and swelling, often with blisters that bleed easily. Though weak and even listless, the person is irritable, lightheaded, oversensitive, disoriented, and a bit fearful, particularly of thunderstorms and being left alone.

Dosing: Use the RED method. Observe and evaluate.

DRUG POISONING AND GLUE SNIFFING

If a person is exhibiting bizarre behavior and you suspect that they have ingested too much of a prescribed or over-the-counter medication or a hallucinogen or designer drug, seek medical help immediately, for many have to be antidoted properly to avoid fatal liver damage. The person should be taken to the emergency room and their healthcare practitioner contacted. If they are incoherent or out of control, dial 911.

IT'S AN EMERGENCY WHEN

- An overdose is suspected. The person must be taken to the emergency room immediately. A remedy can be given on the way to the hospital.
- The person is out of control or severely incoherent.

If you suspect someone has sniffed glue or other inhalants (solvents like nail polish remover, aerosol sprays, gasses like butane, propane, etc.), give a dose of **Arnica** every 15 minutes on the way to the hospital. The solvents in inhalants can contribute to acute respiratory or heart failure, irregular heartbeat, and brain damage.

Remedies to consider on the way to the hospital:

- **Arsenicum**: Burning pain in the throat, esophagus, or abdominal area. Their mouth and throat may be dry, and they are thirsty for sips of water (they may want it cold but do better with warm water). There can be severe vomiting and retching. Paradoxically, although there is much burning with this remedy, warm applications feel good as the person is usually chilly. Characteristically, they are extremely exhausted but anxious with maddening restlessness.

- **Phosphorus**: Burning pains and oversensitivity to chemicals or food containing monosodium glutamate. There may be palpitations or an elevated heartbeat and labored breathing from the least exertion. The lungs are tight, congested, and feel as though there is a heavy weight pressing on the chest. From the throat to the bottom of the rib cage there is a sensation of rawness and burning, which creates a thirst for ice-cold drinks. Skin reactions are mild itching, burning, and swelling, often with blisters that can bleed easily. Though weak and listless, the person is irritable, lightheaded, oversensitive, disoriented, and a bit fearful, particularly of thunderstorms and being left alone.

Dosing: Use the RED method. Observe and evaluate.

ADDITIONAL SUPPORT FOR <u>AFTER</u> DRUG POISONING OR GLUE SNIFFING

- To help the body detoxify, give 2,000 to 5,000 mg. of vitamin C daily - spread out through the day, not all at once - and have the person drink eight glasses of water a day for several days. Sometimes too much vitamin C can cause mild and temporary diarrhea; if it does, reduce the dosage.
- Be aware that poisoning with acetaminophen (Tylenol) can cause fatal liver damage if not antidoted within 24 hours, which requires medical treatment. In addition, depending on how much time has elapsed since ingestion, treatment may also include activated charcoal, NAC (N-Acetyl-L-Cysteine) supplement and gastric lavage (pumping out the stomach). Talk to your healthcare practitioner for appropriate dosing.

FOOD POISONING

See **Chapter 11—Stomach and Abdomen** on **page 130**.

ALTITUDE SICKNESS OR MOUNTAIN SICKNESS

Altitude sickness, also known as mountain sickness, is an illness that suddenly strikes those who venture to higher altitudes without proper acclimation. It typically occurs at about 8,000 feet—or 2,400 meters—above sea level. Hikers, skiers, adventurers, and travelers to lofty mountain ranges where the oxygen is thin can all experience it.

Symptoms may include dizziness or light-headedness, nausea and vomiting, headaches, fatigue, loss of appetite, and shortness of breath on even the slightest exertion.

Most instances of acute altitude sickness are mild and resolve quickly, usually in a few days, once your body adjusts to the higher altitude. But altitude sickness can turn deadly if it affects the lungs, causing pulmonary edema, or the brain, resulting in cerebral edema. If you are anemic, have lung or respiratory issues, or are taking medications that lower your blood pressure, you should consult with your physician before making a trip to a high altitude. Drinking alcohol or using certain medications, especially sedatives, can greatly increase your chances of developing altitude sickness.

IT'S AN EMERGENCY WHEN

- The person experiencing mountain sickness develops high altitude pulmonary edema (HAPE). This is when the lungs start filling up with fluid. Symptoms include excessive shortness of breath that worsen with exertion or when lying down. There is a feeling of drowning/anxiety that worsens when lying down. Dizziness, excessive sweating or chest pain with cold and clammy skin. Don't delay getting them to a hospital as this is a life threatening concern.
- The mountain sickness escalates to high altitude cerebral edema (HACE). This is when the brain starts swelling with fluid. The person is dizzy and nauseous, with mood and cognitive changes. They can experience seizures, lack of coordination, numbness and double vision. In this case it is urgent to get medical attention right away.

COMMON REMEDIES FOR ALTITUDE OR MOUNTAIN SICKNESS

	Arnica	Calcarea carb	Carbo veg
Onset	Ailments from high altitudes. Ailments from ascending.	Ailments from high altitudes. Ailments from ascending.	Ailments from high altitudes. Ailments from ascending.
Symptoms	Headache. Anxiety with vertigo. Difficulty breathing.	Vertigo. Headache. Oppression in chest. Difficulty breathing.	Headache. Difficulty breathing Fainting. Bloating and indigestion.
Mood	Irritable and adverse to company. Says he is well when he is sick.	Anxious and worried about their recovery. Obstinate.	Indifferent and apathetic. Can be irritable at their family.
Indications	Any trauma to the body. Jet lag. Nosebleeds. Bloodshot eyes.	Fear of heights. Even slight ascending causes problems. Out of shape.	Desire for fresh air, and/or to be fanned. Frequent burping. Collapse.
Worse	Exertion. Touch. Being approached. Damp cold.	Ascending. Cold wet weather. Exertion. Looking down from high places.	Being covered. Lying flat. Rich foods. Cold night air.
Better	Lying with head lower. Being outstretched.	Lying down. Breathing fresh air.	Being fanned, Sitting upright. Belching. Elevating feet.

Dosing: Give chosen remedy before ascending then repeat as needed if symptoms return.

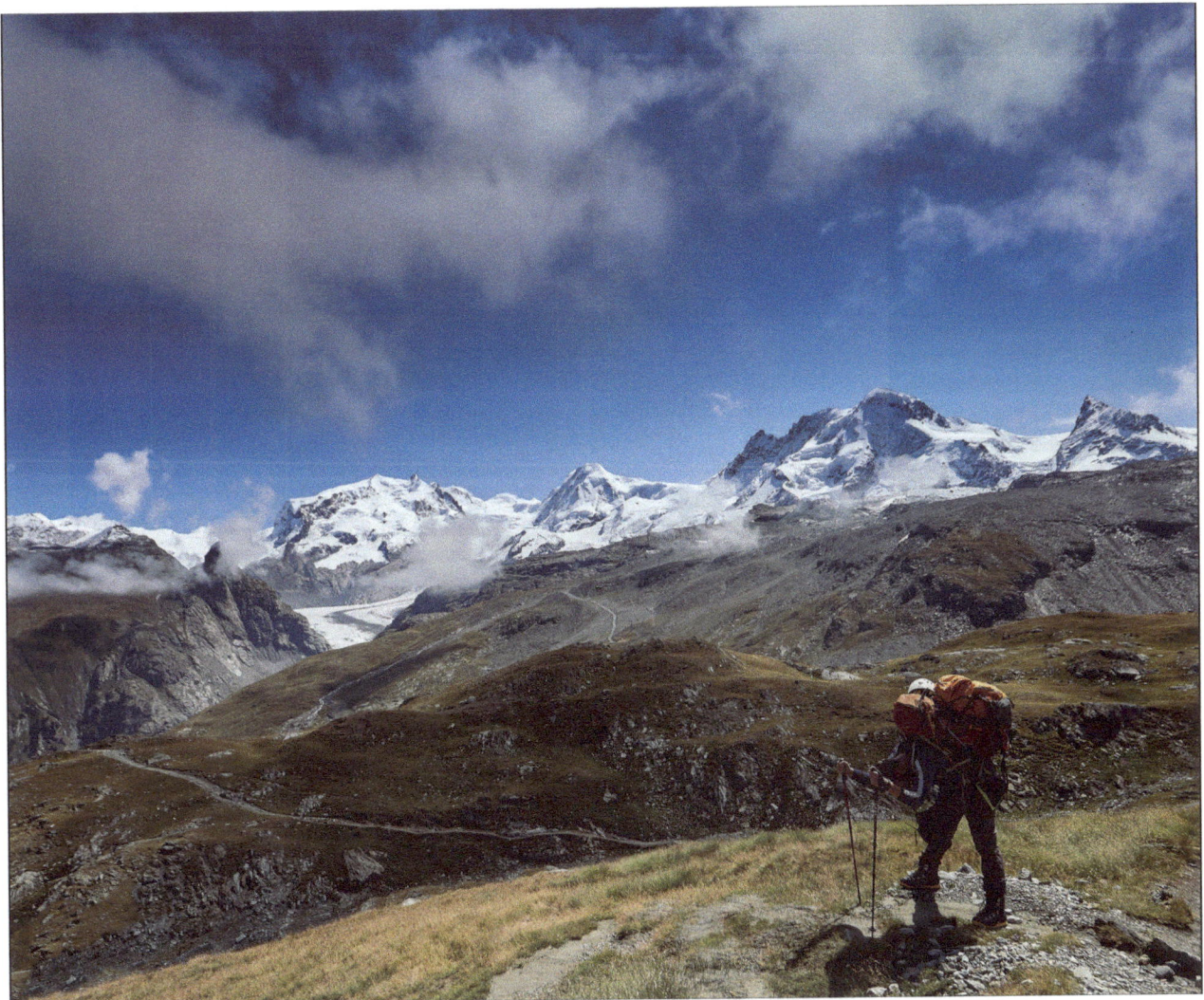

? WHAT'S THE FIRST REMEDY YOU THINK OF WHEN...

1. The person is bleeding after being hit by a baseball on their nose.
2. The person slammed their finger in a car door.
3. There is a painful and hot sunburn.
4. A person burns themselves with a hot skillet.
5. For no known reason the person has itching swollen red hives on their torso and belly.
6. The person got a surf lesson on vacation and now has rib pain that is worse when moving or taking a breath.
7. Someone has gotten too much sun and they have a burning throbbing headache.
8. Someone has water blisters that came on after being in the cold.
9. The person traveled to a location at a high altitude and now has difficulty catching a deep breath.
10. The person ate seafood that caused anaphylactic shock with a swollen tongue and difficulty breathing.
11. There is a suspicion of carbon monoxide poisoning.
12. The person burned their mouth on a very hot piece of cheese pizza.
13. A student drank too much at a college fraternity party and now has a hangover.
14. The two most common remedies for sunstroke and heat stroke are needed.

Answer key on *page 323*.

CHAPTER 5
Head

The human head, with its intricate network of organs and systems, serves as the command center for our bodies. However, just like any other part of our anatomy, the head can experience a range of symptoms that can be both concerning and/or uncomfortable. From fevers and headaches to more specific issues like head lice, blows to the head, and dandruff, these symptoms can significantly impact our overall well-being and quality of life. Let's look at these issues more deeply and what homeopathic remedies might be needed.

FEVERS

A fever is the body's natural strategy for ridding itself of an infection. Fevers may also present for other reasons such as an allergic reaction, heatstroke, or extreme toxicity. Many people have been taught to believe that any fever needs to be immediately brought down, but actually it's the body's way of fighting an infection. Normal body temperature is 98.6 °F (37 °C); anything above that is considered a fever. Fevers above 103 °F (39.4 °C) should be monitored closely and may require medical attention if prolonged.

What happens when you get a fever? A fever causes an increased pulse rate so that the heart can pump blood faster to the organs; faster breathing to increase oxygen in the blood; and chills or perspiration to naturally cool the body temperature. A raised body temperature can help kill invading organisms. It also stimulates the body's defense mechanisms by increasing the production of infection-fighting white blood cells, called leukocytes.

Fevers tend to naturally rise in the late afternoon or early evening and drop or disappear by morning. The fever may rise and fall for a few days. Fevers should be allowed to run their natural course and should not be suppressed using over-the-counter medicine. Hippocrates, the ancient Greek physician and father of Western medicine, said, "Give me a fever and I can cure the child." It is important to allow the self-healing process of a fever to run its course, unless the temperature is extremely high. Be sure to take the temperature with a thermometer, so you know accurately how high the fever is.

A fever in a child often precedes or accompanies an earache, sore throat, common cold, cough, teething, or the flu. It is not the goal of a homeopathic remedy to suppress a fever, but rather to resolve the root cause by addressing the totality of symptoms. This will allow the fever to break naturally. A homeopathic remedy will strengthen the body and help it heal. Children who have had fevers and common childhood illnesses, e.g., chicken pox, tend to be stronger and healthier. In these cases, the immune system has learned how to fight off benign illnesses, because the immune system has not been suppressed with drugs, antibiotics, or vaccines.

Important note: Aspirin should never be given to a young child with a fever as it can cause Reye's syndrome which can cause brain or liver damage.

COMMON REMEDIES FOR FEVERS

	Aconite	Arsenicum	Belladonna	Bryonia	*Ferrum phos	Phosphorus	Rhus tox
Onset	Sudden onset with a high fever, after being exposed to icy winds, fright, shock.	Getting chilled, wet weather, getting overheated, overexertion.	Onset sudden and violent. From getting head wet, cold, dry wind, getting overheated.	Slow onset (may develop over days), from getting chilled by a cold wind especially in spring and autumn.	Onset usually gradual, but can progress steadily. Fears of unknown origin.	Onset is slow and steady from getting drenched in the rain. Ravenous hunger the night before onset.	Getting chilled or wet, sitting on wet ground, getting over-heated after being chilled. Overexertion.
Symptoms	Chills, then dry, burning heat inside and out. Cold sweat, icy coldness of the face. Visible waves of chills passing through the body.	Face hot and body cold, intense high heat and sweating. Chilly on outside and burning inside, but they want heat. Thirst for small, frequent sips.	High fever, bright red, flushed face. Head is hot, hands and feet are cold. Not thirsty during fever, but craves cold water later. Throbbing head pain.	Chills and shivering. Dry, burning heat with extreme thirst for large quantities of cold water. Long fever. Achy pains over whole body. Eyeballs sore.	Early stages of fever, very few or vague symptoms. Person generally doesn't feel well. During heat phase hands are sweaty. Eyes can burn and be bloodshot.	Fever, chills, night sweats. Joints feel stiff. Burning heat up the back with profuse perspiration. Burst of energy followed by weakness. Headache over one eye.	Dry, burning fever alternating with chills. Muscle aches and stiffness. Feels bruised and sore. Constant desire to stretch and move. May get a cold sore.
Mood	During high fever, they become fearful. Can be hard to console. Restless, anxious, tearful.	Restless, anxious, irritable, fussy, oversensitive, needy, demanding.	All senses acute and heightened. Confused, delirious with high fever. Severe agitation.	Intolerant of being disturbed or moved. Wants to just lie still in bed and be left alone. Grumpy.	Irritable, sensitive, talkative.	Needs attention and consolation. Affectionate, fearful, easily upset, irritable.	Anxious, weepy, helpless, mildly delirious, extremely restless.
Indications	Face red, pupils small, eyes glassy. Profuse sweat. Intense thirst for cold water.	Much shivering. Strong chills and cold sweat. They get ill quickly, continue to get weak, then are totally exhausted.	Skin is hot, alternating between moist and dry. Eyes glossy and sparkling with a wild look. Restless sleep.	Profuse sour smelling sweat with the least exertion. Head is hot with a red face. Dry mouth, skin, lips. Eyelids sore, red, swollen.	Chilly, but thirsty for cold drinks. Stretches during chills. This remedy may either abort fever or cause it to be less debilitating.	Craves ice water during chill. At first, may not show how sick they are. Later, it is hard to make any effort. Acute senses. Face pale, then flushed.	Much sweating from slightest exertion. Shivers on any movement or being uncovered. Glands are hard, swollen, tender. Chilly.
Worse	Nighttime around midnight, noise, pressure, touch, cold, dry air.	After midnight, around 2 AM, change of temperature, damp wet weather, cold, exertion, sight and smell of food, cold drinks.	Right side, cold air, touch, noise, jarring, light, around 3 PM.	Movement, 9 PM, touch, warmth, spring, autumn.	Chills at 1 PM or 4-6 AM. Worse on right side, touch, motion, jarring.	Change of weather, wind, thunderstorms, odors, lying on left side, light, morning, evening.	Cold, damp weather, autumn, cold food or drinks, night, being uncovered, drafts, lying still, initial movement after resting.
Better	Fresh air, rest, sweating, warm applications.	Warmth, hot food and drink during hot phase, although there is much burning. Lying down, fresh air, elevating the head.	Rest, light covers, sitting semi-erect, low light, quiet.	Lying completely still, pressure, quiet, being left alone.	Cold applications on head, lying down.	Sleep, sympathy, low light or darkness, eating and drinking cold things, cool applications, open air.	Warm drinks and food. Constant, gentle movement, stretching, sweating, changing position, massage.
Also For	Cold, Cough, Earache, Sore Throat.	Cold, Cough, Earache, Sore Throat.	Cold, Cough, Earache, Sore Throat.	Cold, Cough, Flu, Bronchitis.	Cold, Sore Throat.	Cold, Cough, Flu, Sore Throat, Bronchitis.	Cold, Flu, Sore Throat.

Other common remedies to consider for fevers include: **Apis, Chamomilla, China, *Eupatorium perf, Gelsemium, Mercurius, Natrum mur, Nux vomica, Pulsatilla, *Pyrogen** and **Silicea.**

Dosing: If onset is fast, use the ORANGE level dosing. If onset is slow, consider the BLUE level. If remedy is helping, remember to only repeat with a return of the same symptoms. If no result in 24 hours, then reassess the symptoms for dosing a different remedy. If the symptoms change, then consider changing the remedy.

HEADACHES

A typical acute headache can be caused by many circumstances including stress, eyestrain, overstudying, hormonal imbalances, poor diet, or emotional upset. The symptoms may include a sensation of constriction, soreness, burning, and with many types of pain in the head, neck, or scalp. The pain may be localized or affect the entire head. Sometimes the pain becomes so intense that the person may become nauseated and end up vomiting. Migraine, cluster headaches, and persistent headaches are of a chronic nature and need to be addressed by a professional homeopath or healthcare practitioner. Headaches in a female teen around their period and ovulation can suggest hormone imbalances.

ITS AN EMERGENCY WHEN

- The headache follows a head injury and the person is drowsy, nauseous, and vomiting. Give **Arnica** every 15 minutes until help arrives.
- There is a bad headache, a temperature of over 100.5 °F (38 °C), stiffness in the neck, and intolerance to light.
- The person has a headache with red face, shortness of breath, nosebleeds, lightheadedness, nausea with indigestion, or is easily exhausted. These can be signs of high blood pressure.
- The person is experiencing dizziness with mental confusion, slurred speech, staggering gait, falling, numbness or weakness of a limb, or one side of the whole body; feeling faint, vision disturbance, inability to communicate clearly, or jerky movements. These can be signs of a stroke.
- The head pain comes on suddenly with unusual and incredible pain.

ADDITIONAL SUPPORT FOR HEADACHES

- Make sure the person is fully hydrated.
- Try applying cool compresses to the back of the neck, head, or temples to ease the pain.
- Resting quietly in a quiet, dark place may help reduce symptoms.
- Slow, deep breathing helps calm the nervous system which helps reduce one's reaction to any type of pain.
- Soothing quiet music can be relaxing and take the mind off the pain.
- Taking a hot bath with one cup of Epsom salts can relax and detox the body. If it feels good, gently massaging the scalp, neck, and shoulders can alleviate pain.
- Inviting in what seems to work and letting go of what is causing stress can be very helpful.
- Learning relaxation techniques including meditation and deep breathing practices can alleviate tension and help to make stress more manageable.
- Getting enough sleep is key to being able to deal better with any stressors that arise.

WHEN TO CONTACT YOUR HEALTHCARE PROFESSIONAL

- The person develops a high fever and intense headache.
- The person experiences recurring headaches, or headaches with visual disturbances or dizziness.
- The person has painful and persistent headaches that will not resolve.
- The person has headaches in the temple area with swollen blood vessels, visual disturbances, blind spots, and jaw pain, especially when chewing.

The following is an overview of remedies for headaches by a specific cause:

- anger: **Bryonia, Chamomilla, Lycopodium, Ignatia, Natrum mur,** or **Staphysagria**

- anxiety: **Argentum nit**

- artificial light (as seen in schools or workplaces): **Sepia**

- dehydration: **China**

- emotional upset: **Chamomilla, Gelsemium, Ignatia, Pulsatilla,** or **Staphysagria**

- excessive excitement: **Coffea cruda**

- exhaustion from overactivity: **Arsenicum album, China, Gelsemium, *Nitric acidum, Sepia,** or ***Zincum metallicum**

- menses: **Lycopodium, Sepia, *Zincum metallicum;** before menses: **Bryonia;** just before or after menses: **Natrum mur**

- missing a meal: **Lycopodium, Phosphorous** or **Silicea**

- overeating (rich food): **Nux vomica**

- overeating (fatty food): **Carbo veg, Pulsatilla** or **Sepia**

- overstudying: ***Calcarea phos, Ruta** or **Silicea**

- reading too much: **Natrum mur** or **Ruta**

- sugar (overindulgence): **Argentum nit**

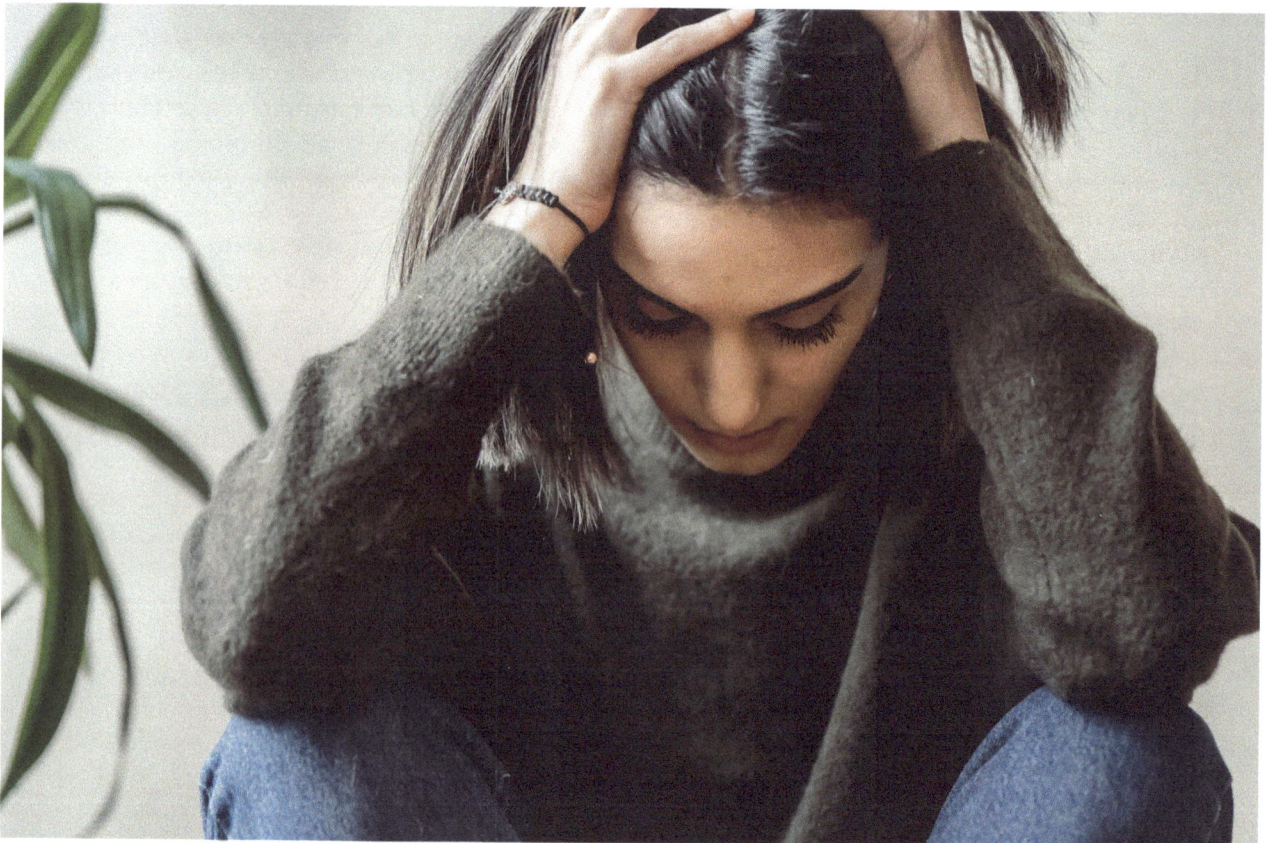

MOST COMMON REMEDIES FOR HEADACHES—part 1

	Aconite	Arnica	Arsenicum	Belladonna	Bryonia
Onset	Sudden onset with high fever, after exposure to icy winds, fright, or shock.	After injury to head, or after exposure to bright lights, sun, or snow.	After getting chilled, wet weather, getting overheated, overexertion.	Onset sudden and violent. From getting head wet, cold, dry wind, getting overheated.	Slow onset (may develop over days), from getting chilled by a cold wind, especially in spring and autumn.
Symptoms	Chills, then dry, burning heat inside and out. Cold sweat, icy coldness of the face. Visible waves of chills passing through the body. Pain feels like a tight band around head, as if the brain is being forced out of the head.	Head feels bruised and congested, vision may be obscured or lost periodically. Occasional sharp, stitching pains. Stooping causes a rush of blood to the head.	Face hot and body cold. Intense high heat and sweating. Chilly on outside and burning inside, but wants more heat. Thirst for small frequent sips.	High fever, bright red flushed face. Head is hot, but hands and feet are cold. Not thirsty during fever but craves cold water later. Throbbing head pain. Face flushed, swollen, hot, with staring eyes and dilated pupils.	Headache with bursting, hammering, and splitting pains. Sinus pressure and pain, nausea, faintness on rising, confusion. Chills and shivering. Dry, burning heat with extreme thirst for lots of cold water. Long fever. Achy pains. Eyeballs sore.
Mood	During high fever, person can become fearful. Hard to console. Restless, anxious, tearful, apprehensive.	Fears touch or being approached, quarrelsome. Desires privacy. Will tell you "I'm fine."	Restless, anxious, irritable, fussy, oversensitive, needy, demanding.	All senses acute and heightened. Confused, delirious with high fever. Severe agitation. Delirium.	Intolerant of being disturbed or moved. Wants to lie still in bed and be left alone. Grumpy, irritable.
Indications	Face red, pupils small, eyes glassy. Profuse sweat. Intense thirst for cold water.	Feeling of bruised soreness, as if from a fall, a beating, or a blow to the head.	Much shivering. Strong chills and cold sweat. Gets ill quickly, continues to get weaker, then gets totally exhausted.	Skin hot. Alternating between moist and dry. Eyes glassy and sparkling with a wild look. Restless sleep. Person may scream in pain or hallucinate.	Profuse, sour smelling sweat with least exertion. Head is hot and face red. Dry mouth, skin, lips. Eyelids sore, red, swollen. Left-sided headache.
Worse	Nighttime, around midnight, noise, pressure, touch. Cold dry air, cold winds, or cold draft.	From movement, being touched or jarred, or excitement.	After midnight, around 2 AM. Change of temperature, damp wet weather, cold, exertion, sight and smell of food, cold drinks.	Right side, cold air, touch, noise, jarring, light, around 3 PM. Heat, bright light. Draft on head, lying down, touch, noise, company, motion.	Movement, 9 PM, touch, warmth, spring, autumn. Slightest movement, including eyes, stooping, coughing, deep breathing. Touch, over-heating, cold drafts, bright light, noise, any annoyances.
Better	Fresh air, rest, sweating, warm applications.	Stillness, lying down, rest, stretching out, or with head low. Privacy.	Warmth, hot food and drink during hot phase, although there is much burning. Lying down, fresh air, elevating the head.	Quiet rest, light covers, sitting semi-erect, stillness, Low light, quiet. Being well wrapped and warm, bedrest, sitting, or with head raised. Pressure.	Lying completely still, pressure, quiet, being left alone. Low light, pressure on painful side, cool drinks, and cool, open air.
Location	Forehead and eyes feels squeezed or bursting. May be more left-sided.	Cold spots on forehead, hot spots on vertex. May be more right-sided.	Pain over left eye, pulsating in forehead, aching in occiput.	Pain in forehead, occiput and temples. Temples throbbing, hammering, sensation of cold in middle of forehead. More right-sided.	Occipital pain; bursting, splitting, crushing. Vertigo felt in occiput. Left eye pressive pain going to occiput.

Dosing: Use the ORANGE method if the onset is fast and there is a need for quick relief. Use the BLUE method if the onset is slow. Observe and evaluate.

MOST COMMON REMEDIES FOR HEADACHES—part 2

	Gelsemium	*Glonoinum	Ignatia	*Kali phos	Natrum Mur
Onset	Acute ailments with slow onset. Common in flu-like states.	After exposure to extreme cold, extreme heat and/or snow blindness. Sunstroke.	Following episodes of anger, grief, also silent anger or grief. Disappointment, fright, reproaches, shame.	Excruciating nervous headache with sensitivity to noise. From overwork or period of intense concentration.	Follows grief, eyestrain, before or after menses, coughing, sunlight.
Symptoms	Head feels full or swollen, as if a tight band is wrapped around it. Face may be flushed, droopy, and congested, with a dull expression, dilated pupils, and heavy eyelids. Person feels weak, dizzy, drowsy, shaky. Leans against things for support.	Violently bursting, throbbing (with every heartbeat), congestive headaches that develop due to extreme cold or heat. Vision impaired as if everything was half-light, half-dark. Can have appearance of sparks before eyes. Ears and teeth may hurt with every heartbeat.	Feels as if a tight band around the forehead, or a nail is being driven through the skull. Head feels hollow and heavy. Vision flickers with zigzagging. Incoordination, dizziness.	Pain and weight at back of head. Empty gone feeling at stomach. Brain feels weary.	May be a migraine. Bursting, blinding headaches as if a thousand little hammers were knocking on the brain. May have disturbed vision before or during.
Mood	Apathetic. Wants to be alone and quiet.	Confusion.	May be emotional, changeable moods.	Weariness, anxiety, worry, and exhaustion.	Nervous, discouraged, broken down, grief.
Indications	Accompanied by fatigue and weakness.	Face is flushed, hot, and sweaty. Vertigo.	Sighing, lack of communication.	Headache of serious students and workaholics. Tension, anxiety and worry.	May have photophobia. Throbbing and heat in head, with red face, nausea and vomiting.
Worse	Excitement, surprise, bad news.	Motion, jarring, stooping. Shaking the head.	Stooping, worry, grief, bad news, tobacco smoke.	Mental exertion. Stress. Before and during menses. Cold dry air and cold drinks.	Morning to evening. Waking up. Coughing, sunlight, motion (even moving eyes), frowning.
Better	Profuse urination, sweating, open air, movement.	Pressure and cold applications, open air, lying still.	Food, changing position.	Warmth, rest, sleep. After rising. Relieved by gentle motion.	Sleep, pressure on eyes, lying with head high, sitting still.
Location	Band-like pain around occiput extending over the eyes. Pain at back of head, from vertex to shoulders. Pain in temples extending to ears.	Pain alternating between temples. Vertex hot, sore and numb. Veins swollen at temples. Deep in head; shock, sensation of explosion or soreness.	Sides of head feel like a nail has been driven in. At back of head, sensation of weight. May be more right-sided.	Back of head and occipital region.	On vertex and/or forehead, hammering and heaviness over eyes.

Dosing: Use the ORANGE method if the onset is fast and there is a need for quick relief. Use the BLUE method if the onset is slow. Observe and evaluate.

MOST COMMON REMEDIES FOR HEADACHES—part 3

	Nux Vomica	Phosphorus	Pulsatilla	Rhus Tox	Sepia
Onset	Too much mental exertion, anger, loss of sleep, digestive upset, over-indulgence in rich food, drugs or alcohol, tension, or stress.	Onset is slow and steady. Following getting drenched in the rain. Ravenous hunger the night before onset.	Abandonment, emotional trauma, grief, fright, overeating, rich food, or overwork.	After getting chilled or wet, sitting on wet ground, getting over-heated after being chilled. Overexertion.	Weekly or monthly headaches. Frequently at menstrual time. With scanty flow or before menses.
Symptoms	Pain at base of skull or pressing pain and heaviness in forehead above the eyes, with a desire to press the head against something. Splitting headache. Brain feels bruised. Can feel as if a nail is being driven into the top of the head. Head may feel expanded.	Fever, chills, night sweats. Joints feel stiff. Burning heat up the back with profuse perspiration. Burst of energy followed by weakness. Headache over one eye.	One-sided headaches mostly on left; however, pain moves around to different parts of the head. Pain is stabbing, piercing, throbbing, with bursting and scalding sensations. Top of head feels heavy with pressure.	Dry, burning fever alternating with chills. Muscle aches and stiffness. Feels bruised and sore. Constant desire to stretch and move. May get a cold sore.	Headaches with nausea and vomiting. Stinging pain over left eye. Shooting and stinging pains. Vertex cold.
Mood	May be driving themselves too hard. Critical, angry, oversensitive to just about everything, impatient.	Needs attention and consolation. Affectionate, fearful, easily upset, irritable.	Weepy, whiny, whimpering, fretful, but affectionate. Wants attention. May feel sorry for self.	Anxious, weepy, help-less, mildly delirious, extremely restless.	Anxious fears over trifles, weepy, sad and gloomy. Shrieks with pain.
Indications	May feel like a band is around the head. Scalp is sensitive. May be dizzy, as if from turning in a circle, with faint feeling or light-headedness. Chilly, with nausea, may vomit. Constipation likely. May press their head into their hands or lean their head into something hard.	Craves ice water during chill. At first, may not show how sick they are. Later, it's hard to make any effort. Acute senses. Face pale, then flushed.	Watery eyes and tears on the side with the most pain. Looking up can make them feel dizzy. Faint feeling or light-headedness. Usually does not have any thirst. May have a sweaty scalp.	Much sweating from slightest exertion. Shivers on any movement or being uncovered. Glands are hard, swollen, tender. Chilly.	Smell of food repulsive. Shooting pains. Stinging pain over left eye. Roots of hair sensitive to combing. Very chilly.
Worse	Cold, touch, anger, motion, noise, odors, sunlight, and morning.	Change of weather, wind, thunderstorms. Odors. Lying on left side. Light. Morning. Evening.	Warm stuffy rooms, during menses, twilight and evening, sunlight lying down, dehydration, excessive joy, rich food.	Cold, damp weather, autumn, cold food or drinks, night, being uncovered, drafts, lying still, initial movement after resting.	Shopping and mental labor. In the evening. Thinking about pain. Lying on painful side.
Better	Warmth, staying wrapped up, napping, firm pressure, hot drinks, moist air, lying or sitting. May want head wrapped.	Sleep, sympathy, low light or darkness, eating and drinking cold things, cool applications, open air.	Intake of liquids, walking in open air or any motion, cool, fresh air, cool applications, pressure, gentle massage, and erect posture.	Warm drinks and food. Constant, gentle movement, stretching, sweating, changing position, massage.	After meals.
Location	Swollen forehead. Frontal headaches.	Ache over one eye, typically right side, with burning temples and throbbing vertex.	Starts in vertex. Occipital ache. Semi-lateral headaches.	Headache in occiput. Forehead pain proceeding backwards. May be more left-sided.	Alternating sides of occiput. Heavy feeling on vertex. More left-sided.

Dosing: Use the ORANGE method if the onset is fast and there is a need for quick relief. Use the BLUE method if the onset is slow. Observe and evaluate.

DANDRUFF

Dandruff is a condition of the scalp that causes flakes of skin to appear. It is often accompanied by itching. Dandruff is a common condition and is not related to hygiene. Symptoms include flakes of skin found throughout hair and itching. Causes of dandruff include:

- over-washing of hair or not shampooing enough

- irritated, oily skin/scalp

- dry skin/scalp

- sensitivity to hair care products

- other skin conditions

- excessive hot showers

- family genetics

- poor diet

ADDITIONAL SUPPORT FOR DANDRUFF

Using appropriate products and changing your hair washing routine can help maintain the natural oil balance:
- Don't wash hair every day. Daily shampooing can cause dandruff by stripping it of needed natural oils.
- Use a shampoo that contains essential oils like tea tree, a natural anti-fungal ingredient that won't dry the scalp like traditional chemically filled dandruff shampoos. This helps to maintain an oil balance on the hair to keep it healthy and growing properly.
- Use a conditioner which contains Aloe Vera and Vitamin E — vital nutrients for your scalp.
- Avoid hot showers or hot water especially on the head as it will exacerbate and prolong the resolution of symptoms.

WHEN TO CONTACT YOUR HEALTHCARE PROFESSIONAL

- If, after a couple of remedies have been taken, the dandruff persists and/or the scalp is red and swollen.

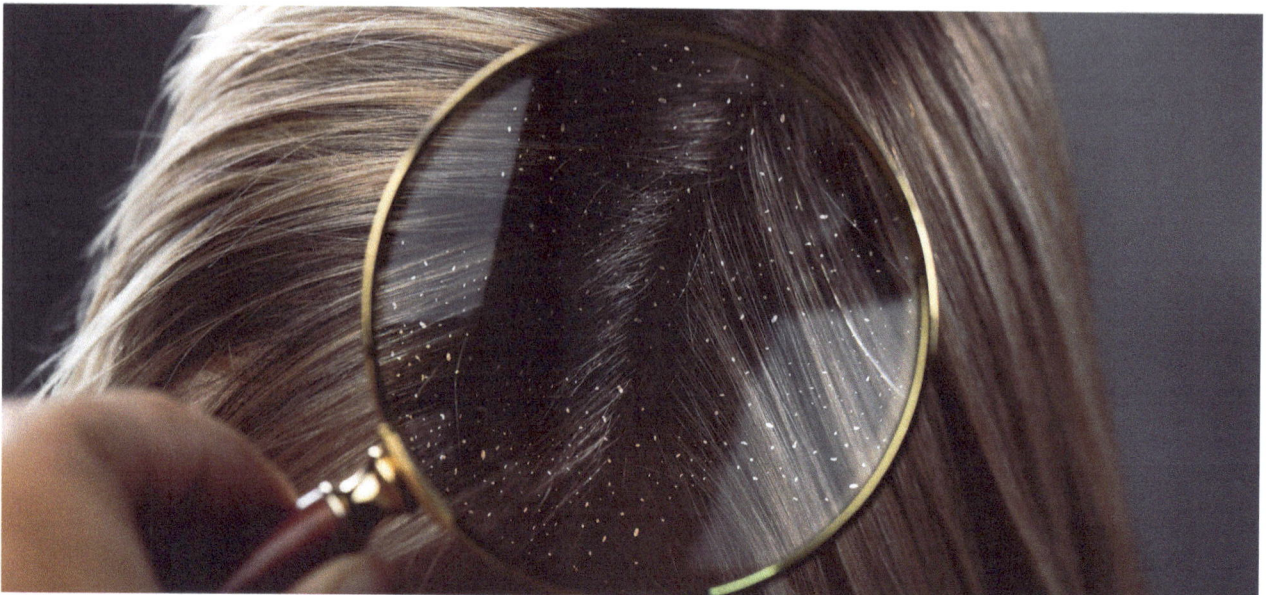

COMMON REMEDIES FOR DANDRUFF

	*Graphites	*Mezereum	Natrum mur	Sulphur	*Thuja
Symptoms	Thick, hard, dry, rough skin that crusts and scales.	Skin intolerably itchy causing thick yellow scabs with pus. Scabs usually scratched off leaves burning sensations, painful marks and possibly scars.	Greasy and oily especially in hair with dry skin and flaking on the margins of the scalp.	Skin or hair dry, scaly. Itches violently at night. Feels hot after scratching. Scratched eruptions with offensive discharge.	Oily or dry hair that sticks up like straw, itching on scalp. Skin burns violently from touch or cold water.
Mood	Difficult to make choices. Anxiety about decisions made, obstinate, discontented, changeable moods, irritability about trifles.	Ill-humored, despondent, censorious, quick to anger about trifles and immediately sorry for it.	Serious, sensitive, objective, overtly responsible.	Aversion to bathing. Offensive personality. Restlessness at night.	Low self-esteem, feels worthless, tries to fit in by imitating behavior of popular or successful people around them.
Indications	Oozes honey-like, thick, sticky, yellow discharges sometimes offensive. Itching is aggravated by heat. Affected most prominently during summer and fall.	Cases of chronic dandruff, skin cold in places where itching is most intense.	Eruptions on the margins of the hairline. Noticeable cracking of the skin.	Itching spots bleed and bite after scratching, spots feel hot after scratching. Sleep disturbed by burning parts on side laid on. Skin excessively sensitive to atmospheric changes.	Helps resistant cases of dandruff. An oily face, with or without acne or pimples, sensitive to cold. Eruptions leave purple spots after healing.
Worse	Cold. Heat of bed, morning, suppression of the discharge.	At night, lying in bed. Cold air, damp.	Worse in the sun or with dampness.	Suppressions by medications, bathing, becoming heated, overexertion, warmth of bed, 11 AM.	Cold, damp, 3 AM or 3 PM, yearly or with the increasing moon.
Better	After taking a walk in the open air. Hot milk, eating.	Wrapping up.	Open air, sweating, fasting.	Open air, motion, dry warm weather.	Warmth, warm wrapping, motion, rubbing, left side.

Dosing: Use the **BROWN** method. Can be taken up to 10 days for this issue. Observe and evaluate.

HEAD LICE

Head lice are tiny wingless insects that infest on the scalp and hair of the human head. Lice feed on blood from the scalp. This infestation is medically called pediculosis capitis. It mostly affects school children and usually results from the direct transfer of lice from the hair of one student to the hair of another. The common symptom is itching of the scalp, neck, and ears. This is a reaction to the saliva that the lice put on the hair shaft to secure the nits (lice eggs). A louse (single adult) is the size of a sesame seed, and an incubating nit is the size of a small flake of dandruff, making them hard to see. They're easiest to spot around the ears and the hairline of the neck.

There are many useful natural options talked about for removing the head lice nits that include using a special lice comb, certain essential oils, other oils like coconut or olive, and more. Since there are many options, consider using an internet search engine to find information about these options by searching "natural treatments for head lice".

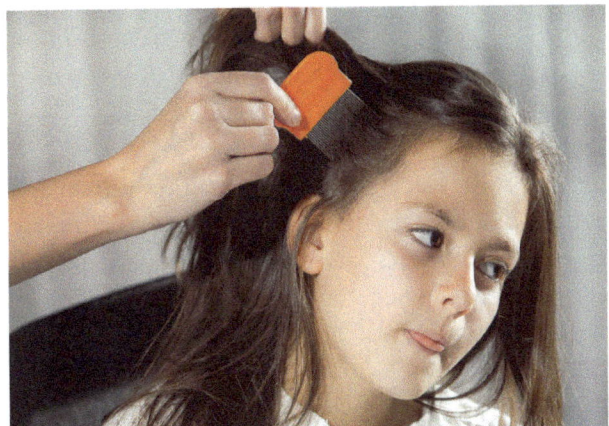

ADDITIONAL SUPPORT FOR REDUCING SUSCEPTIBILITY FOR HEAD LICE

- Eat whole foods, limit sugar, and avoid processed foods. A diet of refined carbohydrates, processed foods, and sugar can depress the immune system making the child susceptible to the lice.
- Reduce allopathic medicines and vaccines when possible as this can lower the body's immune system again, making them more susceptible.
- If the child has had antibiotics (at any time in their life), replace the wiped-out gut flora with daily probiotics. There are many gummy versions for children available in health food stores.
- Increase healthy greens (kale, spinach, etc.) in the person's diet; if needed, add them to fruit smoothies. Also, a super green powder can be added to fruit juice or a smoothie as a substitute for fresh greens.

In addition to these supportive measures, consider these remedies for head lice:

- **Arsenicum**: Chronic recurrence of head lice, the person becomes anxious, restless, and fearful. The scalp becomes intolerably itchy at night with sensitivity when combing and brushing the hair.

- **Lycopodium**: From long-standing anxious anticipation to perform well at school or work. The person's digestion is weak leading to malabsorption and there is a craving for sweets and cakes. Itching aggravated between 4 and 8 PM at night.

- **Sulphur**: Recurring outbreaks. The scalp is dry, the hair brittle, and the head becomes extremely sweaty and moist at night. As soon as the person gets warm in bed, the itching starts with burning and soreness.

BLOWS TO THE HEAD

Head injuries are blows to the scalp, skull, or brain, which are hard enough to cause trauma. Concussions are trauma that happens when the brain is jarred or jolted hard enough to bounce against the skull. A concussion can alter mental functions and disrupt normal functioning of the brain. Being hit directly in the head is not the only way to get a concussion. An impact anywhere on the body can create enough force to jar the brain. Consciousness is not necessarily lost with a concussion. Concussions can be anywhere from mild to severe. The effects may be apparent immediately, or they may not show up until hours, or even days, later. It is important to keep an eye on the person for at least 24-48 hours depending on the severity of the blow.

IT'S AN EMERGENCY WHEN

- The person loses consciousness.
- The person has a convulsion or seizure.
- The person is disoriented, unable to speak, or speaks unintelligibly.
- The person is bleeding profusely from the injury site.
- If a baby has been accidentally dropped and has hit their head.

Give **Arnica** every 15 minutes for any of these conditions on the way to the hospital. If the person is unconscious, you can mix the remedy in water and put it on the pulse point of their wrist or apply it to their face on the lips.

WHEN TO CONTACT YOUR HEALTHCARE PROFESSIONAL

- For any major injuries to the head, always contact a healthcare practitioner even if you have given remedies or been to the hospital.
- If any symptoms linger or are not improving with rest.

ADDITIONAL SUPPORT FOR BLOWS TO THE HEAD

- Keep the person in a quiet, stress-free environment. Watch for signs of a concussion. Give clear liquids with no caffeine or high sugar content. Do not give liquids or solids if they are vomiting. Avoid alcohol.
- If a person has had a concussion, it is important to remove them from any situation where they could hit their head again. Multiple concussions can have long-term negative effects.
- Consider following up with a craniosacral osteopath or cranial sacral therapist.

COMMON REMEDIES FOR BLOWS TO THE HEAD

	Aconite	Arnica	Hypericum	*Natrum sulph
Onset	Injury from hitting a sharp corner or hard surface.	Any blow to the head.	Injury involving nerves of the head and neck.	Blows to the back of the head.
Symptoms	Shock, feeling of pressure in the head, burning, headache, vertigo, sensation as if hair were being pulled.	Shock, sensitivity in the brain, scalp feels contracted, aversion to touch.	Shock to the brain or spinal nerves, dizziness, headache, upward-shooting pains, numbness, and tingling. Head feels heavy, as though there is an icy-cold hand resting on it.	For head injuries, especially to the back of the head. May be dizzy, have headaches in the back of the head, sensitivity to light, or visual disturbances.
Mood	Fear, shock, and insecurity, deer-in-the-headlights look in their eyes.	Dazed, confused and claim, "I am fine," anxious, desire to be left alone.	Anxious and melancholy.	Oversensitive to criticism or scolding, and overly concerned about family members.
Indications	Give this remedy if the person has hit their head quite hard on a sharp corner or a hard surface. The resulting fear, shock, and insecurity call for a dose of this remedy immediately.	Can often bring out bruising very quickly, which is a good sign. Will also help with any swelling internal or external. Will have a blank, dazed, no-one-home look on their face. May not even remember accident.	May have a headache with shooting pains into the cheek that make the eyes feel sore.	Can be given long after a head injury if there is an inability to think or perform mental tasks. Especially helpful when there are emotional changes, including depression, following a head injury. Can undo the lingering effects of a concussion. Music makes them feel sad, the scalp is sensitive, the top of the head feels hot, the brain feels loose when stooping, the head jerks to right side, or they may have piercing pains in the ears. May also have digestive problems, especially recurrent diarrhea.
Worse	Warm room, in the evening and at night, lying on the affected side.	Overexertion, motion, damp, touch.	Jar, exertion, touch, cold, damp, pressure.	Warmth, motion, walking, wet weather.
Better	Open air.	Lying with head low, open air, uncovering, changing position.	Lying on face or abdomen, bending backwards, quiet, rubbing.	Rubbing, eating, stretching, after breakfast.
SPECIAL DOSAGE INSTRUCTIONS				
Special Dosage Instructions	Give remedy and repeat every 10 minutes until the shock and fear have subsided. Then consider **Arnica** if there is any swelling. Repeat if there is a return of symptoms.	If they have been knocked unconscious, put **Arnica** on the inside of the cheek; this can bring them back to consciousness.	If you have a hard time choosing between **Arnica** and **Hypericum**, they can be alternated every 15 minutes until there is an improvement. After the injury, if they seem forgetful or dull, give **Hypericum** three times a week for three weeks. If no improvement after a week, re-evaluate and give a different remedy.	If they are experiencing dizziness, have headaches in the back of the head, sensitivity to light, or visual disturbances after **Arnica** has been given, a dose or two of this remedy will follow **Arnica** well. If symptoms persist after three doses one hour apart, call your healthcare practitioner immediately. For lingering effects of a concussion give remedy three times a week, for up to three weeks. If no improvement after a week, re-evaluate and give a different remedy.

? WHAT'S THE FIRST REMEDY YOU THINK OF WHEN...

1. They were fine when they woke up, but then developed a high fever quickly.
2. There is excessive sweating at night with a fever for multiple days.
3. A spectator got hit in the head by a baseball.
4. A person has symptoms of a concussion.
5. It is taking a long time to heal after experiencing a concussion.
6. Someone has a fever and strangely feels better from all kinds of warmth.
7. A person has an infection with fever and pus on some part of the body without drainage (suspected sepsis).
8. The person always gets a headache when they don't eat.
9. The person has a headache after a relationship break up.
10. A headache comes on after reading a lot either on paper or on a computer screen.

Answer key on page 323.

CHAPTER 6
Eyes

Our eyes are complex and delicate organs, responsible for our sense of sight and visual perception. However, there are various conditions and circumstances that can cause discomfort, disrupting the harmony of our visual experience. From mild irritation to severe pain, these uncomfortable sensations can significantly affect our daily lives and overall well-being. Whether it's a result of external irritants, infections, allergies, or underlying systemic conditions, seeking remedies to alleviate the discomforts is the focus of this chapter.

INFLAMMATION OF THE EYES

Common acute problems with the eyes involve irritation of the mucous membrane that covers the front of the eye and the lining on the inside of the eyelids, also called the conjunctiva. This can be caused by infections, colds, dust, allergies, smoke, pollution, over-squinting, and/or from chemicals in swimming pools.
(Note that for babies and children up to 3 years, there is additional information in **Chapter 20** on **page 243**).

Remedies to consider:
- **Aconite**: After exposure to cold, dust, sand, and swimming pools. Eyes burn and feel better for cold compresses.

- **Rhus Tox**: After overuse of the eyes or change of weather. Eyes are red, especially the left eye, sensitive to light, and feels like sand under the lids. Blinks frequently to make tears.

- ***Euphrasia**: Can be useful during the allergy season. Profuse, hot, burning tears. Eyes look bloodshot and the lids are red as well. Sensitive to light, and possibly itchy; the person blinks a lot.

Dosing: Use the BLUE Method.
Observe and evaluate.

BLOCKED TEAR DUCTS

For infants or young children, see **Chapter 20—First Three Years** starting on **page 243**.

STYES, CHALAZIONS, AND CONJUNCTIVITIS (PINK EYE)

A stye is a small abscess in a gland on the eyelid that looks like a small boil and is usually painful. A condition similar to a stye is a chalazion, a swollen oil gland at the edge of the eyelid. The swelling is red and irritated for awhile before becoming a more hardened lump. Conjunctivitis, also known as "pink eye," is an inflammation of the mucous membrane that covers the front of the eye and lines the inside of the eyelids.

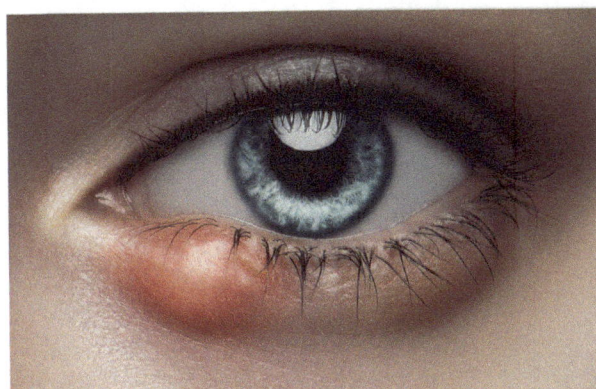

ADDITIONAL SUPPORT FOR EYE INFLAMMATIONS

- Warm and/or cool compresses (depending on what feels best) can be applied to eyes that are caked shut.
- Apply warm compresses with a few drops of **Eyebright tincture** in a ¼ cup very warm water or with a few drops of **Calendula tincture**.
- Do not reuse compresses on eyes with conjunctivitis. Use a fresh compress for each application.
- Wash hands before AND after touching a person's eye if they have conjunctivitis, as it's highly contagious.
- Wash pillowcases and washcloths in hot, soapy water.
- If you are nursing, bathing the baby's eyes in breast milk can be effective.

WHEN TO CONTACT YOUR HEALTHCARE PROFESSIONAL

- If the eyes are bloodshot, or if there is any abnormal vision such as partial loss of sight, blurry vision, or floaters.
- If there is pressure/severe pain in the eyeball, along with sensitivity to light.
- If there are ulcers on the eyelids.
- If the person is constantly squinting.
- The remedies do not resolve the inflammation in 24 hours.

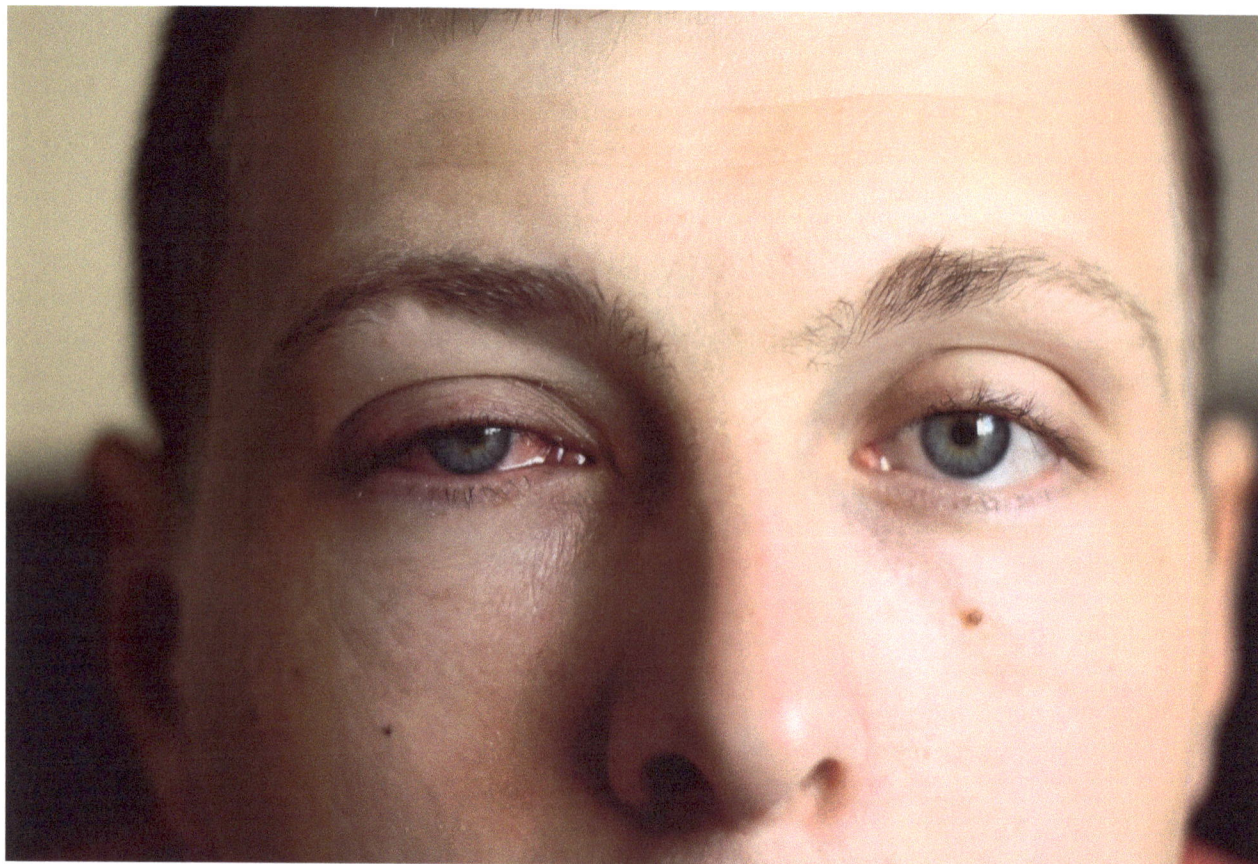

COMMON REMEDIES FOR EYE CONDITIONS

	Apis	Argentum nit	Arsenicum	Calcarea carb	Pulsatilla	Silicea	Staphysagria
Onset	Blocked tear duct, stye, conjunctivitis.	Conjunctivitis or blocked tear duct. Presents shortly after birth.	Conjunctivitis.	Conjunctivitis or blocked tear duct. After exposure to cold.	Conjunctivitis, blocked tear duct, stye. Sticky eyes in newborns.	Blocked tear duct, stye, a foreign body lodged in the eye tissue.	Stye, tumor on eyelids. Cuts or incisions to eye.
Symptoms	Puffiness and swelling around eye. Redness. Hot tears with rawness, stinging, burning.	Eyelid is red, swollen, sore, thick. Discharge is profuse and full of yellow pus. Thick crust on edges of eyelids upon waking; can become glued together.	Burning pain in eyes and eyelids. Hot, acidic tears. Eyes bright red and bloodshot, sometimes with dark rings or puffiness. Eyelids red, crusty and ulcerated.	Sore, watery eyes that ooze yellow or foul-smelling discharge. Eyes glued together after sleeping. Itchy and swollen with gritty sensation.	Profuse, thick, yellow or yellow-green eye discharge which may be smelly. Discharge in corners of eyes, thick upon waking, then watery for rest of the day.	Stye on upper lid, toward the inner corner. Stye emits pus.	Soreness and redness of eyelids. Sometimes there are no complaints.
Mood	Restless.	Irritable, anxious, weepy.	Anxious, restless.	Chilly. May be happy go lucky despite eye issue, not a care in the world Or could be trembling with terror and not want to leave parent's side.	May be weepy, upset and cling to parent.	Mad and upset about eye, demanding attention to clear the issue.	Sweet baby. Can have suppressed anger or anger from insult or humiliation. Family history or multiple griefs.
indications	Discharge clear or full of pus. Much itching, especially at night. Eyes bloodshot.	Swelling, inflammation, redness on inner corner of eye.	Extreme sensitivity to light. Under eyelid may feel gritty. Eyelid may go into spasms.	Sensitivity to light, dilated pupils. May experience fuzzy vision. Baby may be squinting.	Itchy eyes cause a lot of rubbing. Stye usually on upper lid.	Sensitivity to daylight. Eyes very tender to touch, especially when closed.	Stye appears overnight. Itchy, causing extra blinking or scratching of just the stye. Sensation of something in the eye.
Worse	Late afternoon, sun, right eye, heat.	Warm rooms, heat. Upon waking.	Evening, cold damp. Upon waking. Light. On right side.	Open air. Early morning, cold, damp. When accompanied by common cold. Any eye movement.	Evening time. Warm, stuffy rooms, warm wind.	Cold, damp. Fresh air. Touch.	Anger or humiliation.
Better	Cool applications, cool air.	Cool applications. Light pressure. Closing the eyes. Fresh air.	Warm applications. Lying down.	Rest. Warmth.	Temperate fresh air, cool applications.	Heat, warm rooms. Rest.	Cool and warm applications.

Dosing: Use the **BLUE** Method. Could be hourly for the first few doses if very uncomfortable. Observe and evaluate.

Additional remedies to consider for Conjunctivitis (Pink Eye):

- **Belladonna**: For the first stages of conjunctivitis, including the sudden onset of burning, bloodshot eyes, swollen eyelids, and hypersensitivity to light. The eyes are generally hot and throbbing to the touch.

- ***Euphrasia**: Eyes are inflamed with burning or stinging discharges. There is marked redness with intense itching of the eyes. The eyes often water, and there is sensitivity to light and a dry gritty feeling in the eyes.

- **Pulsatilla**: The eyes have a yellow green discharge and itch. May accompany or immediately follow a cold. The eyelids tend to stick together, and symptoms generally improve with cold compresses.

EYE STRAIN AND TIRED OR OVERWORKED EYES

These conditions are brought on by squinting, which can be caused by a person not being able to see clearly—in which case they should be taken to an optometrist. If a teen or an adult has been over-studying, this can cause not only squinting but a weakness of the eyes as well.

Remedies to consider:

- ***Phosphoricum acidum**: for overuse of eyes through reading or study causing a headache and strong desire to close the eyes.

- **Ruta**: for eyestrain from reading or studying accompanied by headache and red eyes.

- ***Zincum metallicum**: for when the eyes are sore and watery with burning tears and itching and soreness of the eyelids.

Dosing: Use the BLUE Method.
In addition to these remedies, consider including **Kali phos 6X** cell salt three to four times a day when eyes are overworked.

ADDITIONAL SUPPORT FOR EYE STRAIN OR OVERWORKED EYES

- Take a break at least once an hour, for about ten minutes of not looking at any screen.
- Allow the eyes to alternatively look at objects far away and then close up to stretch out the eye muscles at least once every 30 minutes.
- Clean eyeglasses, computer screens, and phone screens to avoid having to look through the dust and dirt.
- Practice Palming. Palming is the action of covering the eyes with the hands while resting your eyes from all light stimulation which relaxes the muscles around the eyes and reduces eye fatigue.

To palm,

1. Start by removing your eyeglasses (if applicable).
2. Then vigorously rub your hands back and forth to warm them up.
3. Rest your bent elbows on a surface in front of you.
4. Cup your hands over the eyes while placing the palm of each hand over the corresponding cheekbone allowing your head to rest into your hands so your head and neck are supported by your elbows.
5. Close your eyes to rest.
6. Breathe deeply in this position for five minutes.
7. When ready, open your eyes with your hands still in place and slowly open your fingers to let light in. Take a moment to adjust to the light.
8. Slowly remove both hands from your eyes and take a deep cleansing breath.

BLOWS TO THE EYES

A black eye affects the flesh and orbital bone (the bony structure around the eye). In most cases, a cold compress will feel best.

🏥 **IT'S AN EMERGENCY WHEN**

- The person has two black eyes. Two black eyes at the same time can indicate a skull or a fracture at the base of the skull.
- The person has any visual disturbance, bleeding, severe pain, and/or a persistent headache.
- There is the possibility that the eye itself has been injured or if vision is compromised.

When someone's eye has been injured, it's a good idea to give a dose or two of **Aconite** first before the indicated remedy below. **Aconite** is known as **Arnica** for the eye.

COMMON REMEDIES FOR BLOWS TO THE EYES

	Arnica	*Hamamelis	Hypericum	Ledum	*Symphytum
Onset	Periorbital hematoma (black and blue eye) caused by trauma.	Bloodshot eye.	Scratch on the cornea.	Trauma to eye resulting in purple-colored tissue around the eye.	Orbital bone trauma. If black eye resulted from a fistfight.
Indications	All bruising comes out to the surface, which is what needs to happen. It helps heal the soft tissue in the eye socket.	Painful weakness of the eye. Sensation that the eye is trying to force itself out. This remedy will help absorption of any bleeding inside the eyeball.	Needed if there is severe pain. Especially helpful for a superficial scratch on the cornea.	A black eye where the tissue around the eye feels cold. Cold compresses will feel particularly good. This remedy will absorb serum and blood clots and help if there is pain in the orbital bone.	A black eye with pain in the eyeball. Will also heal any trauma to the orbital bone around the eye. Particularly helpful for a blow to the eye from a ball or fist.
Symptoms	A typical black and blue eye, soft tissue injury.	Bloodshot eyeball and much inflammation around the eye.	Radiating, lancinating or shooting pain in the eye.	Much swelling around the eye, with tender purple tissue. Eye aches.	Eyeball and orbital bone painful even after bruising has disappeared.
Worse	Least touch.	Warm damp air.	Cold and touch.	At night.	Touch, pressure.
Better	Lying with head low.	Gentle pressure on the eyelid.	Bending head backwards.	Cold compresses.	Warmth.
SPECIAL DOSAGE INSTRUCTIONS					
Special Dosage Instructions	Take remedy every hour until symptoms are relieved. If there is no response after three doses, read on to see if other remedies are needed. If the pain is severe, give one dose of **Arnica** and then go on to **Hypericum**.	Take remedy every hour until symptoms are relieved. Repeat only if there is a return of symptoms.	Take remedy every 15 minutes, until improvement. Repeat only if there is a return of symptoms.	After **Arnica**, if indicated, give **Ledum** twice a day for three days.	After **Arnica**, if indicated, give ***Symphytum** twice per day until the pain is gone.

? WHAT'S THE FIRST REMEDY YOU THINK OF WHEN...

1. One wakes up frequently with yellow crust in their eye.

2. They got hit in the eye by a golf ball.

3. The person has a blocked tear duct.

4. There is a splinter or foreign object lodged in the eye.

5. There is overuse of the eyes while studying or reading that causes a headache.

6. An eye has a scratched cornea—to give to the person, on the way to the eye doctor or hospital.

7. Eyes feel irritated, even burning, after swimming in a pool.

8. The person has a black and blue eye from being hit by a baseball.

9. Hot and throbbing eyes are sensitive to the light and touch.

10. Watery eyes are marked with intense itching.

Answer key on page 323.

CHAPTER 7
Ears

Ears are organs that provide two main functions: hearing and balance. For hearing, the eardrum vibrates so that sound waves can enter the ear canal. Balance is achieved through the sensory organ in the inner ear coupled with visual input and other receptors in the body. There are three parts to the ear: the outer ear which includes the ear canal; the middle ear that is composed of three tiny bones, the malleus, incus and stapes; and the inner ear which is the part of the ear that gives us the sense of balance. Ear infections and earaches are common conditions that generally can be addressed by homeopathic remedies.

EAR INFECTIONS

Childhood ear infections are common as children begin teething, have reactions to new foods, and are exposed to the viruses that cause colds and influenza.

When a child or an adult has a common cold, the eustachian tube—the tube that connects the sinuses to the middle ear—can become blocked with excess mucus. Because young children's eustachian tubes are small and more horizontal than an adult's tubes, this makes them more prone to this problem. The pressure from the excess mucus pushes on the eardrum from within and can cause infection with pain and temporary hearing loss. This infection is a type of ear infection called otitis media, or a middle ear infection.

Eighty percent of the time, an earache coming from the middle ear is caused by a virus in the mucus. Antibiotics treat bacteria but not viruses, so the American Academy of Pediatrics (AAP) now does NOT advise antibiotics as a first line of treatment for suspected ear infections. When antibiotics are used to treat otitis media, they tend to suppress the infection, and quite often the ear infection will return after the person completes the course of the antibiotic.

Other possible causes of earaches include pressure from impacted ear wax, a foreign body in the ear canal, or water and chlorine from swimming pools. In addition, it is common for an earache to be associated with fevers, teething, sore throats, or colds.

Some children have a painless condition called "glue ear," when a thick, sticky fluid collects behind the eardrum. This fluid can impair hearing, which can lead to delayed speech and other development. If this is suspected, contact a professional homeopath. A low potency remedy or a constitutional remedy may be needed over a period of weeks to clear the condition.

IT'S AN EMERGENCY WHEN

- The person has a persistent high fever accompanying the earache.
- The person is severely drowsy with the earache.
- There was a recent blow or injury to the ear.
- The ear is oozing any sticky or bloody discharge. This could mean the eardrum has burst.
- The person is vomiting while experiencing ear pain.
- The person has a stiff neck.

ADDITIONAL SUPPORT FOR EARACHES

- Increase fluid intake, especially if there is a fever, to prevent dehydration.
- Use warm or cool applications, depending on what feels good to the person.
- Protect ears from cold or wind with a hat.
- If the person has a head cold, advise them not to blow their nose too hard.
- Avoid getting water in the ear. Do not swim until the earache has resolved completely.
- It is advisable to stop any products made from cow's milk during this condition, because milk and cheese can cause the body to produce more mucus, which raises the level of acidity in the system. (Goat's milk, rice milk, almond milk, or soy products may be substituted for cow's milk products.) Buy raw or organic, when possible.
- Do not attempt to use cotton swabs to clear the wax during an earache. Normal amounts of wax do not cause pain. If an abnormal buildup is suspected, contact your healthcare practitioner. Do not poke anything into the ears; handle the person's head gently, since there might be tender, swollen glands around the neck.
- Consider buying an otoscope (an instrument designed for visual examination of the eardrum). Make sure to have your healthcare provider teach you the correct use to avoid possible injury.
- Sometimes there is such a buildup of mucus that an eardrum may rupture, which may bring relief from the pain. If the eardrum has ruptured, give the remedy **Calendula** internally, three times a day for three days to promote healing. It will usually resolve in about two weeks.

WHEN TO CONTACT YOUR HEALTHCARE PROFESSIONAL

- If the eardrum has ruptured. Multiple ruptures of the eardrum can permanently impair hearing.

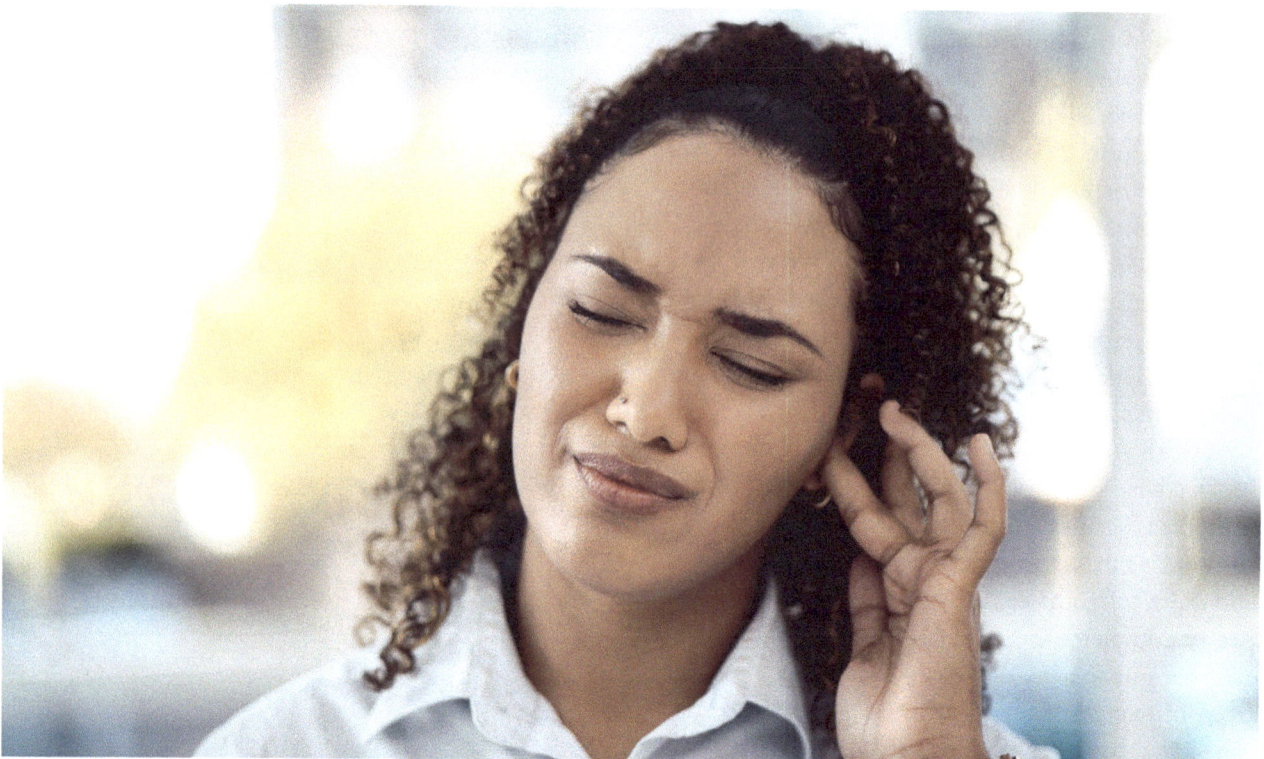

COMMON REMEDIES FOR EAR INFECTIONS AND EARACHES

	Aconite	Belladonna	Chamomilla	Hepar sulph	Mercurius	Pulsatilla	Silicea
Onset	Sudden onset after exposure to cold wind or after a shock. Most useful in first 24 hours at the first sign of symptoms.	Sudden, violent onset from getting head wet and/or being in a cold dry wind.	Onset can be from a cold wind, or anger. Teething.	Slow onset from getting too cold or being out in a cold wind.	Onset from getting chilled.	Onset can be from getting feet wet and becoming chilled.	Slow onset from getting chilled, getting feet wet, or change of weather to cold.
Symptoms	Pains are sharp, piercing, and intense. External ear is usually red or hot to the touch and ear canal opening may look red as well. Ear can be swollen.	Sudden intense throbbing pain which can shoot into throat or neck. Pain is inside and outside of ear. May crave lemonade.	Intense, sharp, intolerable pains. Ears are hot, very sensitive. Holds the painful ear.	Throbbing with unbearable, sharp pains that may radiate into throat or jaw. Usually on right side but can move from left to right. Very chilly.	Pain is boring, pressing, tearing, and extends from teeth or throat to ear. Ear feels blocked and hearing may be impaired.	Pains are aching and sharp and mostly left sided. Ear is hot, red, and ear lobes can be swollen.	Pains pressing outward behind ear. Complaints mostly left sided. Usually itching in ear, wants to bore finger into ear.
Mood	Restless, sensitive, fearful, anxious, and screaming.	Restless, irritable, all senses are acute and heightened. Severely agitated.	Demanding of something then doesn't want it. Frantic with pain. Can't be consoled, fretful.	Extremely irritable, hypersensitive, easily angered, and does not want to be examined or looked at.	Restless, constantly changing mind, and nervous.	Moody, whiny, pathetic, and fretful, yet affectionate. Symptoms change with mood changes.	Subdued, shy, anxious, and nervous. Overly sensitive. Can be stubborn and uncoopera-tive.
Indications	Sensitive to noise. Thirst for cold drinks. Chills come on fast and high fever may follow. Glands usually swollen. May feel like there is a drop of liquid in ear.	External ear red and hot. Usually with high fever, with delirium. Face usually bright red, hot, and flushed. Pupils may be dilated, and eyes may be glassy.	Ears feel plugged. If there is a discharge, it is clear. One cheek may be red and the other pale. Hot, thirsty, and usually has a fever.	Ears sensitive to touch and cold air. Chilly and sweaty. Bony structure behind ear can be painful and inflamed. If there is a discharge, it is thick, yellow, and smelly like old cheese.	Increase in saliva. Usually drools on pillow. Breath and sweat smell foul. If a discharge, it is burning, thick, smelly, gluey, yellow, or green. Glands are swollen. Unstable body temperature (chilly alternates with sweaty).	Ears feel stopped or plugged. Diminished hearing. If there is a discharge, it is thick, creamy, or yellow-green. Usually not thirsty. May feel a pulsing sound in ear.	Ear feels plugged and hearing may be impaired. Sensitive to noise. Neck glands swollen. Offensive discharge, and a thick pus referred to as "glue ear."
Worse	Night, around midnight, midday, noise, pressure, and touch.	Chewing anything, right side, cold air, touch, noise, jarring, light, turning the head, 3 PM.	Usually worse right side. Cold air, touch, teething, music, night, especially around 9 PM.	Touch, uncovering, exertion, cold drafts, winter, solid food, cold dry air, and night.	On right side, night, warmth of bed, sweating, damp cold, drafts, and warm drinks.	Night. Left side. Too warm or stuffy room.	Left side, cold drafts, wind, open air, damp, loud noises, and full moon.
Better	Fresh air, rest, sweating, and hot applications.	Rest, light covering, sitting semi-erect, low light, quiet, and cold water.	Being held, warmth, and mild weather.	Warm drinks, moist heat, wrapping up, damp weather, warm applications, and covering the head and ears.	Moderate temperatures and rest.	Open air. Affection. Being held, hugged, and after a good cry.	Warmth, warm wraps and applications, yawning, and swallowing.

Other common remedies to consider for earaches: **Calcarea carb, *Ferrum phos, *Kali mur,** and **Sulphur.**

Dosing: Start with the ORANGE method, especially if the onset is fast. Observe and evaluate. May need to move onto the BLUE method as the symptoms become less troublesome. Change the remedy if the symptoms change.

SWIMMER'S EAR

Swimmer's ear is a painful condition that is caused when water gets trapped in the ear. If the water is allowed to remain in the ear canal, bacteria and fungal organisms can begin to flourish. This produces inflammation, irritation, or infection. If water is trapped, turn the head back and forth, while lying down on the stomach, to use the force of gravity to drain water from the ear. Gently pulling the ear in different directions can also help. Using a towel, dry the opening of the ear very carefully, as far in as you can.

The most common remedy for swimmer's ear is **Mercurius vivus** (same as **Mercurius** and **Mercurius sol**). This should clear this condition (you may have to give a few doses). If there is no response after giving three doses, try a few doses of **Silicea**.

ADDITIONAL SUPPORT FOR SWIMMER'S EAR

- To prevent swimmer's ear, put two drops of rubbing alcohol in the ear before going swimming.
- Two drops of white vinegar can also prevent the growth of bacteria on the skin in the ear canal.

WHAT'S THE FIRST REMEDY YOU THINK OF WHEN...

1. Your child wakes up screaming, pulling their ear, and is inconsolable.
2. An earache is coupled with increased saliva and bad breath.
3. You get water in your ear after swimming.
4. You get an earache after being exposed to cold wind in your ears.
5. An earache, with itching in the ear, causes the person to bore their finger in the ear to scratch it.
6. The ears are hot from intense, sharp, intolerable pains.
7. Ears feel plugged and stopped up, and you may experience diminished hearing.
8. The discharge from my child's ear is smelly like old cheese.
9. My ears are red and hot, my fever is high, and my cheeks are flushed bright red.
10. You feel chilled and you're getting a fever, your ear is sensitive to noise, and you are craving cold drinks.

Answer key on page 323.

CHAPTER 8
Nose

Your nose plays a crucial role in both maintaining overall health and serving as a gateway for potential illnesses. It acts as a primary air filter, warming, moisturizing, and purifying the air we breathe. It is lined with tiny hair-like structures called cilia and a mucous membrane that help trap dust, allergens, bacteria, and other particles, preventing them from reaching the lungs.

The nasal tissues also contain immune cells that help recognize and fight against potential pathogens, such as viruses and bacteria. This immune response helps protect the body from respiratory infections and maintain overall health. But when the nasal passages aren't functioning properly or become overwhelmed with pathogens, our health can become compromised with several uncomfortable symptoms, especially the common cold, sinusitis, allergies and nosebleeds. Homeopathic remedies can provide needed relief from these uncomfortable symptoms.

COMMON COLDS AND SINUSITIS

The common cold is caused by many different viruses. Each person is different; therefore, symptoms will vary. In the early stages, the body may produce symptoms such as fever, chills, or sweats to fight off the virus. The body may also produce symptoms such as sneezing, runny nose, sore throat, earache, headache, tearing eyes, or cough. These various symptoms all have a purpose. For example, mucus is produced to trap viruses and expel them from the body.

A cold can be the body's way of saying that it's run-down, stressed out, or not getting enough sleep. A cold is like a spring house cleaning; when the cold is over, the lymphatic system is cleaned out and the person usually experiences better energy than before the cold began.

It is key to treat a cold at the first sign of symptoms. Neglected colds can turn into more serious conditions and drag on. At the first sign of symptoms, take the case and give a remedy. The sooner you give a remedy, the symptoms experienced will be less severe and last a shorter time.

It's important to keep in mind that suppressing common cold symptoms with decongestants or nasal sprays—even though they may provide temporary relief—are not beneficial in the long-run and may prolong the illness or drive the symptoms to a deeper organ of the body. Overcoming a cold, without suppressing it, exercises the immune system and helps the body build resistance to future viruses. Homeopathy helps to naturally aid the body in resolving colds, while making the person more comfortable.

Sinusitis may be caused by a combination of viruses, bacteria, fungus, or allergies. The mucus discharge from sinusitis can be clear, yellow, yellow-green, brown, orange, or green. It could also be thick, watery, lumpy, or stringy. Chronic sinusitis is characterized not only by sinus pains, but also by constant post-nasal drip that runs down the back of the throat. If this condition becomes chronic, a visit to a professional homeopath or other natural healthcare practitioner may be needed.

ADDITIONAL SUPPORT FOR COLDS AND SINUSITIS

- Make sure the person is drinking plenty of fluids and getting complete rest. If they get a headache this can be a sign of dehydration. Avoid sugary drinks. Fresh squeezed juice, coconut water or clean water is best.
- Use nasal irrigators to clean the nasal passages several times a day such as a neti pot with a pinch of sea salt added to the warm water or a salt water (saline only) nasal spray.
- If a person is sounding "throaty" ask them to cough. If they feel mucus in the throat, ask them to cough the mucus up and spit it out into a Kleenex and not swallow it again. Keep reminding them to do this. This can help mucus from building up and the person from developing a severe cough.
- Avoid dairy products as they create mucus.
- Give lots of fresh fruit—including oranges, kiwi, pineapple, mango, papaya, etc.—because they contain high amounts of vitamin C which is shown to be an immune booster and antioxidant.
- If you live in a dry climate, you can line the nostrils with organic coconut oil to keep the nostrils moist. A cool mist vaporizer in the bedroom can be helpful to break up thick mucus. Or you can get the bathroom steamed up and have the person breathe in the steam. If it is not too cold or raining, the person can go out into the fresh air for a walk.
- Though you may be tempted to get an over-the-counter decongestant, this will actually prolong the cold and make the person feel worse when it "wears off".

Remedies to consider for specific symptoms of colds:

- colds with the person being very chilly: **Arsenicum, Hepar sulph, Nux vomica, Silicea**

- colds with eye discharges: ***Allium cepa, *Dulcamara, *Euphrasia, Natrum mur**

- extremely sensitive to cold and heat: **Mercurius**

- face flushed bright red and many times eyes are dilated: **Belladonna**

- frequent sneezing: **Aconite, *Allium cepa, *Calcarea sulph, Hepar sulph, Kali Bich, Lycopodium, Mercurius, Natrum mur, Nux vomica, Rhus tox, *Sabadilla, Silicea, Sulphur**

- headache with a cold: **Aconite, Belladonna, Bryonia, Nux vomica, Phosphorus, Pulsatilla, Silicea, Sulphur**

- colds with a loss of smell and or taste: **Calcarea carb, *Calcarea sulph, Hepar sulph, Kali Bich, Mercurius, Natrum mur, Phosphorus, Pulsatilla, Silicea**

Types of Mucus:

- blood-streaked mucus: **Phosphorus**

- burning mucus: **Arsenicum**

- clear/frothy: **Silicea**

- hot mucus: **Aconite, *Allium cepa, Sulphur**

- profuse flow: ***Allium cepa, Arsenicum, *Dulcamara, *Euphrasia** (during the day), ***Kali sulph, Mercurius, Natrum mur, Nux vomica** (during the day), **Phosphorus, Rhus tox**

- watery mucus: ***Allium Cepa, Arsenicum, *Dulcamara** (at the beginning of the cold), ***Euphrasia, Mercurius** (at the beginning of the cold), **Natrum mur, Nux vomica, Rhus tox** (at the beginning of the cold)

- yellow mucus: **Calcarea carb, *Calcarea Sulph, *Dulcamara** (as the cold progresses), **Hepar sulph, *Kali sulph, Lycopodium, Pulsatilla, Sulphur**

- yellow/green mucus: **Kali Bich, Mercurius** (as the cold progresses), **Rhus tox** (as the cold progresses), **Sepia**

- white/grey mucus: ***Kali Mur**

Colds with Strange, Rare, Peculiar Symptoms:

- burning symptoms, but wants warmth and warm drinks: **Arsenicum**

- chilly, but wants the window open at night: **Pulsatilla**

- cold sores with colds: **Natrum mur, Rhus tox**

- colds in female teens that come on just before, during or just after her period: **Sepia**

- colds that come on after getting a haircut: **Belladonna**

- colds with a constant urge to stretch: **Rhus tox**

- craves ice cold drinks or food, but is chilly: **Phosphorus**

- drooling on pillow: **Mercurius**

- has a discharge, but everything feels very dry: **Bryonia**

- has to have every part of the body covered up because they are so chilly: **Hepar sulph**

- mucus tastes salty: **Natrum mur**

- profuse flow of mucus, but feels stuffed up: ***Allium cepa**

- sleeps with feet out from under the covers: **Sulphur**

- sneezing in a warm room or during sleep: **Pulsatilla**

- symptoms are constantly changing: **Pulsatilla**

- wants to keep nose warm by covering it up: ***Dulcamara**

- yawns a lot in open air: ***Euphrasia**

- lots of gas and bloating: **Lycopodium**

Different kinds of colds:

- summer colds: ***Dulcamara**

- autumn colds when there is a sudden change from hot to cold damp: ***Dulcamara**

If the cold symptoms have a SUDDEN onset, here are two common remedies to consider using the ORANGE dosing method:

- **Aconite**: For a cold with sudden onset after being exposed to icy north or east winds, or from shock or fright. This remedy is most useful in the first 24 hours, and at the very first sign of symptoms. Symptoms come on quickly. The person might have shivers followed by a sudden high fever and sweating. The skin is dry and hot, and there's a thirst for cold drinks. There might be frequent sneezing with clear, hot mucus dripping from the nose, or the nose may be dry and stopped up. The eyes feel hot, dry, burn, ache, and may be bloodshot. There may be roaring in the ears and a throbbing headache. The pupils may be contracted. The person is restless, fearful, anxious, and/or screaming, and may have nightmares with restless or difficult sleep.

  Worse from: Nighttime, around midnight, midday, noise, cold drafts, light, and pressure. **Better from:** Fresh air, rest, sweating, and warm applications.

- **Belladonna**: Sudden violent onset, from getting head wet, cold and dry wind, or from getting a haircut. The neck glands are swollen and may be painful. The nose is dry, red, swollen, and may have blood-streaked mucus. The face is flushed bright red, and pupils are usually dilated. The skin is hot and dry. If the person has a high fever, they may be confused and delirious. If thirsty, they crave cold water or lemonade. The eyes may be glassy and sparkling, with a wild look. They may smell imaginary odors. Sleep is restless. They may have a headache. They may be irritable and all senses may be acute and heightened. The person may become severely agitated.

Worse from: noise, light, odors, drafts, touch, sudden motion, and around 3 PM.
Better from: sitting semi-erect or standing up, quiet, and resting in dark rooms with light covers.

Note: After taking **Aconite** or **Belladonna** for a fast onset cold, the symptoms may change to those of a regular cold. You may need to go to another remedy if the cold has not cleared or if the symptom picture changes for the worse. At this point, reevaluate the symptoms.

*See both **Cold Remedy Charts** on the following pages for further remedies to consider.*

If the cold symptoms have a SLOW onset, here are two remedies to consider using the **BLUE** dosing method:

- ***Ferrum phos**: This remedy may be given at the first sign of a cold that doesn't have especially distinctive symptoms and the onset is slow. There may be common symptoms, but if there is nothing distinctive about them, this is the remedy. It is also a remedy for general inflammation, and most useful for the early stages of a fever and/or sore throat. The person is weak, chilly, and thirsty for cold drinks. The face may alternate between being pale and being flushed. The person may complain of a scratchy throat, or a headache in the forehead that is worse on the right side. Some may experience a nosebleed. The eyes can be bloodshot and burning. The mood might be talkative, excited, irritable, and averse to company.

  Worse from: nighttime, especially from 4–6 AM, on the right side, touch, motion, and jarring.
  Better from: cold applications on the head and lying down.

- **Gelsemium**: The person who needs this remedy looks sleepy and weak. The complaints might have started after a strong emotion, such as after hearing bad news, a fright, or after exposure to cold damp weather. They will be tired and yet may not be able to sleep well. There are chills, especially in the back, possibly going up and down the back, perhaps alternating with heat. The person complains of soreness, possible headache, and does not want to drink. The heavy eyelids with listlessness are good indications for this remedy.

  Worse from: 10 AM, emotions, motion, humidity, cold damp weather, hearing bad news.
  Better from: sweating, profuse urination, bending forward, continued motion, reclining with head held high.

Note: After taking one of these remedies, the symptoms may shift to a different remedy type or start the healing process. The person may need another remedy if the cold has not cleared or if the symptom picture changes for the worse. Reevaluate the symptom picture at this point.

See the following two charts for further remedies to consider.

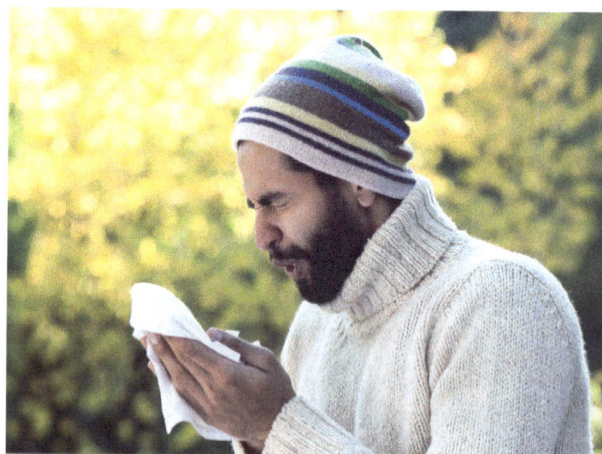

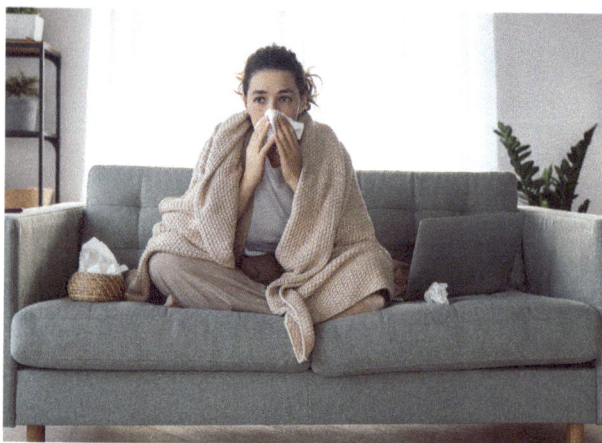

COMMON REMEDIES FOR COLDS—part 1

	*Allium cepa	Arsenicum	Hepar sulph	Kali bich	Mercurius	Natrum mur	Pulsatilla
Onset	Damp, windy, cold weather, getting feet wet.	Getting chilled, wet weather, overheating, overexertion.	Getting cold, or from a cold wind.	Getting chilled.	Getting chilled.	Grief, guilt, disappointment, fright.	Getting feet wet, becoming chilled. After common cold has set in.
Symptoms	Similar to the symptoms of cutting an onion. Frequent sneezing with profuse hot, watery, acidic mucus which burns nose and top lip. Watery non-acidic discharge from eyes which are light-sensitive, burning, and red.	Profuse, burning, watery mucus, especially in the right nostril. Much sneezing, but nose feels stopped up with burning, dry sensation. Nose and top lip sore and red from burning mucus. Raw burning feeling in soft palate.	Catches cold easily and is extremely cold. Glands swollen. Mucus thick, yellow, smelly, and drips down the back of the throat. Nose red, inflamed, swollen. Sneezes a lot when uncovered or in a draft of cold air.	Mucus smelly, acidic, yellow or greenish, sticky, ropy and so thick they can't breathe through their nose or blow it out. Nose feels heavy, dry. Can develop ulcerations and dry crusts in nose, causing bleeding when loosened.	Cold starts in throat or chest and travels up to nose and sinuses. Sneezing with profuse, slimy, watery mucus. Later becomes thick and yellow-green, smelling like old cheese. Mucus burns upper lip and makes nostrils raw. Metallic taste.	Cold starts with much sneezing, worse in morning. Mucus profuse watery discharge, like white of a raw egg. Then nose becomes dry, mucus thickens, and nose gets stopped up. Eyes red, watery, burning with salty or acidic tears.	Symptoms are constantly changing and shifting. Temperature erratic. Mouth dry, but no thirst. Chilly but intolerant of heat. Wants window open. Mucus profuse, bland, thick, creamy-yellow or yellow-green.
Mood	Good temperament, but usually anxious.	Anxious, irritable, oversensitive, needy, demanding. May feel they are dying or will never get better.	Extreme irritability, demanding, sensitive, and does not want to be examined or looked at.	Ill-humored low spirited, indifferent.	Restless, constantly changing their mind, nervous, weary. May tremble.	Easily frustrated, touchy, sulky, easily offended. Oversensitive to noise, odors, lights, hot sun, loud music.	Weepy, whiny, whimpering, fretful, but affectionate. Wants attention. May feel sorry for self.
Indications	Left nostril stuffed up, then moves to right nostril. Sore and tickling throat from acidic post-nasal drip. Sneezing brings no relief.	Strong thirst for small sips. Dull throbbing headache, sensitive to light. Cold can move into chest. Lots of burning sensations, chilly, weak, exhausted. Restless. Face pale with anxious look, may have cold sweat.	May lose sense of smell. Sweating of the head and neck at night. Wants to be wrapped up, kept warm, and stay indoors. Extreme chilliness.	Violent sneezing. Thick post-nasal drip makes voice hoarse. Chilly. Usually loses sense of smell. May feel like there is hair on tongue or in nostrils. Weakness.	Loss of smell or taste. Drools slimy, clear saliva. Bad breath. May have metallic taste. Sensitive to heat and cold. Unstable temperature. Thirst for cold water. Glands in neck swollen and tender.	Mucus tastes salty. Thirst for cold water and salty foods. Loss of taste and smell. Lips dry and cracked. May have ulcers In nose or cold sore.	Mucus profuse in morning and early evening. Sneezing in warm, stuffy room and during sleep. Loss of taste and smell. May crave dairy products. Eyes can be crusty upon awakening. Thirstless.
Worse	Warm stuffy rooms, damp, cold, evening, spring-time.	Physical exertion, after midnight, cold air, cold drinks.	Cold dry air, winter, night, touch, uncovering, exertion, cold drafts.	Sneezing worse morning. Pressure in forehead and maxillary sinus area. Cold, damp, spring, autumn, undressing, 2-3 AM.	Night, drafts, damp weather, sweating, too much cold or heat, lying on right side, warmth of bed, warm drinks.	Exertion, being uncovered, lying on the back, eating, drafts.	Warm stuffy rooms, morning, twilight, getting overheated, fatty or rich foods, dairy products.
Better	Fresh air, cool rooms, cool applications.	Warmth, warm drinks, lying down, fresh air, company. Reassurance they are going to get better.	Moist heat or warm applications, hot drinks, wrapping up the head or ears.	Warmth, wrapping up, pressure, gentle motion.	Moderate steady temperatures, rest, lying on stomach, morning.	Warmth, wrapping up, moist air, hot drinks, belching, quiet, not moving the chest.	Cool fresh air, cold applications and drinks, being uncovered, rest, being consoled, being held or hugged, after a good cry.
Also For	Seasonal Allergies	Sinusitis; Seasonal Allergies	Sinusitis, Tonsilitis	Sinusitis	Tonsilitis	Sinusitis; Seasonal Allergies	Sinusitis; Seasonal Allergies

Note: *Kali sulph is the better remedy if they are worse from heat, better from cold. **Kali bich** is for the opposite of *Kali sulph: worse from cold, better from heat.

COMMON REMEDIES FOR COLDS—part 2

	Bryonia	Calcarea carb	Nux vomica	Phosphorus	Rhus tox	Silicea
Onset	From being exposed to cold winds.	Changes in weather.	Getting chilled in a cold, dry wind or air conditioning.	Getting drenched in rain.	Getting wet, sitting on damp ground, or getting overheated after being chilled.	Getting chilled, getting feet wet, change of weather to cold.
Symptoms	Comes on slowly. Nose is stuffed up but has only a small amount of watery discharge or none at all. Very dry nose, mouth, lips, throat. Eyelids sore, red, and swollen. Eyeballs sore. Bursting headache with shooting pains.	Tends to catch colds easily. Smelly yellow mucus. Nose stuffed up during day but runs at night. Stuffed up nose with loss of smell, however, may complain they smell an offensive odor. Glands are swollen. May have profuse sweating around the head.	Profuse flow of watery mucus in daytime, but nose stuffed up at night or in open air. Stuffiness alternates between nostrils. Violent sneezing, especially in morning. Can be constipated.	Cold can start in throat or chest and travel up to nose and sinuses. Sneezing with profuse, slimy, watery mucus. Later becomes thick and yellow-green, smelling like old cheese. Mucus burns upper lip and makes nostrils raw. Stools usually loose.	Muscles and joints stiff and achy, but better from constant, gentle movement. Aching in bones of the nose. Much sneezing with profuse watery mucus that may turn thick and green. Glands swollen, hard, and tender.	Catches cold quite easily. Nose is either running or alternating between dryness and being blocked. Mucus clear and frothy. Dry, hard crusts form in nose and bleed when loosened. Glands are swollen. Sense of smell is lost. Mouth may have cracked corners.
Mood	Grumpy, irritable, does not want to move. Wants to be left alone. Worries about missing school or work but wants to be home.	Sluggish, stubborn, sensitive, tearful.	Angry, irritable, impatient, easily frustrated.	Affectionate, sweet, fearful, easily upset, but can be irritable.	Anxious, weepy, helpless, mildly delirious, extremely restless.	Subdued, shy, overly sensitive to pain. All senses heightened. Anxious, nervous, can be stubborn or uncooperative.
Indications	Cold often quickly descends into chest. Wants to have room warm, but not hot. Prefers to be still, avoiding movement. Complains of feeling dry everywhere in the body.	Nostrils become dry, sore, ulcerated. Nose and upper lip swollen. Very thirsty. Usually becomes hoarse.	Soft palate feels very full, may have a bloody nose. Chilly at slightest movement. Has dull headache and aches all over. Very little thirst. Throat raw. Sleep restless.	Feels chilly but is thirsty for ice-cold drinks and food. Acute sense of smell. May have headache over one eye. Needs rest until full recovery. Needs consolation and attention.	Dry mouth and throat. Thirsty for sips of water. Tip of nose is red and sore. Usually has red triangle on tip of tongue. Constant urge to stretch. Tosses and turns but cannot get comfortable.	Sweating of head and neck at night. Sneezing in morning and cold air. Chilly. Sensitive to drafts and weather changes. Tires easily, lacks stamina. Ears blocked and itchy with mucus.
Worse	Movement, around 9 PM, touch, warmth, spring, autumn.	Cold, damp, drafts, morning, exertion, fresh air, tight clothes, milk.	Cold dry air, winter, night, touch, uncovering, exertion, cold drafts.	Change of weather, wind, cold, thunderstorms, odors, light, lying on the left side.	Cold damp weather, autumn, cold food or drinks, being uncovered, drafts, lying still, nighttime, first movement, after rest.	Left side, cold air and drafts, being uncovered, morning, damp, being consoled, loud noises, full moon.
Better	Lying completely still, pressure, quiet, cool open air, cool applications and drinks.	Heat, rest, loose clothing.	Moist heat or warm applications, hot drinks, wrapping up the head or ears.	Sleep, sympathy, low lights or dark, eating and drinking cold things, cool applications, open air, massage.	Warm drinks and food, gentle movement, once moving, stretching, warmth, changing positions, massage.	Warmth, being wrapped up, wearing a warm hat, urination, yawning, swallowing.
Also For		Sinusitis	Sinusitis	Sinusitis		Sinusitis

Dosing: Use the BLUE method. Observe and evaluate.

HAY FEVER/SEASONAL ALLERGIES

Seasonal allergies are an allergic response to pollen and mold spores in the air, more commonly known as hay fever. They cause symptoms that include, but are not limited to itchy, irritated, or watery eyes; sneezing, runny nose, congestion, post-nasal drip, throat irritation, sore throat, inflammation of mucous membranes in the nasal passages, sinuses, and airways; cough, congestion of ears, itching in the ears, ear pain, dizziness, ear infection, headaches of various types, wheezing, and asthmatic episodes.

Seasonal allergies are considered an acute condition that occurs due to the presence of high amounts of pollen and mold spores in the air. The symptoms usually go away when the pollen count (the measure of pollen particles held in the air) drops to normal levels.

Pollen is a powdery substance that fertilizes flowers enabling them to produce fruit and seeds. It can be carried from flower to flower by pollinating insects such as bees and butterflies, as well as be released into the air by plants and carried to other flowers by the wind.

Pollen particles come in varying sizes, from very fine to coarse. Generally, it is the smaller pollen particles that cause allergic reactions in humans. The hard-exterior surface of a pollen grain has microscopic projections and sometimes sticky substances that enable the particles to be carried by insects. When inhaled by humans, these particles are detected by the immune system as invaders. The body reacts with an inflammatory response. These projections and sticky goo also enable pollen to stick to clothing and other surfaces. In this way, pollen may be introduced into the home, causing further anguish and suffering for people who have seasonal allergies.

Seasonal allergies can be addressed in several ways. One way would be to limit your exposure to pollen and mold spores during times when plants and mold release their pollen and spores. This occurs mainly in the spring but also, to a lesser extent, in the summer and fall. Pollen is mainly released in the morning on sunny days and wind scatters it.

Avoiding pollen and spores is not an easy task, especially if you live in a climate zone where plants are always in bloom. In those areas, every day is allergy season and people feel no relief.

In allopathic medicine, seasonal allergies are treated with drugs to temporarily mask the symptoms and suppress the immune response. Homeopaths believe that symptoms of allergies occur when the vital force is out of balance. Although it is normal to sneeze and blow out plant pollen from the nose when exposed, this process of the body ridding itself of pollen can become problematic in some individuals. Homeopaths respond by correcting the imbalance with homeopathic preparations of substances that would cause the same symptoms, in a healthy person, as the vital force is expressing in the allergic person.

Homeopathic treatment with the appropriate remedy can be very effective in eliminating the annoying symptoms of seasonal allergies.

ADDITIONAL SUPPORT FOR SEASONAL ALLERGIES

- Stay indoors with windows closed during days with high pollen counts.
- Install HEPA air filters (high efficiency particulate absorbing) on heat and air-conditioning systems or use portable HEPA air filters.
- Use HEPA vacuum cleaner filter bags.
- Find locally made honey and eat one teaspoon per day year-round.
- Delegate outdoor chores to someone else.
- Take clothes off when entering the house and put them right into the wash.
- Remove shoes at the door so pollen and spores are not tracked into the carpet.
- Shower when coming indoors to rinse off pollen and spores.
- Brush, wipe down and/or bathe the dog when it enters the house.
- Dry laundry indoors or use a dryer, rather than drying clothes on an outdoor clothesline.
- Wear a disposable mask if you cannot avoid going outside.
- Clean your house and floors frequently.

WHEN TO CONTACT YOUR HEALTHCARE PROFESSIONAL

- If your symptoms are severe or chronic.
- If none of these common allergy remedies serve to prevent your symptoms from returning.

COMMON REMEDIES FOR SEASONAL ALLERGIES

	*Allium cepa	Arsenicum	*Euphrasia	Gelsemium	Natrum mur	Nux vomica	Pulsatilla
Onset	Left-sided or begins on left side and extends to right. After a cold, wet wind.	From becoming chilled while overheated.	May occur after physical exertion.	May occur after hearing bad news, trauma, or in anticipation of a dreaded event.	May begin with sneezing.	Rapid onset of irritation in eyes, ears, and nose. Small quantity of watery mucus morning and daytime.	Hay fever symptoms most prominent in spring, or hot days of summer and fall.
Symptoms	Profuse colorless watery nasal discharge, dripping like a faucet, which may make the nose or upper lip raw. Nose may be completely obstructed. Violent sneezing. Eyes red and burning, water profusely with bland tears. Tickling in layrnx causes painful coughing without sputum.	Burning watery clear mucus, especially from right side of nose. Nose is completely blocked with post-nasal drip that burns. Sneezing in morning when waking, tickling as if from a feather. Eyes painfully sensitive to light. Chilly, better from warmth.	Profuse bland watery nasal discharge with copious tears that make the skin raw. Sneezing. Eyes inflamed, sensitive to light, may burn, sting, and itch. Annoying tickling cough.	Nonstop sneezing accompanied by watering eyes that are puffy and feeling heavy. Extreme drowsiness and weakness, feels shaky, fatigued, lacks energy. May have dizziness. Nasal discharge that feels hot.	Profuse watery nasal discharge the consistency of egg white. Headache, like many little hammers. Watery eyes may have dark circles under them. Irritation at back of throat.	Irritating sneezing attacks in morning with small amounts of watery mucus. Nose blocked in evening, when trying to sleep. Raw throat from post-nasal drip. Dry, tickling irritated sensations in nose and sinuses. Frontal headache. Chilly when uncovered. Eyes smarting, stinging, light sensitivity. Itching inside ears.	Nose and eye discharges are bland and yellowish. Annoying tearing and itching of the eyes. Desires fresh air, but it worsens symptoms. Feels needy and clings to others, does not want to be alone.
Mood	Absent-minded, weeps.	Worried, restless and anxious. Fearful they will never recover. Anguish, fault-finding, angry.	Dullness, easily frightened or startled. Forgetfulness. Inclined to remain sitting.	Apathetic, lacking energy, exhausted. Brain fog. Desires solitude.	Serious individuals who suppress their emotions, even suppress their sneezes. Does not like to be consoled. Private and does not like others to see their emotions. Worry, anxiety in anticipation of events and may not want to socialize.	Everything and anything may be cause for irritation.	Tearful, clingy, wants constant company in close proximity.
Indications	Hay fever with profuse watery nasal discharge that irritates nose and upper lip, with bland tears. May be accompanied by intense headache relieved when the nose drains.	Chilly, cannot get warm. Burning sensations in nose, throat, eyes. Clear, watery discharges.	Hay fever symptoms predominantly in eyes. Often only one side is affected, usually the right.	Hay fever symptoms accompanied by overwhelming sleepiness. Weakness and apathy.	Mucus discharges like raw egg white that sting irritated membranes. Does not want any form of consolation and tries to suppress the symptoms.	Hay fever symptoms that cause great irritation in person who is short-tempered and irritable.	Hay fever symptoms are bland not irritating, yellowish in color. Uncharacteristically clingy and tearful.
Worse	Late afternoon or evening, in a warm room or indoors. Sharp pains in the larynx, worse coughing. Lying on left side. Very sensitive to flowers, pollens, and peaches.	Cold temperatures. Midnight to early morning.	Morning, rest. Exposure to wind, warm air, fresh air, cold, sunlight, lying on back. May be aggravated by blowing nose.	Becoming overheated. Warm, humid weather.	Open air or wind. Consolation, wine, salty foods, cereal grains, after eating. Physical exertion, bright sun, heat.	Increased nasal discharge in daytime, blocked nasal passages in evening and night. Congestion and throat worse in cold air or drafts.	Becoming over-heated, nighttime, warm room. Cough worse lying down.
Better	Fresh air and cold air.	Cold air improves acute head complaints, warm drinks soothe burning throat.	Nighttime and darkness. Bathing, sinus rinsing.	Rest. Headache better from warm applications.	Fasting, cold, lying down, rest, perspiring.	Warm room or warm drinks can relieve nasal congestion.	Better indoors in air-conditioned room. Cold pack on eyes and bridge of nose.

*Sabadilla and ***Wyethia** are also worth considering for seasonal allergies.
Dosing: Use the BLUE method. Observe and evaluate.

NOSEBLEEDS

Nosebleeds can be alarming, but they aren't usually a sign of anything serious and can often be treated at home. During a nosebleed, blood flows from one or both nostrils. It can be heavy or light and last from a few seconds to 10 minutes or more.

Nosebleeds towards the front of the nose are usually less severe and can be stopped with pressure by pinching the nostrils towards the bridge of the nose. However, if you can taste blood, you likely have a posterior bleed (located towards the back of the nose). These bleeds tend to be more severe and cannot be stopped by pinching your nostrils.

IT'S AN EMERGENCY WHEN

- The bleeding does not stop after remedy and supportive measures have been tried for 20 minutes.
- The person is on blood thinners and bleeding occurs.
- There is unexplained profuse bleeding from the mouth or nose.
- Bleeding or fluid from the nose or ears following a head injury.
- Any time there is bleeding, and you feel you need the help of a medical professional.

ADDITIONAL SUPPORT FOR NOSEBLEEDS

Review and practice universal precautions when handling any bloody situation which includes vigorously washing hands before and after exposure to blood and always wear protective gloves. If available, wear a mask, goggles, and other personal protective equipment (PPE). Limit exposure to potential bloodborne pathogens. Learn more about **Preventing The Spread Of Bloodborne Pathogens** found on the Red Cross website: https://tinyurl.com/d86ac7c.

To stop a nosebleed:
- Sit down and firmly pinch the soft part of your nose, just above your nostrils, for at least 10-15 minutes.
- Lean forward and breathe through your mouth—this will drain blood down your nose instead of down the back of your throat.
- Place an ice pack or bag of frozen vegetables covered by a towel on the bridge of your nose.
- Stay upright, rather than lying down, as this reduces the blood pressure in the blood vessels of your nose and will discourage further bleeding.
- If the bleeding eventually stops, you won't need to seek medical advice unless the occurrence is frequent.

Nosebleed Prevention: If you have frequent nose bleeds, you can strengthen the walls of your nasal blood vessels with these supplements:
- ***Calc fluor 6X (cell salt)**—take it daily Monday through Friday only, skipping weekends.
- Eat food rich in Rutin (part of a vitamin C complex)—the white of the inside of citrus fruit peel; black, green or rooibos tea; buckwheat or kasha (a great source of plant-based protein).
- Take a Vitamin C supplement with bioflavonoids—make sure the label includes Rutin.
- If you live in a dry climate, you can line the nostrils with organic coconut oil to keep the nostrils from drying out, cracking open, and causing bleeding.

COMMON REMEDIES FOR NOSEBLEEDS

	Aconite	Arnica	Belladonna	*Hamamelis	Lachesis	Phosphorus
Symptoms	Shock or fright from a potentially fatal accident. When blood is gushing out.	Pain and swelling after a blow to the nose or from exertion.	Bright red blood. Heat exhaustion, heat cramps, dehydration.	Dark blood. Blood may be clotted or slow moving as from a vein. Instead of menses. More likely to work if the bleeding is dark-colored and slower moving, e.g., as from a vein.	Dark blood. From blowing the nose, boring with finger into the nose. With menopause or instead of menses or when menses are suppressed, e.g., from certain birth control pills.	Bright red blood. Bleeds easily. From and when blowing the nose. Blood-streaked discharges with mucus. More left-sided. Persistent bleeding in young women.

Dosing: Use the ORANGE method. Observe and evaluate.

BLOWS TO THE NOSE

Because the nose sticks out from the face, it tends to sustain injuries frequently, particularly when playing ball sports like basketball, baseball or volleyball. Any trauma to the nose, including blows from accidents and injuries, can cause the blood vessels to rupture.

IT'S AN EMERGENCY WHEN

- There is profuse bleeding that gets worse instead of better.
- The bleeding doesn't stop after well-chosen remedies were given and additional support measures were applied.

The most common remedies for blows to the nose are:

- **Arnica:** The first remedy to use if the nose bleeds after a blow. It will also help with pain and swelling. Give every 10 minutes for up to six doses. If no response, try ***Millefolium achillea**.

- ***Millefolium achillea:** This remedy is needed if the nose continues to bleed bright red blood profusely after being given **Arnica**. Keep the person resting and quiet. Give every 10 minutes for up to six doses.

If no response, try the additional support for nosebleeds in the previous section and/or go to your nearest urgent care.

? WHAT'S THE FIRST REMEDY YOU THINK OF WHEN...

1. You start to get the first signs of a cold.
2. A person has itchy eyes with burning tears and acrid nasal discharge with their allergies.
3. A person has acrid tears and bland nasal discharge with their allergies.
4. A cold produces lots of sneezing in the morning.
5. The person has burning symptoms but wants warmth and warm drinks.
6. Gets frequent and profuse nosebleeds.
7. Someone got an infection in the area where they got their nose pierced.
8. A person got hit in the nose by someone else's elbow causing a nosebleed.
9. An athlete got hit by a basketball while playing in a game.
10. Colds exhibit excess saliva and bad breath.
11. Cold symptoms come on after a haircut.
12. Colds come from a chill after exposure to constant cold air like air conditioning.
13. A person gets frequent nosebleeds and is thirsty for cold drinks.
14. A person gets cold symptoms from getting chilled after being overheated.

Answer key on page 323.

CHAPTER 9
Mouth and Teeth

Did you know that your oral health is interconnected with overall health? Certain conditions, such as cardiovascular disease, diabetes, and respiratory infections, have been linked to poor oral health. To keep the mouth and teeth symptom-free, it is important to practice good oral hygiene habits, including regular brushing, flossing, and rinsing, along with regular dental visits for professional cleanings and check-ups. Additionally, maintaining a balanced diet, avoiding tobacco products, and limiting sugary snacks and drinks can further contribute to oral health. Even with good hygiene, however, you can still have some oral issues. Let homeopathy help with your prevention and healing.

EXCESSIVE TOOTH DECAY

The most common cause of excessive tooth decay is poor dental hygiene—lack of frequent brushing and/or flossing—but it can be also caused by a number of other reasons including genetic predisposition and excessive sugar intake. You can help prevent this by maintaining a good dental routine as instructed by your dentist as well as seeking regular dental checkups where a trained professional can catch early damage before it becomes a larger problem.

Because tooth decay is typically a chronic situation, it can be a challenge to know which remedy to take and for how long. Consulting with a professional homeopath might be helpful.

Also, consider homeopathic cell salts—a combination of **Calc fluor 6X, Calc phos 6X** and **Silicea 6X**—twice a day to stem the incidence of cavities. *Learn more about **Cell Salts** in **Chapter 3**.*

TOOTHACHES

A toothache is usually a sign of inflammation in the nerve root – the result of decay, tooth trauma, or gum disease.

WHEN TO CONTACT YOUR DENTIST

- If you have a continuous toothache that prevents sleep.
- If you have a fever with a toothache.
- If you have a tooth that is very sensitive to heat, cold, or sweet things.

In the meantime, try one of these remedies to ease the pain, but be sure to follow up with a dental exam.

COMMON REMEDIES FOR TOOTHACHE

	Belladonna	Calcarea carb	Chamomilla	Hypericum	Magnesium phos	Mercurius	Pulsatilla
Onset	Sudden.			Injury to a nerve.		Toothache from an abscess or decaying tooth.	
Symptoms	Throbbing pain and dry mouth. Very red gums. Sharp, shooting, cutting pains that suddenly come and go.	Drawing, throbbing, pricking in teeth; with red swollen gums.	Pain is unbearable, may radiate to the ears.	Pains are excessive and sharp, shooting, tearing, or drawing. Tingling, burning, and numbness may also be present.	Pain like an electric shock or muscle cramping.	Pains are pulsating, tearing, shooting. May extend to the ears, may have bad breath or metallic taste in mouth with excessive salivation. Teeth feel elongated and sore.	Sharp, shooting pains in teeth. Desires open, cool air. Mouth dry, but thirstless.
Mood	Irritable, excitable.	Despairing, irritable.	Irritable and over-sensitive, nothing soothes.	Irritable.	Moody; silent.	Changeable.	Weepy and clingy, desires company.
Indications	Feverish with a flushed, hot face and great nervous excitability.	Cold air striking body goes right through teeth.	Intolerable pain worse for warmth but not relieved by cold. Teething in children.	Can be used for pain and sensitivity after root canals, teeth extractions or other procedures that impact the nerve.	Shooting pains.	Painful ulcerations at the roots of teeth and for pain in hollow teeth.	Feels as if teeth would be forced out.
Worse	At night, from touch or motion such as chewing. Right side.	When exposed to hot or cold air. Noise. Wakes at night with pain.	Entering a warm room. Eating or drinking anything warm. Especially after drinking coffee. Nighttime.	Drafts and cold.	Cold.	From warmth or cold.	Having anything hot in the mouth.
Better	Pressure on area.	Touching teeth with tongue.	Dipping finger in cold water and applying to affected area.	Warmth. Lying on face.	Warmth and warm fluids, better from pressure.	Gentle rubbing of the face.	Relieved by cold water in the mouth. After a good cry.

Dosing: Use the BLUE method. Observe and evaluate.

BROKEN TOOTH

With age and time, teeth can become brittle and frail, making damaging them easier. Decay-induced breaks start as simple cavities, but they can develop to eventually cause a tooth to split or crumble from the inside out. You can help prevent this by maintaining a good dental routine as instructed by your dentist as well as seeking regular dental checkups where a trained professional can catch early damage before it becomes a larger problem.

WHEN TO CONTACT YOUR DENTIST

- If you have experienced a tooth injury as a result of an accident or injury.
- If your teeth are cracked or broken.
- A homeopathic remedy can help relieve pain or symptoms until you are seen by your dentist.
- Following a broken tooth, **Hypericum** is the first remedy to consider if you suspect the nerve has suffered trauma.

COMMON REMEDIES FOR A BROKEN TOOTH

	Arnica	*Calcarea fluor	Hypericum	Lachesis	*Sulphuric Acid
Symptoms	Cracked teeth. Painful or bruised feeling.	Broken teeth ache if food touches them. Also from cold.	Numbness, tingling, electric shock pains following a broken tooth.	Tearing, drawing, and shooting pains in roots of teeth (of lower jaw); from warm and cold drinks, sometimes with swelling of the cheeks, and a sensation as if the teeth were too long.	Teeth are dull and chalky looking with frequent painful tearing on the teeth, primarily on the left side of mouth.
Indications	Low throbbing pain, soreness.	Hollow teeth appear prematurely in children. Enamel of teeth is rough and uneven. Teeth break easily. Loose teeth.	If you suspect the nerve has suffered trauma.	Pieces break off. Brittleness and looseness of the teeth.	Defective enamel. Pains increase slowly and stop suddenly.
Worse	Pain worse from any touch, from any pressure applied.	Pain worse from cold.	Hot or cold drinks and food.	Touch. Evening.	Pain worse in evening and after lying down.

Dosing: Use the BLUE Method. Observe and evaluate.

TOOTH ABSCESS

An abscess is a pus-filled cavity in the root of a tooth. The bacteria in the abscess produces toxins which can then cause a gum boil, felt as swelling, as the infection seeks an outlet.

ADDITIONAL SUPPORT FOR A TOOTH ABSCESS

- Rinse the mouth gently with one teaspoon sea salt to ½ cup boiled water as needed. Make sure water has cooled off before gently rinsing.
- Rinse the mouth out every four hours with a mouthwash created with a few drops each of **Hypericum** and **Calendula Tinctures** (also pre-made in a product called **HyperCal mouthwash**) mixed in a glass of warm water. DO NOT SWALLOW.

> *To make a **calendula/hypericum solution**, purchase a "mother tincture" of each remedy. A mother tincture is made from a mixture of the original herb and alcohol or glycerin. Unlike the homeopathic form, which is drastically diluted, a mother tincture is a concentrated form of the active element of the herb.*
>
> *To prepare the solution, use a clean jar or bottle and distilled or spring water. Using very clean utensils, measure out one-part **Calendula tincture**, one-part **Hypericum tincture**, and eight-parts distilled water. Close the container and shake gently to blend.*

WHEN TO CONTACT YOUR DENTIST or HEALTHCARE PROFESSIONAL

- The affected tooth will hurt when chewed on, and there can be a throbbing pain.
- A painful boil or swelling on the gum might be visible.

COMMON REMEDIES FOR TOOTH ABSCESS

	Belladonna	Bryonia	Hepar sulph	Mercurius	Silicea	*Pyrogen
Symptoms	Mouth dry, gum is very hot and swollen.	Acute inflammation or pricking pain.	Tooth is hypersensitive to touch and cold.	Profuse saliva and a bad taste in mouth. Burning sensations.	Abscess at the root of teeth. Slow or incomplete process of development and healing.	Fever and pus without drainage, suspected sepsis.
Indications	Bright red or purplish color. Sudden pain, throbbing, extreme sensitivity to touch, thirstless.	Dry mouth, excessive thirst, bitter taste	Chronic abscesses with suppuration.	Bleeding ulcers or gums, pains radiate to the ears, metallic taste in mouth, edges of tongue wavy or indented.	To promote discharge of a gum boil; teeth may feel loose.	Tongue red, smooth and shiny. Restless.
Worse	Touch. Heat.	Rapid motions, stooping, upon rising, deep breathing.	Least draft of air and worse from cold.	At night, heat or cold aggravates.	Eating warm food. When cold air gets into the mouth. At night.	Cold and wet, foul or sweet taste.

Dosing: Use the **BLUE** Method. Observe and evaluate.

GINGIVITIS

Gum disease can be very painful and is a major cause of tooth loss. Infected or bleeding gums are usually caused by a buildup of plaque on the teeth, poor dental hygiene, or because the saliva is too acidic. In less common cases, vitamin deficiency, blood disorders, excessive sugar intake, or drugs may be the cause. Women sometimes find more gum sensitivity due to hormonal shifting during and after a pregnancy and during perimenopause. Treatment can be complex, and a visit to a dentist or periodontist (someone who specializes in gum health) is recommended. In addition, you can use a homeopathic remedy.

COMMON REMEDIES FOR GINGIVITIS

	China	*Ferrum phos	Hypericum	Mercurius	Nux vomica	Phosphorus
Symptoms	Sensation of swelling, teeth throb.	Gums that bleed after brushing.	Tender gum tissue with shooting pains.	Offensive odor from the mouth with excess salivation. May have coated tongue and metallic taste in mouth.	Gums swollen, white and bleeding. Back of the tongue has a whitish coating.	Gums bleed easily and there is an over-production of mucus.
Indications	Swollen gums, mouth dry, possible night sweats.	Poor gum tone.	Injuries to dental nerves. Gums receded into tooth roots.	Gums are swollen, ulcerated and retracted from teeth.	Swollen, painful gums. Dry mouth. Easily angered by any stimulus.	Swollen gums.
Worse	Least touch, open air, cold.	After eating food, night or early morning.	Cold.	Heat or cold.	After eating. Washing face with cold water. Coffee, alcohol, drugs.	Open air. Cold food or drink.
Better	Pressing teeth together firmly, warmth.	Cold.	Warmth.	Rubbing cheek.	External warmth.	Warmth.

Dosing: Use the **BROWN** method. Observe and evaluate.

ORAL SURGERY

For pain and discomfort following any invasive dental procedure, homeopathy can offer healing assistance.

COMMON REMEDIES FOR ORAL SURGERY

	Apis	Arnica	Chamomilla	Hypericum	Magnesium phos	Phosphorus	Staphysagria
Onset	Give immediately after procedure.	After dental surgery. Any invasive dental or gum work.	Give one hour prior to appointment if irritable.	After any tooth extraction if pain presents.	After dental surgery.	Bleeding after dental surgery.	After dental surgery.
Symptoms	The site is red, puffy and stinging.	Feels as if roots were scraped. Soreness or swelling of gums. May bleed excessively.	Teeth feel too long.	Shooting pains.	Muscle cramping with stiff, sore jaws. Violent shooting pains that come in waves.	Swelling with excessive or easy bleeding. Pale around mouth/nose. Palate itchy.	Pain at site of incision. Gums bleed when pressed on.
Mood	Sensitive, irritable, despondent.	Physically restless but mentally apathetic. Says, "I'm fine," when actually not.	Fear of the procedure. Sensitive to pain. Hard to please.	Irritable.	Complaining.	Depressed, sad.	Can be angry with the pain.
Indications	Soreness at injection site.	Feels bruised. Swelling and pain.	Low pain threshold.	Injury to nerve. Severe aching in tooth.	Prolonged dental work, more right-sided.	Following tooth extraction.	Soft tissue surgery.
Worse	Heat.	Inhaling fresh air or warm applications.	Night. Entering warm room. Talking.	Night.	On going to bed. Cold things, cold air, lying on right side.	Open air, anything cold. Chewing. Lying on left side.	Cold air. Cold drinks.
Better	After a little exercise. Lying on back or side.	Better for open air. Cold food or drinks.	Dipping finger in cold water and applying to affected area.	Lying on affected side. Keeping quiet.	Heat and hot drinks.	Warmth applied to outside of mouth.	Hard pressure and heat.

Special Dosing Instructions: Take **Arnica** after the procedure hourly, then after novocaine wears off, decide which remedy fits your symptoms best. If in a lot of pain, you can alternate hourly (or more frequently) with **Arnica** and another chosen remedy until symptoms subside. Consider using the **PLUSSING** method of dosing (*see Chapter 2 on page 36*).

BRACES & OTHER ORTHODONTICS

The following are the most commonly indicated remedies to give following an orthodontic procedure:

- **Chamomilla**: For tooth pain from the pressure of braces or dentures.

- **Rhus tox**: For cramping pain in the jaw from holding the jaw open for an extended length of time.

- **Arnica**: For pain and swelling following an extraction; general soreness.

MOUTH SORES

Mouth sores are caused by a virus in the herpes family. The common name is a fever blister. Many factors can be involved with these annoying outbreaks along the chin, nose, or lip area.

Note: a sore inside the mouth is a canker sore, which is not the same thing as a cold sore but responds to remedies with similar symptomatology.

ADDITIONAL SUPPORT FOR MOUTH SORES

- The amino acid supplement, lysine, can be given along with zinc and bioflavonoids.
- Washing hands is important as is avoiding touching, scratching, or picking at the sore.
- Cold sores are highly contagious so do not share anything that touches the infected area.

WHEN TO CONTACT YOUR HEALTHCARE PROFESSIONAL

- If the problem persists, consider consulting a professional homeopath or healthcare practitioner.

COMMON REMEDIES FOR MOUTH SORES

	Arsenicum	*Dulcamara	Hepar sulph	Mercurius	Natrum mur	Rhus tox	Sepia
Onset	Dry, tingling, burning, itchy skin preceding blister outbreak.	Stinging pain, pinching sensation with blister outbreak.	Prickly sensation. Stinging sensation with blister outbreak.	Profuse saliva, tender, burning, stinging.	Inflamed and dry skin, tingly, stinging, and itchy.	Restless, skin tingles, violent itching.	Dry, red, itchy skin.
Symptoms	Burning, red, crusty blisters. Thirst for small sips.	Thick, brown, crusted blisters.	Bleeding of blister. Bad odor of blister.	Thin oozing, yellow-green fluid from blister, crusty layer.	Peeling or raw skin.	Crops of blisters, oozing water fluid, moist crust later.	Weak, tired, clear oozing, slightly milky liquid in blisters.
Mood	Fearful, anxious.	Impatient, quarrelsome.	Irritable.	Changeable.	Wants to be left alone.	Restless.	Sad.
Indications	Blister eruption.	Stinging, pinching sensation.	Bleeding blister.	Bad odor.	Common to see on lower lip.	Could look like poison ivy.	Thick crusts on blisters.
Worse	Cold, right side, after midnight.	PMS, cold, wet weather.	Cold, sweat, pain, touch, draft.	Chill, overheating, nighttime.	Sun, emotions, hurt feelings.	Cold, staying quiet, getting wet while sweating, evenings.	Before menses, spring, dampness, cold air.
Better	Warm compress, warm weather.	Cool applications.	Quiet. Warm applications, warm cloths. Wet weather.	Moderate temperature, quiet and rest.	Warm compresses, stretching, warmth, movement.	Warm compresses, stretching, warmth, and movement.	Warmth, dancing, music.

Dosing: Use the BLUE method. Observe and evaluate.

BLOWS TO THE MOUTH, LIPS, JAW AND TEETH

Blows to the mouth, including the lips, jaws and teeth, can cause a lot of pain and/or bleeding.

ADDITIONAL SUPPORT FOR BLOWS TO THE MOUTH/LIPS/JAW AND TEETH

- Apply ice to the injured area to reduce the immediate swelling.
- Keep the injured area clean.

WHEN TO CONTACT YOUR DENTIST or HEALTHCARE PROFESSIONAL

- If you cracked or knocked out a tooth.
- If your lip is split and may need stitches.
- If your jaw was dislocated.
- If the pain isn't resolving after a few remedies, consult your dentist.

The most common remedies for blows to the jaw, lips, mouth, and teeth are:

- **Arnica**: This remedy relieves soreness and bruising after a blow to the teeth. Give two to three times per day for three days to aid in healing and prevent soreness.

- **Hypericum**: A good remedy for blows to the mouth because the lips are rich in nerves, and this remedy helps relieve nerve pain. Give every 15 minutes until there is relief. It can also help nerve pains in injured teeth, when the teeth are excessively tender and sensitive. Give two to three times a day for three days to help with the sensitivity. Re-dose as needed if it continues after three days. A broken tooth will most likely need both **Arnica** and **Hypericum**, as well as a trip to the dentist.

- **Chamomilla**: This remedy will relieve unbearable pain from a broken or injured tooth. Give every 15 minutes for four doses and then hourly until relieved if there is a response. If not, re-evaluate and give another remedy.

Note: For a blow to the teeth, alternate **Arnica** and **Hypericum** every two hours until the pain has subsided. Repeat only if pain returns.

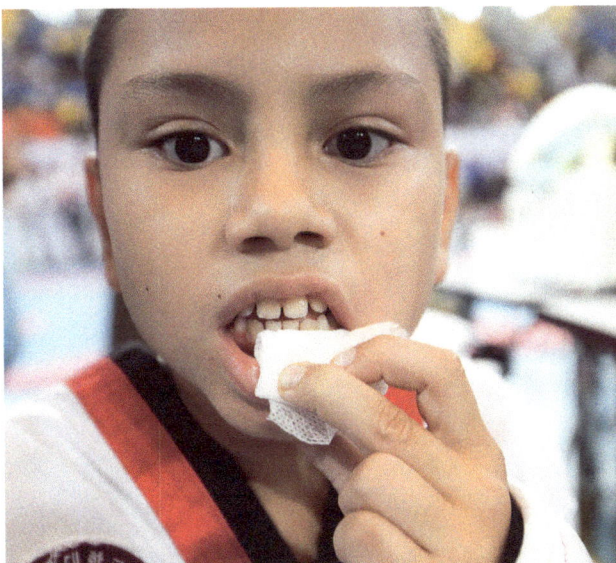

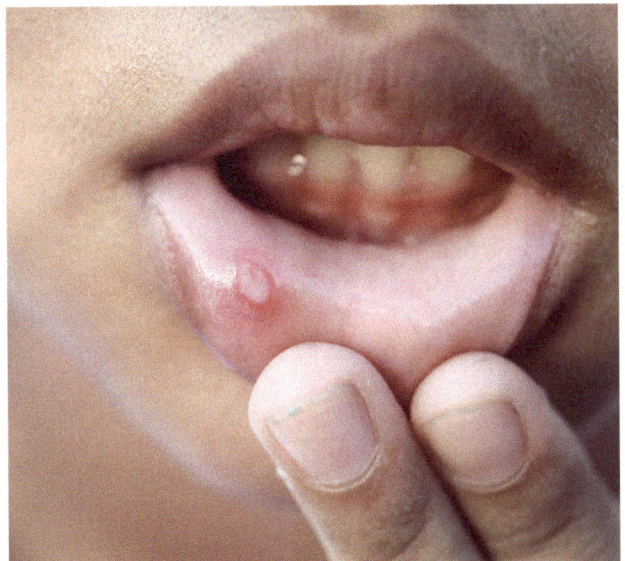

? WHAT'S THE FIRST REMEDY YOU THINK OF WHEN...

1. A cold sore that is crusty, burns, but feels better with the application of a warm compress.
2. Tooth pain comes from the pressure of braces or dentures.
3. Shooting pains in the gums and the mouth may have an injury to nerves.
4. Soreness, swelling and pain occur AFTER dental surgery.
5. Achiness from a broken tooth is worse when food touches it or from the cold.
6. Gingivitis causes gums to swell and become retracted from teeth, causing bad breath and increased salivation.
7. A tooth abscess causes increased saliva, burning, a metallic taste in mouth, bleeding gums that are worse at night along with pain radiating to ears.
8. Relief of soreness and bruising is needed after a blow to the mouth and teeth.
9. Someone has cavities and excessive tooth decay (along with a regular dental visit).
10. A person fears upcoming dental procedures and has a low threshold to pain. Meant to be given 1 hour before the procedure.
11. A toothache comes on suddenly with throbbing pain.
12. Cramping pain occurs in the jaw after an orthodontic procedure from having the mouth open for a long period of time.
13. A tooth has just been pulled.
14. A tooth having just been pulled is now experiencing shooting nerve pains.
15. A tooth infection has pus discharging along with swollen tender gums.

Answer key on page 323.

CHAPTER 10
Throat and Chest

A healthy throat is a vital component of overall well-being, as it plays a pivotal role in our ability to communicate, breathe, and swallow. The throat serves as a gateway to both the respiratory and digestive systems, making it susceptible to various infections and conditions. Among the most common ailments that can afflict the throat are chest infections, which can cause discomfort, pain, and hinder our daily activities and sleep. Learning about possible homeopathic remedies for these symptoms is useful for taking good care of our throat health, ensuring proper breathing, and promoting overall physical wellness.

SORE THROATS AND TONSILLITIS

A sore throat is an inflammation with pain, difficulty swallowing, and sometimes swollen glands. Tonsillitis is a swelling of the tonsils, the two lymphatic sacs behind the base of the tongue, on either side of the top of the throat. They are an integral part of the lymphatic drainage system. Swollen tonsils are part of the normal eliminative process for getting rid of an invading bacteria or virus. Acute tonsillitis produces swelling, inflammation of the tonsils, a sore throat, and fever that may be low-grade, medium, or high. The person may also have headaches or stomachaches.

The adenoids, which are made of the same lymphatic tissue, are located above the soft palate (roof of the mouth). These may also become swollen, impeding speech and nose breathing. Chronically swollen tonsils or adenoids should be treated by a healthcare professional and/or a professional homeopath. In some children the uvula can become swollen as well. The uvula is a small, conic piece of flesh extending down from the soft palate at the entrance to the throat.

People of any age may develop a sore throat. Vomiting may occur if a lot of mucus is being swallowed. The person may have excess mucus or saliva, bad breath, and an odd taste in their mouth. If a baby develops this condition, they may refuse to eat, cry while nursing, or rub the ears, which might lead you to think they have an earache or are teething. This is why it's important to choose a remedy based on the person's individualized symptoms.

IT'S AN EMERGENCY WHEN

- A child has a temperature over 103 °F (39.4 °C).
- A person is unresponsive, has trouble breathing, repeated vomiting, convulsions, or is listless or limp.
- There is stiffness and pain in the neck along with fever.
- There is great difficulty swallowing, with severe pain.
- There is difficulty breathing because of severely swollen and enlarged tonsils.
- There is a high fever and rapid swelling in the larynx.

ADDITIONAL SUPPORT FOR <u>ALL</u> SORE THROAT SYMPTOMS

- Consider taking ***Ferrum phos 6X cell salt** up to four times a day for the inflammation (To learn more, see **Chapter 3—Cell Salts**).
- Drink plenty of fluids, especially if there is a fever, to prevent dehydration.
- Discontinue or keep dairy products to a minimum, because they cause excess mucus and raise the level of acidity in the system. Goat's or sheep's milk, or products made from these milks, may be substituted for cow's milk and products containing it. Plant based milks may also be substituted. Using organic is best.
- Gargle with one teaspoon of **Calendula tincture** in one cup of warm water, three times a day.
- Gargle with warm saltwater several times a day.
- Try some elderberry syrup to coat the throat.
- Use lozenges that do not contain camphor, menthol, or eucalyptus. Try blackcurrant pastilles or lemon drops instead.
- Humidify the room if your home has forced-air heat.
- If warm drinks feel better, make a tea with 2-3 fresh lemons by cutting, squeezing, and boiling them for 15-20 minutes in a saucepan full of water. Drink it like a hot tea, add honey and sip.
- If cold drinks feel better, fresh carrot juice is soothing to a sore throat.

WHEN TO CONTACT YOUR HEALTHCARE PROFESSIONAL

- A baby under three months old has a rise in temperature.
- A child under two years of age has a fever for more than 24 hours.
- The person has had a fever for more than three days.
- A rash appears on the body at the same time as the sore throat.
- A child's tongue looks like a strawberry; this can indicate scarlet fever.
- The person has had laryngitis for longer than seven days.
- Glands swell or health decreases; also, if laryngitis becomes chronic.
- The person has recurring sore throats not helped with homeopathic remedies.

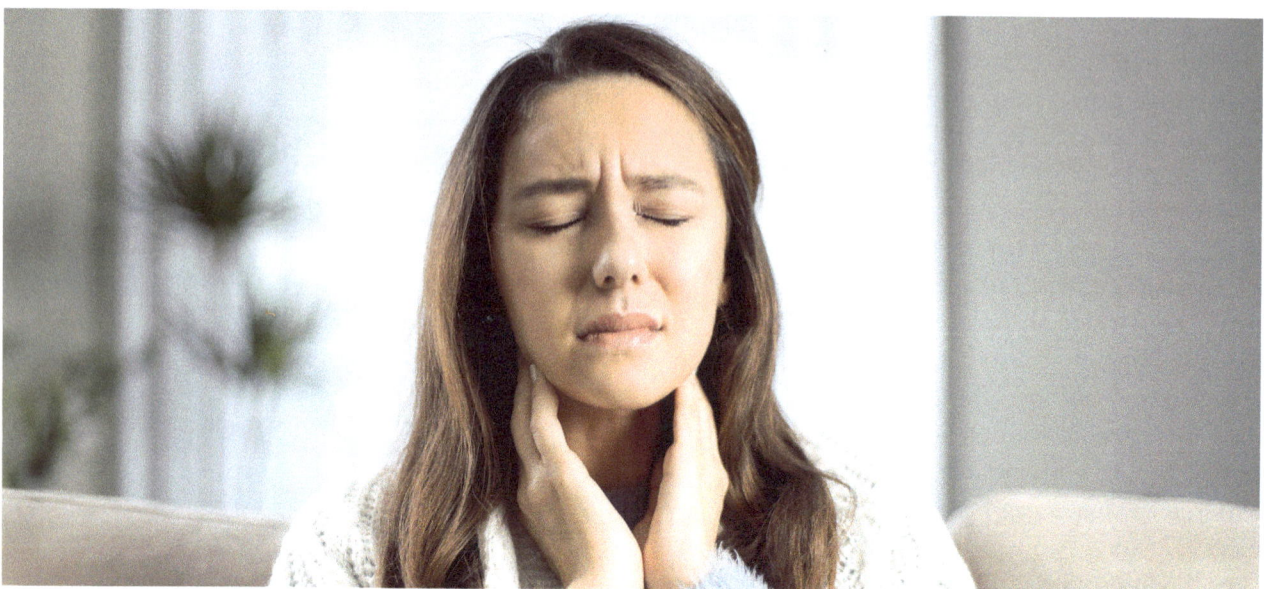

COMMON REMEDIES FOR SORE THROATS AND TONSILLITIS

	Aconite	Apis	Belladonna	Hepar Sulph	Lachesis	Mercurius	*Phytolacca
Onset	Sudden high fever after being exposed to icy winds, fright, or shock.	Onset from anger, fright, or grief.	Sudden onset, with severe symptoms, after getting chilled or overheated.	Slow onset, from getting too cold or cold wind.	Onset in spring and cloudy weather. Pain begins on left side but may move to middle or right side.	Getting chilled, brings on a sore throat at every change in the weather.	Onset from exposure to cold, damp weather.
Symptoms	Throat constricted, red, dry, and hot. Burning and needle-like pains that shoot into ears. Difficulty swallowing.	Swollen, dry, constricted, and inflamed throat. Sensation as if splinter in throat. Stinging and burning pains. Tongue and uvula swollen.	Fine in the morning, but by 3 PM have a high fever with a sore, bright-red throat that is burning, dry, hot, raw, tender, and constricted.	Severe, sharp splinter-like pains that shoot up into ear on swallowing or yawning. The right side is the most painful, but both sides can be affected.	Tearing pains extending to ear. Sensation of constriction and choking. Feels like lump moving up and down in throat which causes constant desire to swallow.	Throat feels sore, swollen, raw, and burning. Red or bluish-red with white or yellow coating. Needle-like pains shoot into ear or neck on swallowing.	Throat is dark red or bluish-red. Feels hot, too narrow, raw, and burning. Root of tongue and soft palate ache. Pain comes and goes on the right, shoots into ear.
Mood	Restless, fearful, and anxious. May have a fear of death. May have nightmares.	Restless, sleepy and very irritable when disturbed or touched. Weepy.	Restless and irritable. Severe agitation.	Extremely irritable, hypersensitive, easily angered. Does not want to be examined or looked at.	Anxious, nervous, excitable, very talkative, rambles on and on. Sensitive to touch and pain.	Restless, constantly changing mind, nervous.	May moan a lot. Very little interest in anything. Sensitive and restless.
Indications	Tonsils swollen and feel dry. Feels as if something is stuck in throat. Strong thirst for cold drinks.	Right side is worse. Tongue is fiery-red and raw. Mouth is dry. Throat is red or purple. Skin feels sore and sensitive. Wants cold water to soothe throat but is not thirsty.	Throat muscles sensitive, making it hard to swallow, but constant desire to do so. Pains severe, needle-like, and worse on right side. Glands usually swollen.	Sensation as if plug or fishbone stuck in the throat. Glands swollen. Solid food hard to swallow. Very chilly with smelly sweat and breath.	Throat swollen, dark red or purple. Tries to cough up sticky mucus. Tongue burns, swells, trembles when protruded.	Right side usually worse. Drools clear saliva on the pillow. Coughs up lumpy mucus. Constant desire to swallow. Breath smells bad. Weary and may tremble.	Sensation as if lump or red hot ball in throat. Thick and choking greyish-white or yellow mucus. Cannot swallow hot things. Swollen glands in neck and under ear.
Worse	Nighttime around midnight, or midday. Noise, pressure.	From 3-5 PM. Warmth, touch, heavy blankets, pressure, swallowing solids, hot or sour food.	Around 3 PM. Swallowing liquids, cold air, touch, noise, jarring, light, turning the head, sudden motion.	Touch, uncovering, exertion, cold drafts, winter, solid food, cold dry air, night.	Slightest touch to front of neck, on waking, lying down, nighttime, or falling asleep. Swallowing hot drinks, on left side, heat.	Evening, drafts, damp weather, sweating, too much cold or heat, lying on right side, warmth in bed, warm drinks.	Cold damp weather, changes in weather, hot drinks, touch, pressure.
Better	Fresh air, rest, sweating, hot applications.	Cool applications, cold liquids, air. Uncovered or lightly covered.	Rest, light covers, sitting semi-erect, low light, quiet.	Warm drinks, moist heat, being wrapped up, damp weather.	Open air, cold drinks, swallowing solids, eating fruits. Wearing loose clothing, especially around neck.	Moderate, even temperatures. Rest, lying on stomach, morning.	Warmth, cold drinks, rest, lying on stomach or left side.
Also For	Laryngitis	Tonsillitis	Tonsillitis	Laryngitis, Tonsillitis	Laryngitis, Tonsillitis	Tonsillitis	Tonsillitis

Dosing: Use the **BLUE** Method. Observe and evaluate.

LARYNGITIS AND VOICE LOSS

Acute laryngitis is an inflammation and swelling of the vocal cords in the area of the larynx (the portion of the throat from the mouth to just below the Adam's apple, sometimes called the voice box). Laryngitis produces a change in the voice that results in hoarseness, huskiness, loud whispering, a high pitch, or a complete loss of the voice. The swelling and inflammation are due to dry mucous membranes, or an accumulation of thick mucus from post-nasal drip down the back of the throat. The larynx area is rich in lymph glands that can become swollen while fighting off infection. Mucus from a cold can then get stuck around the swollen vocal cords.

The cause of laryngitis with a cold can be either viral or bacterial. It is usually triggered by getting chilled or wet. Laryngitis may also be caused by overstraining the voice, allergies, secondhand smoke, pollutants, or prolonged coughing. In some cases, it can be caused by chronic suppression of emotions or resisting the need to cry.

See **Additional Support for ALL Sore Throats** earlier in this chapter on **page 110**.

COMMON REMEDIES FOR LARYNGITIS AND VOICE LOSS

	*Arum triphyllum	Belladonna	*Causticum	Gelsemium	Ignatia	Phosphorus
Onset	Hoarseness, especially from overuse of voice, talking, screaming, singing. Also called "clergyman's sore throat".	Ailments from excitement, fright, fear, anger. Affinity for the mucous membranes.	Hoarseness from overuse.	Weakness on all levels from overuse.	Ailments from anger and disappointment.	After being chilled or changes in temperature.
Symptoms	Hoarseness of a public speaker who, after a long exertion, gets cold (as from a draft), and suddenly is unable to finish. Excitable and irritable in mind and body. Bores head into pillow or hands.	Violent symptoms with heat, redness, burning. Symptoms appear and disappear suddenly. Narrow sensation when swallowing.	Hoarseness after exposure to cold air, with stress. Feels very strongly about things and wants to be heard.	Laryngitis loss of voice from fright or emotions. Slow onset. Great weakness and trembling.	Disappointments with silent grief and brooding. Involuntary sighing. Emotional outbursts very quickly controlled: only tears, short sobs; constant swallowing, twitching mouth, biting inside the cheek, etc. Tendency to eat away stress, especially anger and grief.	Hoarse voice, cannot talk. Larynx is dry, raw, rough and sore. Chilly with burning pains in throat and chest.
Mood	Irritable, excessively cross and stubborn.	Impressionable, sympathetic, connected, open, extroverted. Reacts intensely. When ill can become "devilish", irritable, rude, not amenable to discipline, accusing, complaining.	Melancholy, anxious, irritable. Hysterical, whining.	Apprehension, anticipation, and timidity. Dread of ordeals, examinations, new situations. Lack of will power, mental and physical.	Conflict with inner self. Bitterness. Ailments from disappointment. Inner conflict. Self-reproach.	Wants company, attention and sympathy. Fearful. Restless and fidgety.
Indications	Loss of voice from speaking, e.g., teacher, lawyer.	Loss of voice after excitement. Redness and heat of face, pulsating carotids.	Constant desire to clear throat.	Weakness, stage fright. Left sided colds.	Ailments from strong emotions. High ideals and expectations.	Sore throat. May have nosebleed and/or diarrhea with it.
Worse	Talking, singing, cold winds, cold-wet, heat, lying down.	Heat of sun, when heated in general. Afternoon (3 PM). Drafts on head. After taking cold.	With cold, in cold morning, in times of high stress, e.g., exams, stresses of life.	Fear, fright, surprise. Excitement from bad news. Shock. Ordeal. Weather. Heat. Periodicity. Summer. Thinking of ailments.	Emotions. Air. Odors. Touch. Coffee, Tobacco. Consolation. Slight touch. Winter, Walking fast. Morning, on waking.	Odors, strong light, noise, cold air, left side, open air.
Better	After eating, motion.	Resting voice. After sleep, eating. Light covering. Bending backwards. Dark room. Standing or sitting erect. Warm room.	Rest voice. Cold drinks.	Rest voice. Profuse urination. Perspiration. Mental effort. Bending forward. Closing eyes. Open air.	Rest voice. Physical exertion. While eating. Warm stove. Change of position. Profuse urination. Warmth. Swallowing.	Warmth, eating, cold food or drinks, lying on right side, massage.

Dosing: If the onset is fast, use the ORANGE Method. If the onset is slow, use the BLUE Method. Observe and evaluate.

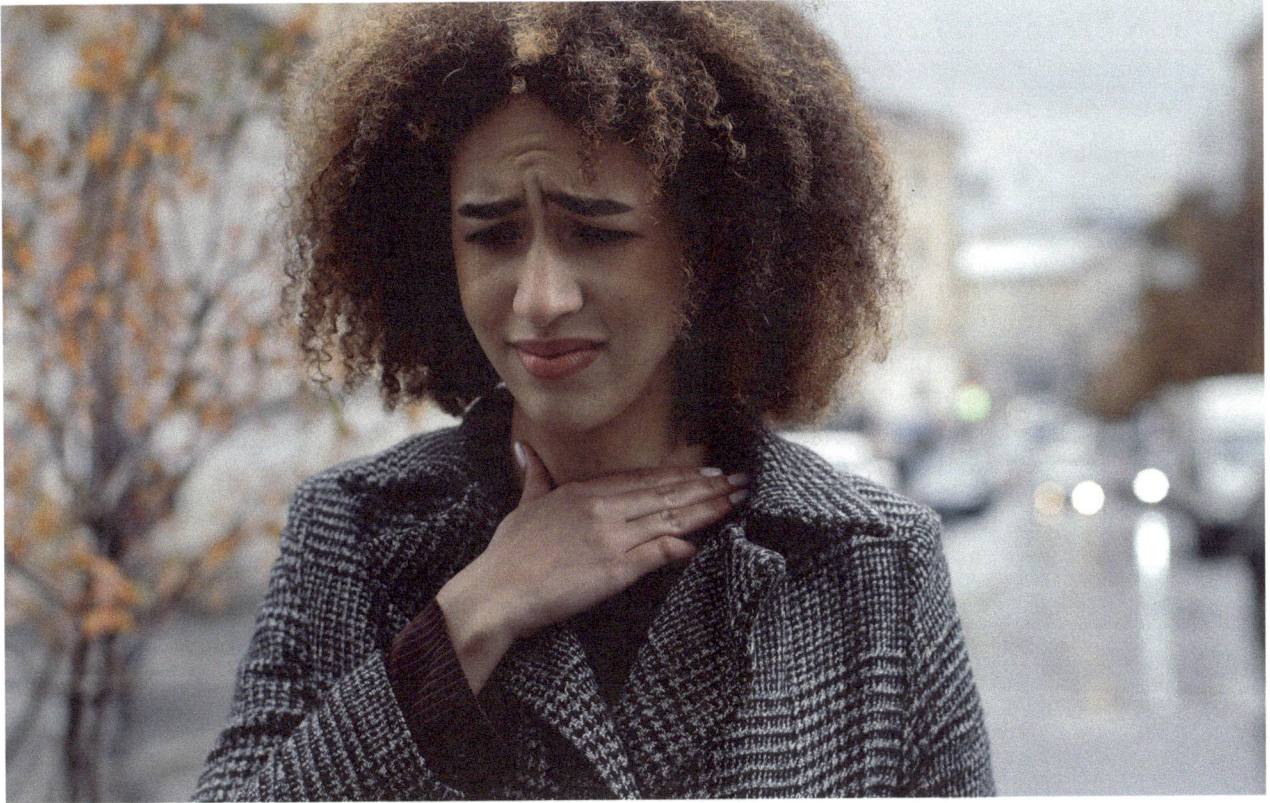

STREP THROAT

Strep throat is a contagious disease caused by infection of streptococcal bacteria. The throat becomes inflamed with a swelling of the mucus lining in the back of the throat. This condition can come on fast and can range from mild to severe. The symptoms usually begin between one to four days after initially acquiring the infection. Dehydration due to lack of adequate fluid intake can become a problem, especially in children. Strep throat and a sore throat can often have similar overlapping symptoms. However, strep throat may have some of these additional symptoms:

- fever
- throat feels inflamed, painful, with difficulty swallowing
- tonsils and the back of the throat appear red and swollen with white patches or spots
- swollen and tender lymph nodes on the sides of the upper neck
- headache
- abdominal pain
- nausea and vomiting
- loss of appetite
- small red spots on the soft or hard palate of the roof of the mouth
- skin rash and a tongue that looks like a bright red strawberry (indicating scarlet fever)

Note: If the person had a positive strep culture from the healthcare provider, another culture should be taken after they have recovered to make sure that the strep is gone. Know that 15% of people are carriers of strep and may not exhibit any symptoms but still have a positive strep test.

WHEN TO CONTACT YOUR HEALTHCARE PROFESSIONAL

- If you suspect the person has scarlet fever and is not responding to remedies after 24 hours.

See **Additional Support for ALL Sore Throats** earlier in this chapter on **page 110.**

COMMON REMEDIES FOR STREP THROAT

	Arsenicum	Belladonna	Hepar sulph	Mercurius	*Phytolacca
Onset	From getting chilled, overexertion, being overheated, or in wet weather.	Sudden onset with severe symptoms after getting chilled or over-heated.	From cold air.	From getting chilled or overheated.	From cold damp weather.
Symptoms	Throat is swollen, constricted, and burning. Great difficulty swallowing anything; food feels stuck in esophagus.	May feel fine in the morning, but by 3 PM have a high fever with a sore, bright-red throat. Throat feels burning, dry, hot, raw, constricted, and tender to the slightest touch. Hard to swallow but a constant desire to do so. Pains are severe, stitching, and worse on the right side.	Yellow pus on the tonsils. Sensation of a splinter, fish bone, or plug in the throat.	Throat is very raw and sore with pain extending to the ear from the throat. Excessive saliva and bad breath. Swollen cervical glands.	Shooting burning pain in the throat with swollen throat and tonsils. Throat dry and rough. Pain shoots to ears when swallowing.
Mood	Cannot settle down and does not want to be left alone. Anxious, irritable, fussy, over-sensitive, needy, and demanding. An older child or adult may fear they are dying or will not recover. May become delirious with high fever.	Restless and irritable, and all senses are heightened. Can become agitated to the point of biting, screaming, and hitting.	Sad, irritable, weepy. Depressed. Contrary. No appetite, no thirst, sleepless the whole night, with groaning and moaning.	Changeable. Easily agitated. Irritable. Forgetful, weak memory.	Hard to talk, hoarseness. Indifferent to life. Melancholy, gloomy. Over-sensitive, pain intolerable.
Indications	A lot of burning pain, oddly enough relieved by heat. Face is hot pale with an anxious look, and the body is cold yet covered with cold sweat. Will feel better under covers, but forehead will feel better with cool application. Thirst for drinks, but in sips. Weak, chilly, and exhausted, but restless.	Glands in the neck and throat are usually swollen. Only want cold water or lemonade in sips but are not generally thirsty. Will hold head forward and take sips of liquids in order to help them swallow solid food. Face can alternate between pale and red. Can have spasms in the throat. Tongue may look like a strawberry.	Much mucus in the throat. Painful even swallowing saliva. Scraping in the throat. Possible tickling and suffocative cough.	Increased perspiration. Tongue is swollen and scalloped on its edges. May have canker sores in the mouth or on the tongue. Burning sensation in the throat. Greenish color mucus. May have stabbing pains that spread out into the ears.	Throat very dry, rough, and sore with a feeling of a lump. Tonsils and palate congested, and of a dark red or dark purple color. Excruciating pains that shoot through ears on attempting to swallow.
Worse	Physical exertion, after midnight, cold air, the sight or smell of food, and cold drinks.	Swallowing liquids, cold air, touch, noise, odors, jarring, light, turning the head, sudden motion, and around 3 PM.	Swallowing food. Dry cold air, slightest draft. Night.	Night. Perspiration. Drafts. Blowing nose.	Anything hot, right side, stepping down, looking down. Night.
Better	Warmth, hot food and drinks, lying down, fresh air. Assurance they are going to get better, and company.	Rest, light covers, sitting semi-erect, low lights, and quiet.	After eating, warmth, moist heat, damp weather.	Rest. Morning. Moderate temperature.	After breakfast, Eating. Warm, dry air.

Dosing: If the onset is fast, use the ORANGE Method. If the onset is slow, use the BLUE Method. Observe and evaluate.

CHEST INFECTIONS

A chest infection is an ailment of the lungs or bronchial tubes. Some chest infections are mild and clear up on their own, but others can be severe and life threatening. Almost all chest infections have fever as a symptom. The viruses and bacteria can take hold of the body due to prior susceptibility—being run down, highly stressed out, severely depressed, poor eating habits, deeply grieved, out of balance, or sleep-deprived.

Chest infections (colds, coughs, etc.) can quickly turn into serious conditions in those who are hereditarily susceptible, in a weak person, someone who smokes or is on long-term medication. A chest infection can develop and is often the result of not getting enough rest or not taking enough care in the initial stages of an acute respiratory illness. It is typically characterized by a cough with mucus in the lungs.

A course of antibiotics is the preferred conventional treatment for a chest infection. Even if the condition is viral rather than bacterial, antibiotics are prescribed to prevent opportunistic bacteria from colonizing the already compromised lungs. This may be avoided with a well-chosen homeopathic remedy.

COUGHS

A cough is the body's way of clearing the delicate air passages of irritants—usually mucus. The body produces this sticky substance to carry viruses, bacteria, inhaled particles (dust and pollen) and dead white blood cells out of the body. It is best to avoid using over-the-counter cough medicines because they interfere with coughing, which is the natural protective mechanism of the lungs to rid themselves of mucus. If suppressed, a cough can lead to deeper infections; or it might take longer for the person to get rid of the cough completely.

Homeopathy aids the body in ridding itself of the need for the cough and making the person more comfortable. Coughs can be hard to treat because of the wide variety of symptoms. There are many aspects of coughs that need to be considered. When treating a cough, try not to get discouraged, as you may need to re-evaluate the person's symptoms two or three times. You may also need to repeat a remedy a few times a day over the course of a few days.

It's important to note that a neglected, persistent cough can lead to or indicate other problems, so it is advisable to get an evaluation by a healthcare practitioner if the cough is not resolving.

There are many different types of coughs. The most common ones include dry, loose, spasmodic, whooping and croupy coughs. In addition, a cough might be painful or not painful. Below is an in-depth explanation of each type of cough.

A quick guide to identifying different types of coughs and their indicated remedy(s):

- "machine-gun coughs" that repeat frequently in rapid succession: **Drosera, *Coccus cacti, *Corallium rubrum**

- spells of rapid coughing: ***Rumex crispus**

- barking sound like a seal: **Aconite, Hepar sulph, *Spongia**

- sounds like a saw being driven through a pine board: ***Spongia**

- hissing, with hoarseness: **Antimonium tart**

- with rattling in the chest: **Antimonium tart, *Coccus cacti**

- dry cough: **Aconite, Arsenicum, Belladonna, Bryonia, *Causticum, Chamomilla, Ignatia, *Iodum purum, Kali bich, Lachesis, Nux vomica, Phosphorus, Pulsatilla, *Rumex crispus, *Spongia,** and ***Sticta pulmonaria** (a remedy comparison chart is provided in this section)

- loose coughs: **Antimonium tart, Hepar sulph, Ipecac, *Kali sulph, Lycopodium,** and **Pulsatilla** (a remedy comparison chart is provided in this section)

- spasmodic coughs: **Carbo veg, *Coccus cacti, *Cuprum, Drosera, Ignatia,** and **Ipecac** (a remedy comparison chart is provided in this section)

- whooping sound: **Antimonium tart, Bryonia, Carbo veg, *Coccus cacti, *Cuprum, Drosera, Ipecac, Lycopodium, Nux vomica, Phosphorus,** and ***Spongia**

- croup: **Aconite, Hepar sulph,** and ***Spongia**. If there are no results from these remedies, consider: **Arsenicum, Belladonna, *Iodum purum, Ipecac, Kali bich, Lachesis, Phosphorus,** or ***Rumex crispus**.

An important note about conventional/allopathic cough and cold products for children: The American Academy of Pediatrics (www.aap.org) states that over-the-counter cough and cold medicines should NOT be given to children under the age of four years old, because they do not work and can have dangerous side effects. There are warning labels on these products that state they should not be given to children under two years old.

🫱 ADDITIONAL SUPPORT FOR **ALL** TYPES OF COUGHS

- Lemon, honey, and glycerin are soothing for coughs that are tickling and teasing. Squeeze half a lemon into a half-cup of warm (not boiling) water. Add one teaspoon of honey and two teaspoons of glycerin. Use pharmaceutical-grade glycerin from a pharmacy. Give one-teaspoon doses as needed.
- Thyme is traditionally used for coughs and lung problems. Make a tea by pouring one cup of boiling water over one teaspoonful of leaves and flower tops. Brew for ten to 15 minutes. You can add a pinch of rosemary as well. Strain off the leaves and add honey to taste.
- Ginger tea is good for moist coughs. Boil three to four slices of fresh ginger in two cups of water; simmer for 15 minutes.
- Licorice root tea is also good for moist coughs.
- Cut four lemons into quarters, squeeze the juice into a saucepan, then fill the rest of the pan with water. Boil the lemon water for at least 15 minutes. Drink hot like tea, adding honey to taste. The lemon will help break up the mucus.

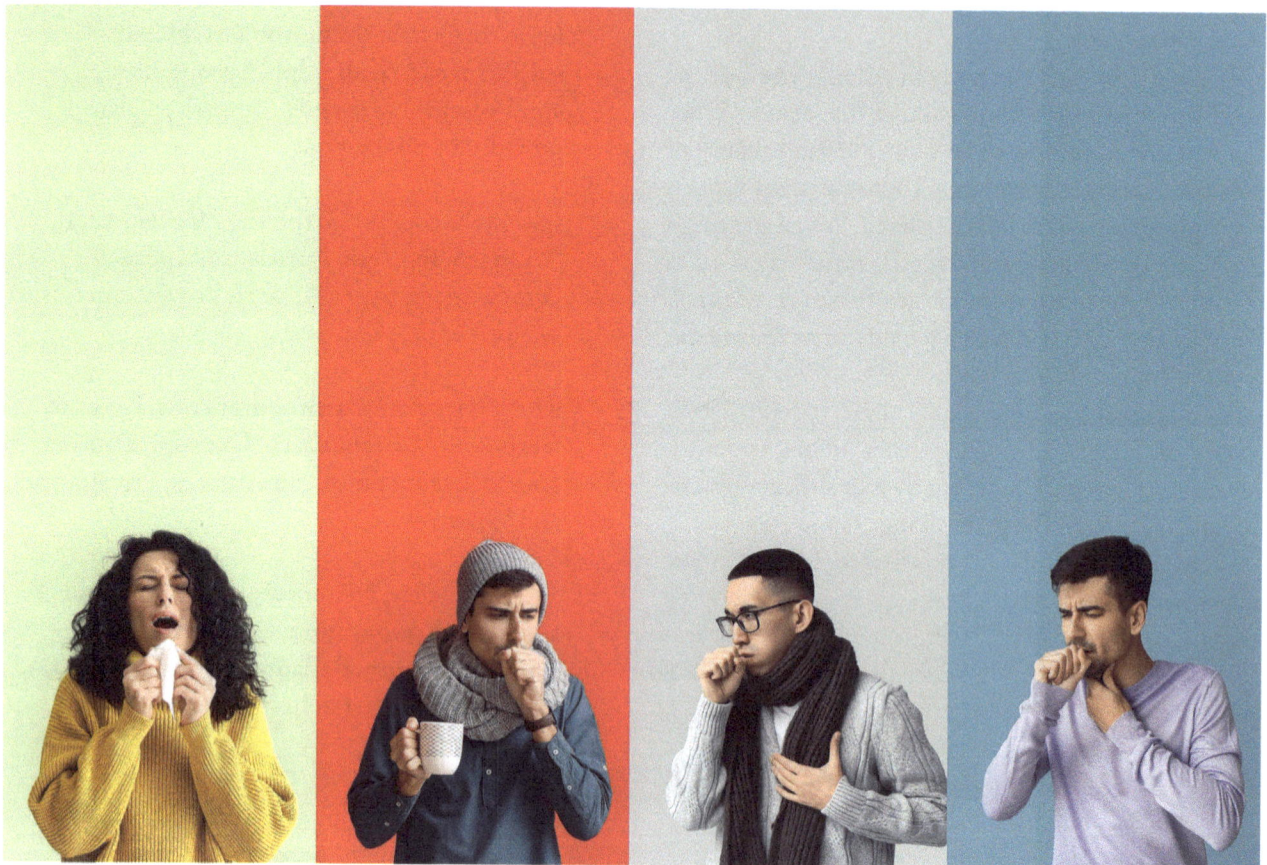

DRY COUGHS

A dry cough is usually hacking, raspy, or tickling, because the mucous membranes are dry, or the mucus is tough and sticking to the air passages. The chest usually feels tight. A cough can be a symptom of an upper respiratory infection (URI), allergy, or even gastric reflux (the chest won't necessarily have any symptoms or sensations). See **Additional Support for All Types of Coughs** above.

COMMON REMEDIES FOR DRY COUGHS

	Arsenicum	Belladonna	Bryonia	Nux vomica	Phosphorus	*Rumex crispus	*Spongia
Onset	Getting chilled, wet weather, getting overheated, overexertion.	Sudden onset from cold, dry winds. Getting chilled when head is wet.	Slow onset. Getting chilled from a cold wind, especially in spring and autumn.	Getting chilled in cold, dry, windy weather.	Onset slow and steady, from getting drenched in rain.	Onset from changes in weather, from getting chilled in cold air.	Getting chilled from dry, cold winds. Getting overexcited.
Symptoms	Cough from tickling in the larynx or deep in the chest.	Violent, hacking, tormenting, exhausting cough that comes in fits. Tickling in the trachea.	Painful, tickling cough that makes the stomach sore. Aggravated by movement. Sits up to cough, may hold chest.	Violent, tickling, exhausting cough with an intense headache.	Cough is dry then later loose, painful, racking, tickling, and exhausting. Wakes at night and must sit up to cough. Tickling sensation in throat triggers coughing.	Cough is painful, tickling, suffocative, and choking. Short, fitful spurts, or constant hacking that prevents sleep.	Cough is constant, deep, violent, hollow. Barking, like a saw going through dry wood. Feels as if breathing through a dry sponge.
Mood	Restless, anxious, irritable, fussy, over-sensitive, needy, demanding. Wants company but only for reassurance.	Severely agitated. May grind their teeth.	Grumpy, intolerant of being disturbed or moved. Wants to just lie still in bed and be left alone.	Easily frustrated and offended, touchy. Over-sensitive to noise, odors, light, loud music.	Needs attention and consolation, affectionate, fearful, easily upset, irritable.	Serious, indifferent to surroundings, restless in evenings, low-spirited.	Easily excitable, anxious, with a feeling of heaviness.
Indications	Wheezy breathing. Chest burns or feels cold. Chilly. Does not have a lot of mucus.	Breathing is short, shallow, rapid. Pains are sharp and needle-like. Face red and everything is hot. Dry nose and throat. Eyes dilated.	Shortness of breath. Needle-like pains in chest. Great dryness of mucus membranes. Need to press hands against head or chest to limit motion when coughing.	Breathing is shallow and difficult. Torn loose, raw, tight feeling in chest. Thick, sour mucus. Shivering. Hoarseness.	Cold has moved into the chest. Tightness in the chest, with sensation of a weight on the chest.	Sore, raw, burning in chest and throat. Tickling in throat, with thick, stuck mucus. Coughing from even the slightest pressure on the throat. Averse to talking.	Gasping for breath, fear of suffocation, feeling of constriction. Much dryness. Soreness and burning in larynx. Stuck mucus. Sweating.
Worse	Physical exertion, after midnight, cold air. Sight and smell of food, and cold drinks.	Night, yawning, deep breathing, cold air, touch, noise, jarring, light, fine dust, and 3 PM.	9 PM, touch, movement, after eating or drinking, warm room, spring and autumn.	Morning, between midnight and waking. Cold air, exertion, uncovering, lying on back. After eating or after mental work.	Change of weather, wind, cold, thunderstorms, motion, odors, lying on left side, light, morning, evening.	11 PM, 2 AM, 5 AM. Touching pit of the throat, lying on the left, talking, deeply inhaling cool air, going from cool to warm, motion, being uncovered.	Lying down in a warm room, dry cold wind, touch, excitement, ice-cold drinks, swallowing, after sleep, sweets, talking, movement.
Better	Warmth, hot food and drink, lying down, fresh air, company.	Rest, light covering, sitting semi-erect, low lights, quiet.	Lying completely still, pressure, quiet, being left alone.	Warmth, being wrapped up, moist air, hot drinks, belching, quiet, not moving the chest.	Sleep, sympathy, low lights or darkness, eating and drinking cold things, cool applications, open air.	Covering mouth and nose, daytime, wrapping up, sucking on non-mentholated lozenges.	Warm drinks, food in small amounts, calm, quiet, lying with head low, moist heat, bending forward.
Also For		Whooping Cough	Whooping Cough		Whooping Cough and Croup		Croup

Dosing: Use the BLUE method. Observe and evaluate. Using the plussing dosing can also be helpful.
*See **page 36** for instructions.*

LOOSE COUGHS

A loose cough is one with a lot of mucus in the air passages. There is a loose rattling and bubbling sound in the chest that can be heard in the cough or the breathing. Even though there is a lot of mucus, it may be hard for the person to cough it up. This kind of cough can take a while to clear. A loose cough can be from post-nasal drip also, not always a cough from chest congestion.

*See **Additional Support for All Types of Coughs** in this chapter on **page 116**.*

COMMON REMEDIES FOR LOOSE COUGHS

	Antimonium tart	Hepar sulph	Ipecac	Lycopodium	Pulsatilla
Onset	After a long bout with cold or flu. Getting angry.	Getting too cold, getting chilled from a cold wind.	Warm, moist weather. Weak or frail, catches cold easily.	Getting chilled in wet weather.	Getting feet wet. Getting chilled.
Symptoms	Develops gradually. Suffocative, loud, rattling. Sits up or bends head backward to cough. Too weak to raise the mucus up.	Choking, rattling cough that comes in fits and ends in gagging. Frustrated before coughing. Sweats during cough.	Incessant and wheezy cough that frequently leads to retching, gagging, or vomiting. Spasmodic cough.	Deep, rattling, hollow cough with much tickling. Coughs day and night. Cannot cough up stuck mucus.	Irritating, racking cough that comes in fits. Dry, tickling cough at night; loose, moist, rattling cough during day. Symptoms keep changing.
Mood	Whiny, moaning, irritable. Wants to be left alone, not touched, looked at, or examined.	Angry, irritable, oversensitive, especially to pain.	Anxious, demanding, easily frustrated. Difficult to please.	Sensitive to noise and strong smells. Irritable, temperamental, does not like to be contradicted.	Weepy, moody, whiny. Changeable mood.
Indications	Gasping for air and panting. Rattling in chest with each breath—both in and out. Lots of mucus in lungs. May vomit from mucus.	Difficulty breathing. Rattling in chest. Hoarseness or loss of voice. Thick, yellow mucus that smells like old cheese. Chilly, weak, sneezes at exposure to cold air.	Short of breath, gasping for air. Sneezing, with much mucus in chest. Constriction in chest and larynx. Sensitive to heat and cold. Hot inside house, but cold outside. May have bloody nose. Nausea.	Short and rattling breath with irritation in trachea. Chest is tight and burns. Much thick, salty tasting, yellow or greenish mucus. Gassy, bloated, weak, chilly.	Loud, rattling breathing at night. Fear of suffocation if they lie down. Lots of thick, gooey, yellow or green mucus on waking.
Worse	Night, warm rooms, anger, sleep, eating, cold, damp, lying down, warm drinks.	Evening until midnight, cold drinks or food, cold dry air, drafts, lying on left side, uncovering, pressure, touch.	Least motion, breathing out, overeating, warm room, dampness, lying down, rich foods, vomiting.	Between 4-8 (both AM and PM), falling asleep, lying on back, deep breathing, wet weather, warm rooms, after naps, on waking, from sleep.	Lying down, especially on left side. Warm stuffy rooms, evening, nighttime, getting overheated, fatty or rich foods.
Better	Getting the mucus out, sitting erect, motion, burping, vomiting, cool open air, lying on right side.	Heat, wrapping up, bending head back, moist heat, damp weather.	Rest, inhaling cool air while wrapped warmly, open air, pressure, closing eyes, cold drinks.	Warm drinks and food, motion, early afternoons, cool applications.	Cool, fresh air, cold applications, sympathy, gentle motion, attention. Propped up in a semi-erect position.
Also For	Whooping Cough	Croup	Whooping Cough		

Note: If there are no results from these remedies, consider: **Arsenicum, Belladonna, *Iodum purum, Kali bich, Lachesis, Phosphorus,** or ***Rumex crispus.**

Dosing: Use the BLUE method. Observe and evaluate. Using the plussing dosing can also be helpful.
*See **page 36** for instructions.*

SPASMODIC COUGHS

Spasmodic coughs come in fits of uncontrollable, violent, and prolonged spasms of coughing.
See **Additional Support for All Types of Coughs** in this chapter on **page 116**.

COMMON REMEDIES FOR SPASMODIC COUGHS

	Carbo veg	*Coccus cacti	*Cuprum	Drosera	Ignatia
Onset	Onset from frosty air, extreme temperatures, warm damp weather, wind on the head. Failure to completely recover from a previous illness.	Onset from cold air, cold wind.	Onset from cold air, cold wind.	Any irritation of larynx.	May come on after a major emotional upset like grief or shock, or from getting overly angry. Often comes on after a sore throat.
Mood	Indifferent to everything, a bit confused. Weak, irritable, sluggish.	Feels sad, lethargic.	Nervous, uneasy, possible rage, biting and tearing things apart, convulsive laughter.	Anxious, irritable, extremely restless. Easily angered but wants someone with them.	Moody, quarrelsome, tearful. Wants to be alone, does not want to be consoled.
Indications	Rattling in chest with itching in throat. Burning in chest behind sternum. Gagging, choking, vomiting of mucus. Feels cold but wants to be fanned. Thirsty. Hoarseness, worse in evening. Exhausted by even slightest exertion.	Paroxysms (frequent, violent) of cough. Tickling in larynx. Constantly clearing throat. Feels as if a thread hangs down the back of the throat. Much internal heat with perspiration. Brushing teeth causes cough. Thick ropy mucus can cause retching or vomiting.	Sudden attacks of suffocation. Painful constrictions in chest. Voice hoarse especially in cold air. Metallic taste in the mouth. Breathing can be fast and may pant. Hands and feet usually cold. Restless in bed.	Tickling throat, dry trachea. Holds chest with hands when coughing due to pain in throat, larynx, chest, and maybe stomach. Face may turn blue. Cough can end with gagging. Mucus is stringy, yellow, may have streaks of blood. Chilly with cold sweats and shivering.	Sighing, yawning, takes deep breath for relief. Sleepy after a coughing fit. Constriction, aching, shooting pains in chest. Feels as if a weight is on chest. Speaks in whispers. Tickling in throat. Very sensitive to pain.
Worse	Warmth, damp weather, lying down, walking, eating, talking, changes in temperature. Fatty foods, wine, coffee, milk.	6 AM or 11 PM. On waking, nighttime in a hot bed, heat, warm drinks, lying down, brushing teeth, wind.	Bending backwards, laughing, deep breathing in cold air, 3 AM, eating, hiccups.	Laughing, talking, crying, cold food or drink, becoming too warm in bed, lying down, vomiting, evenings, after midnight.	Evenings, emotions, worry, fright, grief, touch, cold fresh air, walking, lying down.
Better	Being fanned vigorously, elevating feet, cold, belching.	Cool open air, cool drinks, walking, washing in cool water, light covers, yawning, leaning forward to clear mucus.	Sipping cold drinks, perspiring, lying quietly.	Pressure, and fresh air.	Deep breathing, swallowing, eating in general, eating sweets, changing positions, warmth, being left alone.
Also For	Whooping Cough	Whooping Cough	Whooping Cough	Whooping Cough	Whooping Cough

Dosing: Use the BLUE method. Observe and evaluate. Using the plussing dosing can also be helpful.
See **page 36** for instructions.

CROUP

Croup is a viral infection of the vocal cords and the trachea (windpipe). The air passages become narrowed by swollen mucous membranes. This gives the cough a croupy, metallic, wet or barking sound. It may or may not be accompanied by a fever. Croup is usually much worse at night and less severe during the day. It requires careful watching in the very young because the symptoms can change rapidly.

The cough is frequently described as the sound of a barking seal, or a high-pitched, hoarse dog barking caused by the opening of the vocal cords becoming more narrow. It's like the space between the vocal cords went from being that of the diameter of a straw to that of being the diameter of a coffee stirrer. It's really hard to push air through something that narrow, and that's when you hear the bark when they're trying to take a deep breath in and cough that air out very forcefully. If the cough is severe, they may gag or choke.

It is usually brought on by a cold or flu typically in children ages six months to four years old. It can also be in children as young as three months old and as old as age 15. This is rare in adults.

IT'S AN EMERGENCY WHEN

- The person has serious trouble breathing with the cough.
- The person doesn't respond to remedies or additional support.

ADDITIONAL SUPPORT FOR CROUP

- Get the bathroom steamed up by closing the bathroom door and turning on the hot water shower to create the steam. Then bring the person into the bathroom because warm, moist air can work best to relax the vocal cords. After 10 minutes or so breathing in the steam in the bathroom, find some cold air either outside or in front of an open freezer door and let the person take multiple deep breaths of that air. This process can be repeated as often as needed to open up the airways.
- A cool mist humidifier, not a hot vaporizer, also will help with getting the swelling down.
- Try warm fluids for the coughing spasms.

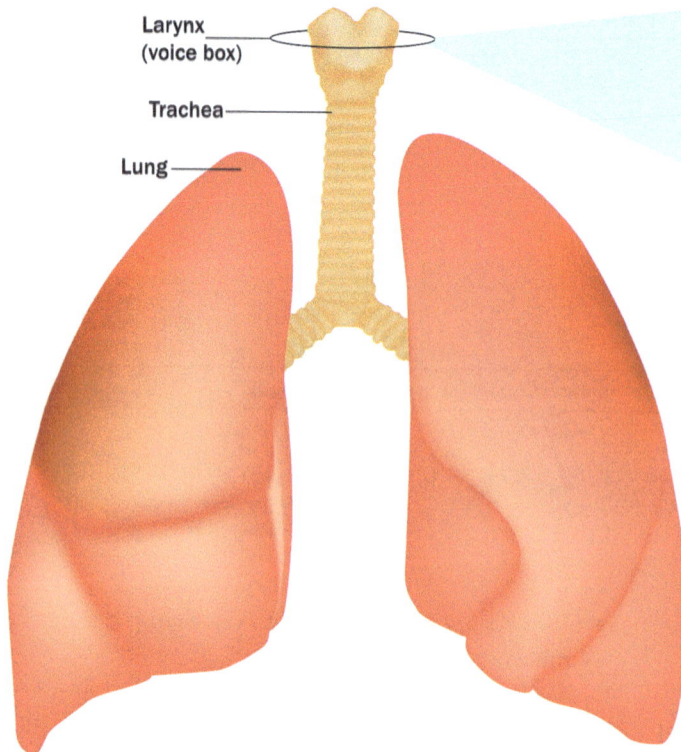

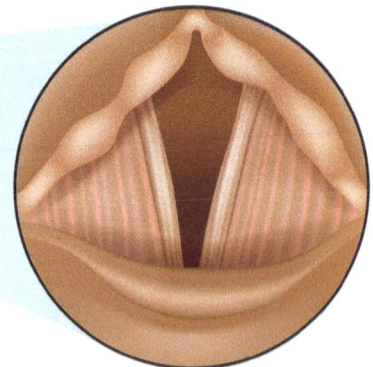

Larynx (voice box)

Trachea

Lung

Normal vocal cords

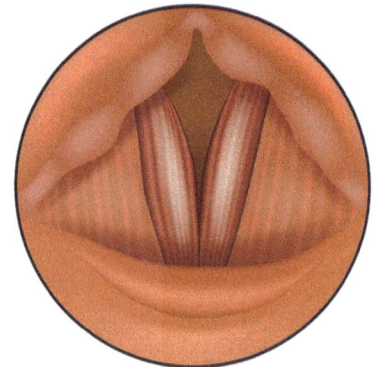

Inflamed vocal cords

COMMON REMEDIES FOR CROUP

	Aconite	Arsenicum	Belladonna	Hepar sulph	*Iodum purum	Phosphorus	*Spongia
Onset	Sudden, getting chilled by cold air or wind, shock, or great fright.	Onset from getting chilled, after overheating or overexertion. Wet weather.	Sudden onset from cold, dry wind. Getting chilled when head is wet.	Getting too cold or getting chilled from a cold wind.	Nervous shock.	Onset from getting drenched in rain or changes in weather.	Getting chilled from dry, cold winds. From getting overexcited.
Symptoms	Hoarse, dry coughs with a loud, sharp quality. Shortness of breath, oppressed breathing on least motion.	Short, dry, hacking, loose cough. Very little frothy mucus that may be flecked with blood and tastes salty. Rapid, whistling, wheezy breathing with shortness of breath.	Violent, hacking, tormenting, exhausting cough that comes in fits. Tickling in the trachea.	Choking, rattling cough that comes in fits and ends in gagging. Frustrated before coughing. Sweats during cough.	Dry, barking, spasmodic, hoarse, tickling cough with rawness, dryness in trachea and chest. Larynx is tight, painful and constricted. Grasps throat while coughing. Feels too hot.	Cough is hard, dry, tight, painful, racking, tickling. Dry cough at first, then becomes loose. Rawness, burning from throat to bottom of ribcage. Very strong thirst for ice-cold drinks.	Cough is constant, deep, violent, hollow. Barking like a saw going through dry wood. Feels as if breathing through a dry sponge.
Mood	Anxiety, fear, especially of dying. Worry, panic.	Restless, anxious to the point of fearing death. Wants order and tidiness.	Severely agitated. May grind teeth.	Angry, irritable. Oversensitive, especially to pain.	Anxious, worried, restless, weak, in a bad mood, tearful.	Affectionate, sweet, fearful, easily upset, irritable.	Easily excitable, anxious with a feeling of heaviness.
Indications	Restless. Panic during coughing fit because taking a breath is difficult. Tingling in chest after coughing attack.	Cough dry at night, loose during day. Chest burning or cold. Must sit up to cough. Tickling sensation in larynx. Wants frequent sips of water to lubricate dry mouth and throat.	Breathing is short, shallow, rapid. Pains are sharp and needle-like. Face red, and everything is hot. Dry nose and throat. Eyes dilated.	Difficulty breathing. Rattling in chest. Hoarseness or loss of voice. Thick, yellow mucus that smells like old cheese. Chilly, weak, sensitive to cold air.	Hoarseness, loss of voice. Breathing difficult with much wheezing. Mucus hard to expel, may be blood streaked. After coughing feels weak, may tremble. Glands in neck are swollen and hard. Sweats easily.	Mucus frothy, yellow, may have blood streaks. Dry cough at night. Chest feels heavy with tight, burning, dry heat. Hoarse. Body trembles with coughing fit. Labored breathing on least exertion. Nosebleed from coughing.	Gasping for breath, fear of suffocation, feeling of constriction. Much dryness. Soreness and burning in larynx. Stuck mucus. Sweating.
Worse	Night and after midnight. Noise, pressure, motion, light, warm rooms, touch, dry cold air.	2 AM, lying down especially on back, drinking, laughing, odors, cold damp air, ascending.	Night, yawning, deep breathing, cold air, touch, noise, jarring, light, dust, and 3 PM.	Evening until midnight, cold drinks or food, cold dry air, drafts, lying on left side, uncovering, pressure, touch.	Heat, exertion, wet weather, warm room, too many covers, touch, pressure, lying on back, morning.	Change of temperature, thunderstorms, evening, strong fumes, light, exertion, lying on left side, talking, laughing.	Lying down in a warm room, dry cold wind, touch, day, excitement, swallowing, after sleep, sweets, talking, movement.
Better	Fresh air, rest, hot applications.	Sitting up, propped up with lots of pillows. Hot drinks, heat, dry hot applications, sweating.	Rest, light covering, sitting semi-erect, low lights, quiet.	Heat, wrapping up, bending head back, moist heat, damp weather.	Cold fresh air, must have cool surroundings, walking in open air, sitting up, eating, bathing.	Sleep, attention, sympathy, light massage, open air, low lights or dark. Eating and drinking cold things, cool applications, lying on right side.	Warm drinks, food in small amounts, calm, quiet, lying with head low, moist heat, bending forward.

Special Dosing Instructions:

- If this is an emergency and you're heading to the hospital, you can still give a remedy along the way.
- If the croup does come on around midnight, this indicates **Aconite** as an initial remedy. It can be accompanied by heat, anxiety, restlessness, or hoarseness. The cough is usually dry and barking like a seal; breaths are short and difficult. One dose will often ease the symptoms immediately. If symptoms persist, repeat in half an hour.
- If the **Aconite** provides no relief, and the child's breathing sounds harsh, is becoming more labored, and the cough persists, give one dose of ***Spongia**. If the person is not sleeping, breathing is still not easy and coughing continues, give one dose of **Hepar sulph**. Take the person to the hospital if breathing continues to be uneasy.

WHOOPING COUGH/PERTUSSIS

Information about whooping cough is included here because there have been many cases where a person/child develops whooping cough even after having been immunized with the DTaP vaccine or TDap booster (Diphtheria, Tetanus and Pertussis—the medical term for whooping cough).

Whooping cough, or pertussis, is caused by Bordetella pertussis bacteria. The "whoop" sound is a hoarse intake of breath at the end of a bout of coughing. The bacteria emit toxins that paralyze the cilia — the tiny hairs that line the respiratory opening of the lungs. Because of the paralysis, inflammation sets in, interfering with the clearing of normal mucus. Thick, sticky mucus builds up and produces a gagging cough. The incubation period of whooping cough is seven to ten days. Infected people, typically children, are contagious from onset up to 21 days after coughing has begun. Whooping cough was once known as the "100-day cough" because that was the typical period from onset to full recovery.

This cough is more likely to occur in the spring or summer. It usually starts with a low-grade fever, sneezing, a runny nose, and a loose cough that is worse at night. This may continue up to two weeks. The person may also be achy, have low energy, a loss of appetite, watery eyes, and earaches. The mucus becomes thick and the person cannot cough it up. The coughing fits often end in gagging and vomiting. There may be eight to ten coughs per breath. The person's face can become blue, due to the long coughing bouts and shortness of breath. There may be a look of terror on the person's face because of the severity of the cough, being unable to catch their breath, or the pain of coughing causing fear. This stage can last up to six weeks.

Whooping cough requires calm observation and patience. It's a long and tiring condition for caregivers and patients. Remedy pictures can change unexpectedly and it's best to have expert help if the coughing persists. It's rare for complications to occur in a child over one year old; however, it's important to monitor symptoms very carefully to avoid damage to the lungs. In the very young, it can also cause a hernia in the navel or a bowel prolapse. Complications can include pneumothorax (collapsed lung which requires emergency hospital treatment), pleurisy (inflammation of tissue membranes that line the chest cavity and surround the lungs), or pneumonia.

IT'S AN EMERGENCY WHEN

- A person with a cough has a temperature over 103 °F (39.4 °C).
- There is a lack of reaction, trouble breathing, repeated vomiting, or convulsions.
- Pains in the chest become persistent, especially if they are present when not coughing.
- Sharp pains shoot through the chest area when the person is moving around.
- Wheezing and rattling in the chest causes difficulty breathing.
- Hyperventilation (rapid breathing) or sleep apnea (pauses in breathing during sleep).
- The face becomes blue with coughing or breathing.
- There may not always be a cough in children with pneumonia. Go to the hospital if a child has a fever and is breathing rapidly, erratically or with difficulty, or is limp, lethargic, and very pale.
- There is a high fever, rapid swelling in the larynx, or excessive drooling on the pillow because the person cannot swallow.

WHEN TO CONTACT YOUR HEALTHCARE PROFESSIONAL

- Coughing spells that aren't improving.
- A child has a fever over 102 °F (38.8 °C) with the cough.
- Signs of dehydration that include dry mouth, no tears, sunken eyes, strong smelling urine or no urine for 6 hours.
- Sharp decrease in appetite.
- The person is weak and difficult to wake up.

COMMON REMEDIES FOR WHOOPING COUGHS

	Antimonium tart	Bryonia	*Coccus cacti	*Cuprum	Drosera	Ipecac	Phosphorus
Onset	After a long bout with a cold or flu. Getting too angry.	Slow onset. Getting chilled from a cold wind, especially in spring and autumn.	Onset from cold air and cold wind.	Onset from cold air and cold wind.	Can be caused by smoking or drinking. Cough with measles.	Warm, moist weather. Weak or frail, catches cold easily.	Onset slow and steady, from getting drenched in rain.
Symptoms	Cough excited by anger, and after eating. Rapid, short, labored breathing with much gasping for air. Loud sounds of mucus rattling in chest. There is so much mucus that you can even feel it when touching their chest.	Dry and spasmodic cough that makes the entire body shake. Eating and drinking lead to gagging, retching, and vomiting. Short of breath, but deep breaths bring on coughing fits.	Spasmodic cough on first waking, ending in vomiting long, clear strings of mucus that hang from mouth. Holds breath for fear of another coughing attack.	Prolonged coughing fits that leave person exhausted and breathless. Violent spasms in the larynx. Gasps repeatedly, to the point that face may have a dark blue tint. Skin can have a bluish tint generally. Mucus in trachea.	Coughing causes breathlessness and comes in quick succession. Yellow mucus is coughed up in morning. Fever with headache. May have nosebleeds with the cough. Every attempt to bring up mucus ends in severe retching and vomiting.	Violent, hollow cough that creates shortness of breath. Turns pale, whole body goes rigid and stiff. Face is blue. Cough ends in gagging and vomiting of mucus that may be blood streaked.	Cough is dry then later loose. Painful, racking, tickling, exhausting. Wakes at night and must sit up to cough. Tickling sensation in throat triggers coughing.
Mood	Whiny, moaning, irritable. Wants to be left alone, not touched, looked at, or examined.	Grumpy, intolerant of being disturbed or moved, wants to lie still in bed and be left alone.	Sad, lethargic.	Nervous, uneasy, possible attacks of rage, biting and tearing things apart, convulsive laughter.	Anxious, irritable, extremely restless. Easily angered, but always wants someone around.	Anxious, demanding, easily frustrated. Almost nothing pleases them.	Needs attention and consolation. Affectionate, fearful, easily upset, irritable.
Indications	Nausea, vomiting, and gagging with the cough eventually bringing up mucus that has been swallowed. Bends head backwards when coughing.	Needs to have small quantities of food and drink at a time. Needs to be encouraged to eat and drink very slowly. Does not want to be touched.	Headache feels as if head will split open. Needs cool room. Wants cold water nearby to prevent a coughing attack.	Can be so intense that person stops breathing, stiffens, and goes into convulsions or seizures. Seek medical help immediately.	Area below the ribs becomes very sore from coughing. Chest feels tight and seized up, unable to talk or exhale.	Much nausea, especially at smell of food. Can bleed from nose or mouth.	Cough may end in retching, causing pain in abdomen and exhaustion. Must sit up to cough. Suffocative breathing.
Worse	Night, warm rooms, anger, sleep, eating, cold, damp, lying down, warm drinks.	9 PM, touch, movement, warmth, spring, and autumn.	On waking, nighttime in a hot bed, heat, lying down, brushing teeth, morning, wind.	Bending backwards, laughing, deep breathing in cold air, 3 AM, eating, hiccups.	Laughing, talking, crying, cold food, becoming too warm in bed, lying down, vomiting, evenings, after midnight, cold food or drink.	Least motion, overeating, warmth, dampness, lying down, rich foods, vomiting.	Change of weather, wind, cold, thunderstorms, odors, lying on left side, light, morning, evening.
Better	Getting the mucus out, sitting erect, motion, burping, vomiting, cool open air, lying on right side.	Lying completely still, pressure, quiet, being left alone.	Cool air, cold drinks, walking, washing in cool water, light covers, yawning. Leaning forward to clear mucus.	Sipping cold drinks, perspiring, lying quietly.	Pressure, fresh air.	Rest, inhaling cool air while wrapped warmly, open air, pressure, closing eyes, cold drinks.	Sleep, sympathy, low lights or darkness, eating and drinking cold things, cool applications, open air.

Note: There are many remedies for whooping cough, and it is not unusual for a person to need more than one of them. If there are no results from the above remedies, also consider **Carbo veg, Lycopodium, Nux vomica,** and ***Spongia.***
Dosing: If the onset is fast, use the ORANGE Method. If the onset is slow, use the BLUE Method. Observe and evaluate.

WHAT'S THE FIRST REMEDY YOU THINK OF WHEN...

1. A very dry cough is accompanied by a dry mouth and thirst for cold drinks.
2. Someone went to bed feeling fine, then woke up with a very painful and burning sore throat.
3. A person has laryngitis with an illness.
4. A spectator loses their voice screaming at a rock concert.
5. There is sudden right-sided burning and a red sore throat that is worse at 3pm along with high fever.
6. A slow onset sore throat with splinter-like pains occurs with a strong aversion to being touched.
7. A very sore dry throat produces pain extending to ears when swallowing, with excess saliva and bad breath.
8. A child wakes in the middle of the night with a barking cough.
9. The person has a dry cough that ends with gagging or vomiting (without nausea).
10. The loss of their voice happens from strong anger or disappointment.

Answer key on page 323.

CHAPTER 11
Stomach and Abdomen

The stomach plays a crucial role in one's overall health by serving as a vital organ in the digestive system. Its primary functions are to break down food into smaller particles, mix it with digestive juices, and facilitate the absorption of nutrients. When it is functioning well, we feel well. However, when it malfunctions, we may experience symptoms such as indigestion and gas, heartburn, vomiting or the uncomfortable effects from food poisoning. It's also important to know when a lower stomach pain is indicating something more serious such as appendicitis. The information in this chapter will help guide you to know more about each uncomfortable condition and possible remedies to help.

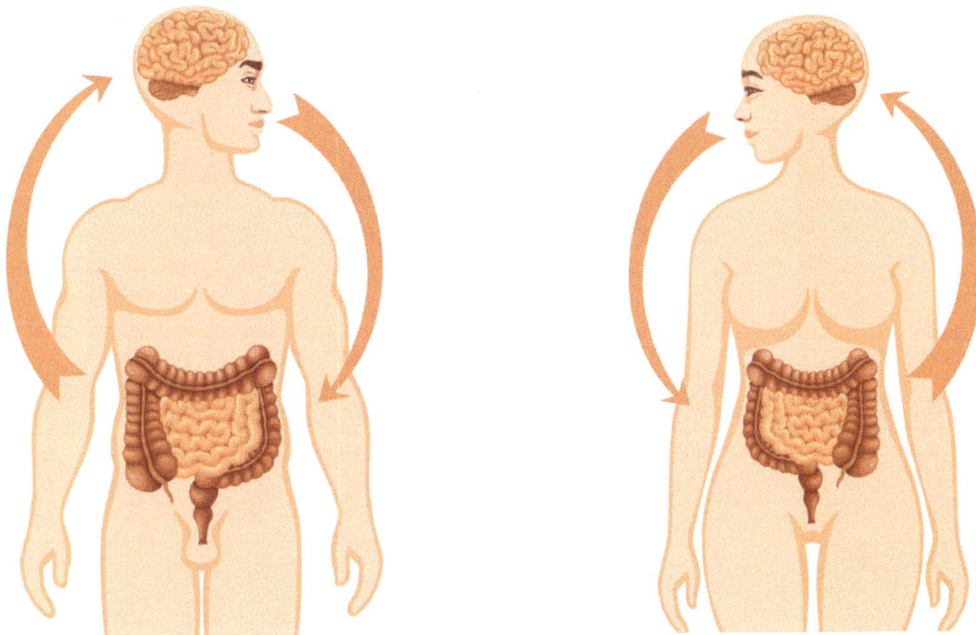

INDIGESTION AND GAS

Indigestion, also known as dyspepsia, refers to discomfort or pain in the stomach that is often accompanied by bloating, belching and passing gas, and a feeling of fullness. It can be caused by a multitude of factors including but not limited to one's anxiety or stress levels, mental or physical tension, overeating or eating too fast, consuming spicy or fatty foods, or having an underlying medical condition like gastroesophageal reflux disease (GERD) or irritable bowel syndrome (IBS). There can be aches and pains, cramping, gas, bloating, heartburn, unusual stools, and/or nausea and vomiting from the pain.

ADDITIONAL SUPPORT FOR INDIGESTION AND GAS

- Try to isolate offending foods and remove them from your diet. Some common offenders are tomato sauce, tomato juice, orange juice, chocolate, red wine, alcohol, spicy foods, fatty foods, cruciferous vegetables and gluten and dairy.
- Consider taking an Activated Charcoal supplement to absorb the harmful substances. Be advised that your stool may turn black for a few days from the charcoal.

> **Important note:** *Activated Charcoal can interrupt the absorption of supplements or prevent a medication from being absorbed, so make sure to take it two hours before or after taking medication or supplements.*

- Avoid chewing with your mouth open, talking while you chew, or eating too fast. This makes you swallow too much air, which can add to indigestion.
- Drink beverages after, rather than during, meals. Let your stomach's juices work on digesting the food first.
- Avoid overeating.
- Avoid late night eating or finish eating at least three hours before bedtime.
- If you smoke, seriously consider quitting.

COMMON REMEDIES FOR INDIGESTION AND GAS

	Bryonia	Carbo veg	Chamomilla	Lycopodium	Nux vomica	Pulsatilla
Onset	After eating rich or fatty foods.	After eating anything offensive to the body.	Before, during, or after episode of anger.	After eating and anticipating an ordeal.	Overindulgence of food or drink after prolonged mental or emotional stress.	After eating too much fruit, greasy or rich foods. After ingesting cold drinks or after emotional upset.
Symptoms	Food lies in the stomach undigested and feels like a lump.	Belching, cramping pains, aversion to meat, milk, and fatty food.	Gas won't come up or go down. Bitter taste, cramping. Cold sweat after eating or drinking.	Rumbling of gas. Feeling full, bloating, discharge of flatus.	Belching and nausea. Abdominal distension, heartburn, headache.	Dry mouth with bitter taste. Belching, heartburn, stomach pain.
Mood	Ill-tempered. Doesn't want to be disturbed.	Sluggish.	Angry, irritable, demanding. Asks for things and then refuses them.	Melancholy. Annoyed by little things.	Irritable and over-sensitive.	Highly emotional, weeps and has changeable moods.
Indications	Burning and cutting pain in abdomen. Nausea and faintness upon standing up. Pressure feeling in stomach.	Gas and belching 1/2 hour after eating. Desire for loose clothing.	Restlessness. Abdomen sensitive to touch. Nothing satisfies. Passing gas does not satisfy.	Heartburn. Craving for sweets. Doesn't like tight clothing around waist.	Sour taste in mouth, sour and bitter eructations.	Wants loose clothing. Worst bloating at night after dinner. Frequent belching.
Worse	Warmth, motion, eating, hot weather. Light touch.	Evening, open air, cold, warm damp weather, tight clothing.	Heat, anger, open air, night, warm drinks.	Right side, 4-8 PM, cold drinks, heat or warm room.	Morning, mental exertion, spices, stimulants, cold.	Twilight, lying on left or painful side, rich fatty food, after eating, warm room.
Better	Lying on painful side, rest, pressure, and eating cold things.	Being fanned, from burping, loose clothing.	Warm wet weather, warm applications on abdomen.	After midnight, warm food or drink, motion, getting cold, uncovering.	Evening, strong pressure, uninterrupted nap, warmth, passing gas.	Motion, open air, cool air, cold applications.

Dosing: Use the BLUE method. Observe and evaluate.

HEARTBURN

Heartburn, also known as acid reflux, occurs when stomach acid flows back into the esophagus causing a burning sensation in the chest and throat. It can cause nausea, vomiting and/or anxiety. Common factors that cause heartburn can include eating high calorie or spicy food, sedentary lifestyle, lying down after eating, slow digestion, or constipation. Chronic heartburn can lead to more serious complications if left untreated.

IT'S AN EMERGENCY WHEN

- Extreme weakness, breathlessness, and/or sweating accompanies heartburn.
- If any dizziness, and/or distress in the heart region, is felt with heartburn.
- If there is any tingling sensation felt on either side of the body with heartburn.

ADDITIONAL SUPPORT FOR HEARTBURN

- Try to isolate offending foods and remove them from your diet. Some common offenders are tomato sauce, tomato juice, orange juice, chocolate, red wine, alcohol, spicy foods, fatty foods and gluten and dairy.
- Baking soda can help reduce heartburn by neutralizing stomach acid. Dissolve a ¼ teaspoon of baking soda in four ounces of cool water and drink the mixture slowly. If needed very often, consider consulting with your healthcare provider or with a professional homeopath.
- Eating some apple sauce or a cupful of apples sprinkled with cumin powder, salt and black pepper reduces heartburn.
- Take a gentle walk after meals to aid digestion.

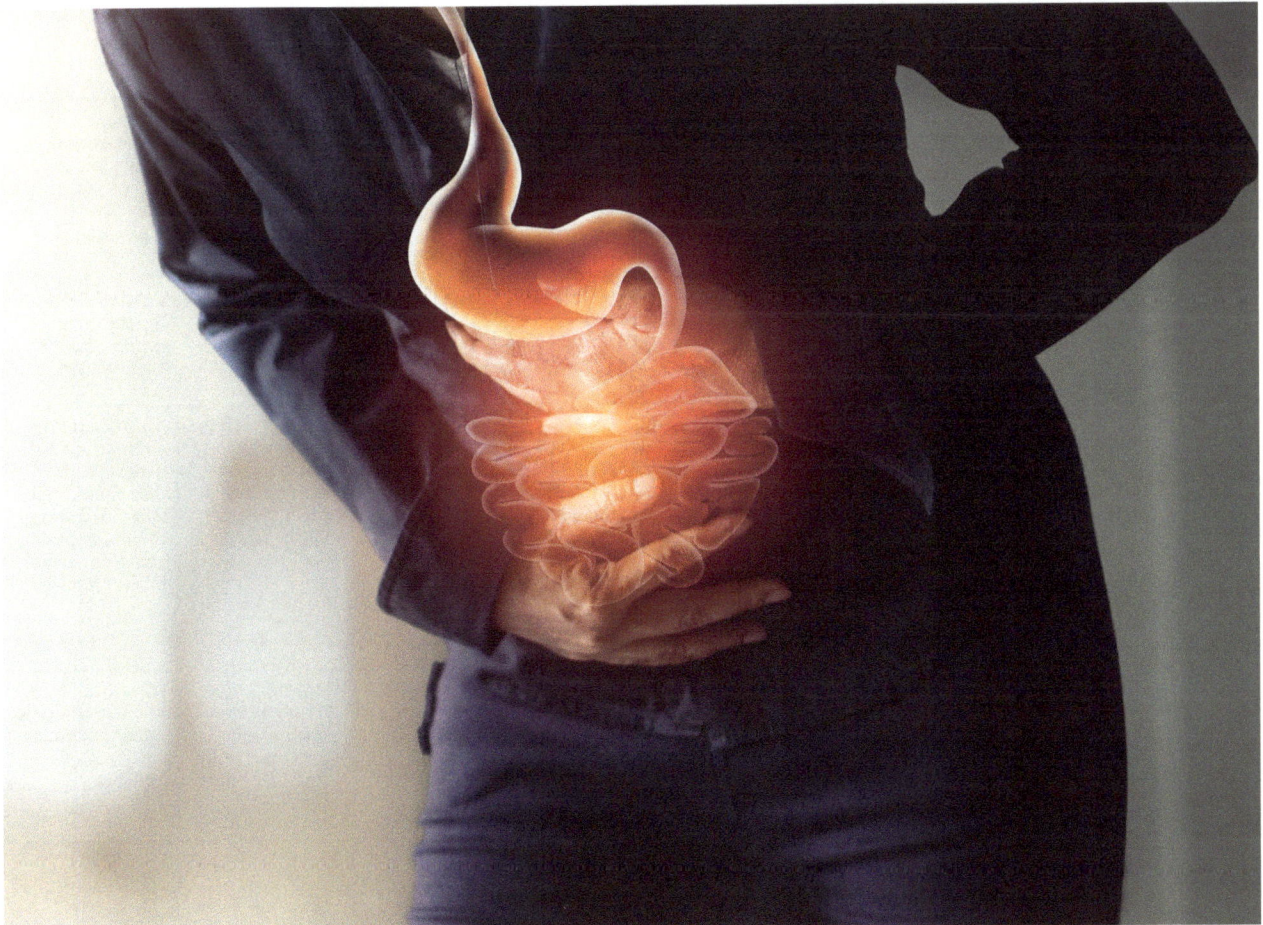

COMMON REMEDIES FOR HEARTBURN/ACID REFLUX

	Arsenicum	Bryonia	Carbo veg	Lycopodium	Nux vomica	Pulsatilla	Sepia
Onset	May result from intestinal flu or food poisoning due to cold food in hot weather, or spoiled food.	Cold drinks when getting overheated. Inactivity of digestive process. After wine, sweets.	Overloading digestive system with a variety of food, eating offensive things to the body.	After high calorie or fermented food. Overwork, anticipating ordeals. Fright, mortification.	Continued overindulgence of food, drinks, toxins, strong coffee. Irregular schedule, sedentary habits. Overworking.	After too much fruit, greasy or rich food. Having cold food or drinks right after a meal. Emotional upset.	When forced to do something. Late stages of pregnancy and lactation. Worry about career, over-work. After drinking milk, fatty foods.
Symptoms	Water brash, vomiting and diarrhea may appear together, burning sensation in the stomach and/or throat.	Bitter or sour belching tasting of food. Flatulence, distended stomach. Burning pains near diaphragm, constipation, dry stools.	Water brash, sour belching, bitter taste. Excessive gas trapped in stomach and intestines. Burning in stomach extending to back along spine.	Fullness, rumbling, bloating. Difficulty passing flatus. Sour eructations, heartburn, waterbrash with burning in stomach.	Nausea with headache. Sensation of weight in stomach with pain, upward pressure. Constipation. Gastric distension after eating, belching, heartburn.	Dry mouth, bitter or greasy taste with belching, heartburn. Stomach pain and tightness. Frequent burps tasting of eaten food. Waterbrash with cold sweat.	Heartburn from stomach to throat with sour taste and scraping sensation. Water brash after eating or drinking. Sinking emptiness at pit of stomach.
Mood	Restless, fearful, fussy, exhausted, and demanding care.	Anxious about business, money, career. Irritability. No desire to answer, instead gets angry.	Mentally, emotionally, physically exhausted. Sluggish. Indifferent yet easily angered.	Defiant, melancholy and easily annoyed. Sensitive, cries when thanked. Cross when awake. Suspicious, fault-finding.	Irritable, quarrelsome, spiteful, fault-finding. Impatient in slight illnesses. Over-sensitive to noises, smells, light, loud talking.	Mild, gentle, yielding, highly emotional, weepy, changeable moods. Indecisive, hasty.	Indifferent to loved ones, dreads being alone. Cannot let go, discontented. Feels unfortunate. Anxious about health.
Indications	Chilly. Desires warm drinks, extremely thirsty yet sips little, but often.	Burning and cutting abdominal pain. Stomach sensitive to touch. Thirsty for much cold water. Stone-like weight in stomach.	Burning, tightness in stomach. Feels suffocated, desires air on face, loose clothing. Gas and belching due to sluggish digestion.	Heartburn, craving for sweets. Doesn't like tight clothing around waist. Right sided discomfort, may move to left. Desires hot food.	Sour taste, sour or bitter burps with difficulty belching. Causeless hiccups. Heartburn with heat rising. Offensive breath.	Wants loose clothing due to bloating. Frequent burping. Hungry, knows not for what. Thirstless. Seeks open air. Moist white tongue.	Pressure with bearing down felt in uterus with constipation. Noisy gas in stomach. Acidity and burning in stomach, after eructations. Wants sour or savory food.
Worse	Cold food, cold drinks, cold applications. Cold, wet damp weather. Smell or sight of food. Drinking alcohol. 1-2 PM/12-2 AM.	From slight motion. Becoming hot. Morning, on rising or sitting up. After eating.	Before sleep, being warm, wet weather, summer, hot air. High calorie or spoiled food. Tight clothing, any slight pressure or exertion.	Right side. 4-8 PM. Cold drinks, wheat, dairy, oysters, even smallest amount of food. Heat or in a warm room.	Morning, waking at 4 AM. Before breakfast, spices, stimulants. An hour or two after eating. Cold, dry weather. Mental exertion.	Lying on left or painful side, rich fatty food, after eating. In a warm close room. Twilight.	Afternoon, evening. Sexual excesses. At rest. Sultry moist weather, before thunderstorms. Left side. Sweat. Before menses.
Better	Warmth, warm food and warm drinks. Being cared for. Keeping head high in bed.	Lying on painful side. Rest, being quiet. Cool things, cool temperature. Belching.	From eructations, passing wind. In cold air, being fanned.	After midnight. Warm food. Motion. Cool damp weather. Uncovering, loose clothing.	Evening, wet weather. Strong pressure. Uninterrupted nap. Warmth. Passing gas.	Motion. Open air, cool air, cold applications, cold food and drinks, though not thirsty.	Warmth of bed, hot applications. Violent exercise, vigorous walking.

Dosing: Use the **BLUE** method. Observe and evaluate.

VOMITING

Vomiting, or emesis, is the forceful expulsion of stomach contents through the mouth. It's the body's way of getting rid of toxins and germs and eliminating food the stomach can't or shouldn't digest. Nausea usually precedes vomiting and serves as a warning to not feed the digestive system until it feels better. Vomiting can come on as a result of a multitude of reasons including, but not limited to, concurrent illnesses such as ear infections and stomach flus, pregnancy, excessive alcohol consumption, migraines, kidney stones, urinary tract infections, gallbladder attacks, food poisoning, motion sickness and vertigo. Vomiting is a protective mechanism to eliminate harmful substances from the body, but persistent or severe vomiting can lead to dehydration and electrolyte imbalances. **Note:** If you suspect food poisoning, see the following section in this chapter on *Food Poisoning*.

IT'S AN EMERGENCY WHEN

- After continuous vomiting, the eyes or mouth are very dry with little or no saliva or tears.
- The person is dehydrated as evidence of the Skin Pinch Test. Pinch the skin either on the back of the hand or arm for a few seconds and then let go. If the skin returns to normal immediately, the person is fine, but if it takes a moment, the person may well be dehydrated. Seek medical attention if so.
- After continuous vomiting, the eyes are sunken.
- In babies, if the fontanel (soft spot on top of head) is sunken.
- After continuous vomiting, urine production is greatly reduced.
- Nausea and vomiting are accompanied by severe abdominal pain lasting more than an hour.
- There is any blood in the vomit or the vomit looks like coffee grounds.
- There is profuse projectile vomiting.

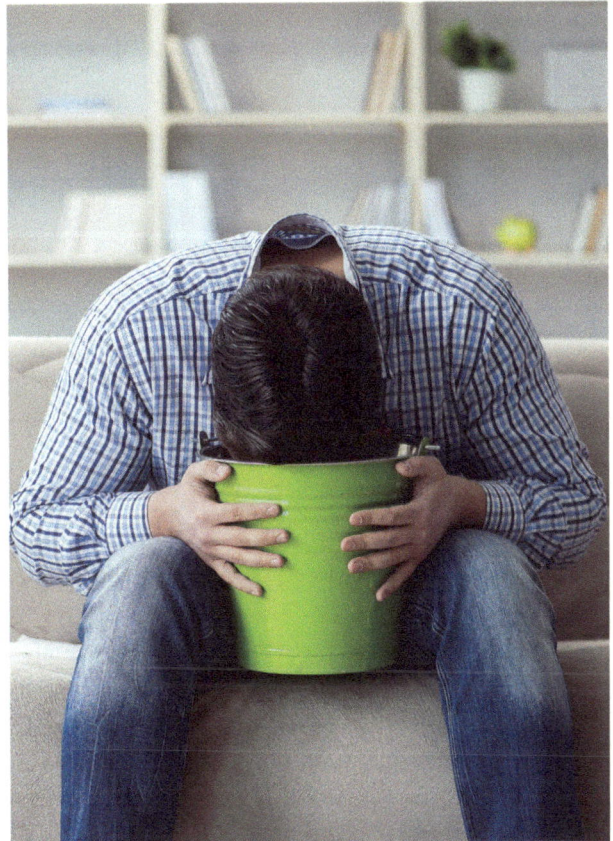

ADDITIONAL SUPPORT FOR VOMITING

- Repeated vomiting without fluid replenishment is dehydrating. Giving fluids, even a little and often at first, and avoiding solids for a day or so will help recuperation.
- Consider drinking electrolyte solutions that don't contain refined sugars.
- Suck on an ice cube or frozen fruit pop if you aren't able to drink.
- Try sipping on some miso soup or coconut water for electrolyte replacement.

COMMON REMEDIES FOR VOMITING

	Arsenicum	Bryonia	Ipecac	Nux vomica	Phosphorus	*Veratrum
Onset	From spoiled or highly seasoned food.	After eating something that tasted good. After eating bread.	After a coughing attack. After cold drinks. After smoking.	From overindulgence. Rich food and drink.	From dietary indiscretion.	Vomiting with violent retching.
Symptoms	Extreme exhaustion.	Bitter risings. Stomach feels heavy. After eating, stomach sensitive to touch. Vomiting of bile or water, vomiting of warm drinks.	Great amounts of saliva, gripping pain. Vomiting after cough with no nausea.	Nausea, copious retching.	Nausea, vomiting frequently with diarrhea. With chills and cold sweat.	Cramps. Purging. Thirst for cold water. Cold sweat.
Mood	Irritable, anxious, oversensitive.	Irritable, ill-tempered.	Irritable.	Irritable and over-sensitive.	Restless.	Melancholy. Effect of grief.
Indications	Cannot stand sight or smell of food. Burning pains in abdomen relieved by heat.	Thirsty for large amounts of cold drinks. Stitching, tearing pains.	Clean tongue. Vomiting with constant nausea. Not better after vomiting.	Feeling of pain and weight in stomach.	Vomits as soon as water or food warms in the stomach. Thirsty for cold drinks. Pains in the epigastric region (above bellybutton).	Cold perspiration on the forehead. Copious vomiting and nausea. Frequently with diarrhea.
Worse	Cold drinks, cold, highly seasoned food.	Morning. Eating. Motion. Touch. Warm drinks which may be vomited immediately.	Slightest motion.	Morning, after eating. Cold. Narcotics. Spices. Stimulants. Open air.	Eating or drinking.	Drinking. Least motion. At night. Wet, cold weather.
Better	Head elevated. Heat. Warm drinks.	Lying on painful side. Eating. Firm pressure. Rest.	Open air, rest, pressure, closing eyes, cold drinks.	Evening. Strong pressure on belly. Uninterrupted nap. Warmth.	Open air. Moving about.	Warmth. Walking.

Dosing: Use the **ORANGE** method. Observe and evaluate.

FOOD POISONING

Food poisoning is caused by consuming contaminated food or beverages that contain harmful bacteria, viruses, parasites, or toxins. It usually comes on violently anywhere from 30 minutes to eight hours after ingesting the offending food or drink. Various viruses and bacteria including salmonella, E. coli, or another pathogen can be associated with the symptoms of severe diarrhea, nausea, abdominal pain, and vomiting. A low-grade fever and/or headache may also be present. These incidents are usually over in six to twelve hours but leave a residual weakness. Vomiting and diarrhea are the body's way of getting the offending poison out. Homeopathy will not suppress or stop this necessary response, but it will lessen the duration and severity. Hydration and rest are important in managing food poisoning, and severe cases might require medical attention.

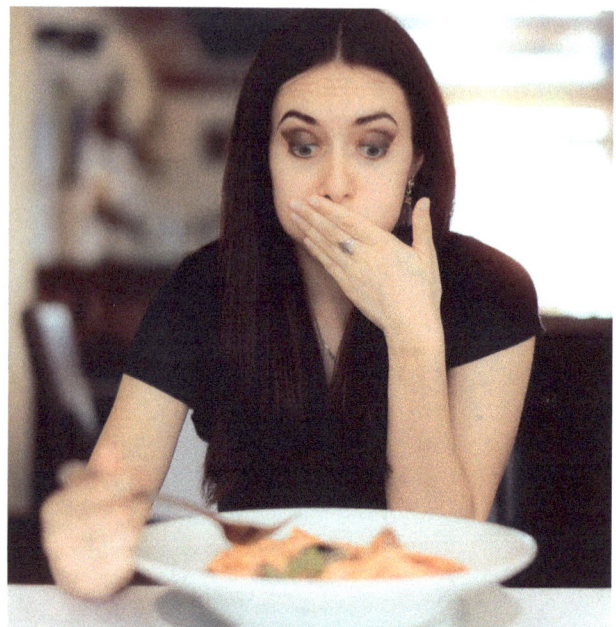

IT'S AN EMERGENCY WHEN

- The person is nonreactive, has trouble breathing, has convulsions, or is listless or limp.
- The person is refusing to drink. You must ask for professional help, as shock and collapse with dehydration can cause severe damage to brain cells.
- The person is dehydrated as evidence of the Skin Pinch Test. Pinch the skin either on the back of the hand or arm for a few seconds and then let go. If the skin returns to normal immediately, the person is fine, but if it takes a moment, the person may well be dehydrated.
- You suspect the person may have a parasite causing the issue.
- After continuous vomiting, the eyes or mouth are very dry with little or no saliva or tears.
- After continuous vomiting, the eyes are sunken.
- After continuous vomiting, urine production is greatly reduced.
- Nausea and vomiting are accompanied by severe abdominal pain lasting more than an hour.
- There is any blood in the vomit or the vomit looks like coffee grounds.
- There is profuse projectile vomiting.

ADDITIONAL SUPPORT FOR FOOD POISONING

- Consider taking an Activated Charcoal supplement to absorb the harmful substances. Be advised that your stool may turn black for a few days from the charcoal.

> **Important note:** *Activated Charcoal can interrupt the absorption of supplements or prevent a medication from being absorbed, so make sure to take it 2 hours before or after taking medication or supplements.*

- Ensure hydration with good water, coconut water, and/or miso soup.
- A homemade fluid replacement can be made with a fifty-fifty mix of apple (or any clear, pulp-free) juice and water. Fresh, pulp-free watermelon juice and water is one of the quickest and most natural ways to replenish electrolytes.
- Even if the person is vomiting, encourage them to drink small sips frequently.
- Giving bananas, applesauce, white toast, and white rice will give binding power to the intestines and slow diarrhea. These foods can be slowly reintroduced after vomiting. It is better for them to eat small amounts frequently.
- Cut out all dairy products and fruit, with the exception of bananas or applesauce. Use organic foods when possible.
- Get plenty of rest.
- After a heavy loss of fluids from vomiting and diarrhea, expect improvement to be gradual. Do not overtax the system by reintroducing any rich or fatty foods too quickly. If the person has no appetite, they need to be encouraged to eat just a little.
- Some young children want to stop eating for fear of vomiting if the symptoms have been severe. Reassurance may be needed.

WHEN TO CONTACT YOUR HEALTHCARE PROFESSIONAL

- The person is depleted, in pain, or becomes dehydrated.
- There has been no improvement in 24 hours.
- The person cannot stop vomiting.
- Blood repeatedly appears in the stool or vomit.

The following is an overview of remedies for food poisoning from eating specific foods:

- beef: **Arsenicum, Carbo veg, China**
- chicken: **Arsenicum, Carbo veg**
- fish: **Arsenicum, Carbo veg, China, Pulsatilla**
- fruit—spoiled: **Arsenicum, China, *Zingiber** (especially melon)
- fruit—too much: **Bryonia, China, Ipecac**
- fruit—unripe: **Ipecac**
- impure water: ***Zingiber**
- pork: **Ipecac, Pulsatilla**
- shellfish: **Arsenicum, *Urtica urens**

China may be needed if the person is weak, exhausted, and can't seem to get their energy back. Give remedy every two hours until improvement. If there is no improvement after 24 hours, call a healthcare practitioner. Other remedies to consider for food poisoning include **Belladonna** and ***Lobelia**.

COMMON REMEDIES FOR FOOD POISONING—part 1

	Arsenicum	Bryonia	Carbo veg
Onset	After eating spoiled chicken, beef, shellfish, fish, or fruit.	For distress after eating too much fruit or drinking ice-cold drinks. After overheating.	From eating spoiled chicken, beef, or fish.
Symptoms	Retching after eating or drinking ice-cold water. Anxiety, burning, and rawness in pit of stomach. Vomiting and diarrhea give temporary relief and may be simultaneous. Vomit burns throat. Abdomen is sensitive to touch. Only wants small amount of food.	Nausea and faintness on rising. Vomits solid food, bile, and water.	Any food disagrees with digestive tract. Extreme burning pains. Sour belches. Restricted breathing. Faintness. Cannot bear sight or thought of food. Severe bloating. Cannot bear anything tight around waist. Bad breath. Pale face can have bluish tint. Feels faint on standing up, low vitality, exhaustion with chilliness or cold sweats, and feeble pulse. May bend over from pain. Wants fresh air, cold to the touch with cold sweat.
Mood	Anxious, restless, can't lie still. Exhausted but has enough energy to be demanding. May fear they are going to die.	Very grumpy, irritable. Does not want to move, and wants to be left alone.	Anxious, confused, indifferent, irritable, and sluggish.
Diarrhea	Very watery, burning, slimy, brown, yellow, or black stools that may contain undigested food. Foul-smelling stools in small quantities, which burn anus. Cramping in abdomen. Great weakness follows stool. Chilly, but wants sips of cold water to wet mouth, or might refuse water for fear of vomiting. Can't bear the thought of food.	Stools are loose, yellow, and mushy. Anal area burns. Usually little or no cramping. Worse in the morning after getting up and moving around. Stomach is sensitive to touch.	Lots of gas and burning on the anus when passing acidic, foul-smelling stools.
Worse	Midnight to 2 AM. Cold food or drinks. Getting chilled. Cold.	Movement. Morning. Hot weather. Eating cabbage.	Drinking ice water. Loss of fluids. Butter, fats, and milk. Lying down.
Better	Heat. Warm applications to the abdomen.	Pressure. Rest. Being quiet and left alone. Cool drinks.	Cool, fresh air. Being fanned. Elevating their feet. Passing gas. Burping.

Dosing: Use the ORANGE method. Observe and evaluate.

COMMON REMEDIES FOR FOOD POISONING—part 2

	China	Ipecac	Pulsatilla	*Zingiber
Onset	For food poisoning from eating spoiled beef, fish, or fruit, or too much fruit.	From eating unripe fruit, too much fruit, or spoiled pork.	From eating spoiled pork or fish.	Eating spoiled melon or impure water or bread.
Symptoms	Frequent vomiting of undigested food. Sour-smelling vomit. Very swollen, painful abdomen with lots of gas, and belching that gives no relief. Sore and cold feeling in the stomach. Hiccups, and abdominal rumbling. Thirst for cold water.	Constant, unyielding nausea. May want to vomit but can't. Vomiting does not relieve nausea. Vomits food, bile, green mucous, and/or bright red blood. Usually has a headache, increased salivation, horrible cutting and cramping pains. Face is pale. Cannot stand smell of food. May twitch and have hiccups. May have violent itching of skin.	Vomits food long after it was eaten. Feels as if there is a stone lodged in the stomach just below the ribs. Can still taste the food that caused the problem. Gas and belching.	Feels exhausted and weak. Face is red and hot. May feel hot and chilly at the same time. Confused, irritable in the evening. Nervous, fidgety. Stomach feels heavy and empty, with rumbling, gas, and acidity. Taste of food remains for a long time. Dry mouth and much thirst.
Mood	Irritable and oversensitive to touch and drafts. Nervous and may have problems sleeping.	Angry when they don't get their way. Complain, scream. Nothing pleases. Depressed, dejected, irritable, scornful, impatient, fretful.	Tearful and moody, weeps easily, wants lots of sympathy and company. Will feel sorry for themselves.	Nervous and fidgety.
Diarrhea	Pale, frothy stools, acidic and profuse, with undigested food. Painless. Gas pains can make them bend double. Involuntary. For dehydration from diarrhea and vomiting. Weak with much sweating. May feel faint, and/or have ringing in the ears. Dehydration may cause a feeling of weakness after there is no longer vomiting or passing diarrhea.	Stools are yellow or green, streaked with blood, and very offensive smelling. Stools can be bright green.	Watery, green stools, but do not pass as much as they would like. No two stools look alike. Rumbling in the gut, and low appetite. Rarely thirsty.	Accompanied by lots of gas and belching. Cutting pains. Feeling anus is loose and hot, with much soreness. Stools are extremely loose.
Worse	Drafts. Tea. Nighttime. Eating.	Eating ice cream, rich foods, pastries, sweets, and berries. Stooping. Heat. Motion. Overeating.	Heat, after fright. Twilight. Warm, stuffy rooms. Rich food, fats, and ice cream.	After eating (especially bread). From touch. Lying down. In the evening and at 3 AM. From cold, damp air.
Better	Much quiet rest. Hydration. Firm pressure. Bending double. Warmth.	Open air. Rest. Closing the eyes.	Cool, fresh air. Hydration. Slow, gentle movement.	Sitting. Standing. Being covered.

Dosing: Use the ORANGE method. Observe and evaluate.

APPENDICITIS

Appendicitis is the inflammation of the appendix, a small pouch attached to the large intestine. It often presents as sudden and severe pain in the lower right abdomen. The pain can begin around the belly button and migrate to the lower right side. Additional symptoms, including nausea and/or vomiting, diarrhea, loss of appetite and fever, can accompany the abdominal pain. A health professional will suspect appendicitis based on symptoms and a physical exam (testing for rebound tenderness), then confirms the diagnosis with a blood test, urine analysis, and/or an imaging test (such as X-ray, ultrasound, CT scan, or MRI). If left untreated, an inflamed appendix can rupture, leading to a serious infection.

IT'S AN EMERGENCY WHEN

Left untreated, an inflamed appendix may burst or perforate, spilling infectious materials into the abdominal cavity and cause a very serious infection or even death. If you suspect appendicitis, DO NOT WAIT to see if a remedy will resolve the symptoms; go IMMEDIATELY to the hospital and give the most appropriate homeopathic remedy on the way to help alleviate discomfort.

COMMON REMEDIES FOR APPENDICITIS (GIVEN ON THE WAY TO THE HOSPITAL)				
	Belladonna	**Bryonia**	**Lycopodium**	**Phosphorus**
Symptoms	Sudden throbbing pain. Face flushed, red with fever. Pains are worse with gentle touch, but better with firm pressure.	Sharp, right-sided pain, better from firm pressure or lying on the painful side with knees drawn up to chest. Feels much worse with the release of any pressure and fears the slightest movement. Likely feels best in quiet room with fresh air. May have a dry mouth with thirst for cold drinks.	Sudden or dull and progressing right-sided pain starts on the right, often between 3-8 PM. Feels better with gentle rubbing of belly. Must loosen clothing. Person may feel chilly, but feels better in open air. Shivering with flatulence.	Sudden onset of sharp pain on right, made worse from lying on right. Shivering, headache, flatulence. Desires cold drinks. Pains are made worse from talking, odors, light touch. Feels worse in open or cool air.

Special Dosing Instructions: Give one dose of the chosen remedy **every 10 minutes** for up to six doses. If no effect, re-evaluate and give another remedy.

? WHAT'S THE FIRST REMEDY YOU THINK OF WHEN...

1. Someone ate too much at their friend's wedding.
2. A person has projectile vomiting with powerful diarrhea.
3. You suspect appendicitis with your son's complaint of sharp pain on the right side with knees drawn up, after you have called 911.
4. You start to vomit after a fried chicken dinner and it burns your throat.
5. You just got home from a party where you ate and drank too much and now you're vomiting.
6. A bloated stomach causes rumblings and release of gas improves the sensation.
7. The person vomits the minute water warms in their stomach.
8. Someone suspects they've gotten food poisoning.
9. A cough causes gagging with vomiting.
10. Eating something offensive causes excessive gas or belching with a need to be fanned afterwards.

Answer key on page 324.

CHAPTER 12
Stool Issues

Stool issues such as diarrhea, constipation and the potential development of hemorrhoids, can cause significant discomfort and disrupt daily routines. Whether it's the sudden urgency and frequent bowel movements of diarrhea, the struggle to pass stools due to constipation, or the subsequent formation of painful hemorrhoids, having some knowledge about homeopathic remedies for these conditions is quite useful.

Reminder: The symptoms and remedies presented in this chapter are meant for acute prescribing. If any of these conditions are chronic (meaning lasting longer than 3 months), consider contacting a professional homeopath.

DIARRHEA

Diarrhea is the body's way of rapidly eliminating germs, bacteria, and toxins from the intestinal tract. Though this is helpful, excessive diarrhea can cause dehydration, anemia, and/or malnourishment.

Diarrhea is loose or watery stools (bowel movements), sometimes accompanied by stomach cramping, gas, rumbling or pain. It can be caused by eating spoiled food, drinking contaminated water, food intolerances such as milk or gluten, experiencing stress, or having poor hygiene habits. Diarrhea can also accompany a stomach virus and can simply be frequent loose stool.

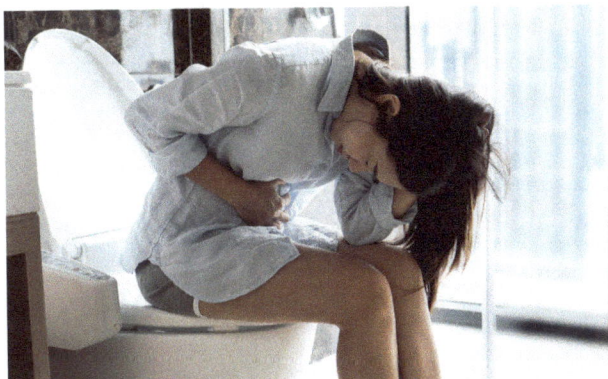

♡ ADDITIONAL SUPPORT FOR DIARRHEA

- Make sure the person is sufficiently hydrated as diarrhea takes a lot of water out of the body.
- Consider drinking any clear liquid (not made with fat) such as watered-down fruit juice, freshly made vegetable broth, or rice water (excess water after boiling rice).
- The BRAT diet (Bananas, Rice, Applesauce, Toast) can be used for just 1-3 days. It is no longer recommended for children's use over an extended period of time as malnutrition can occur according to the American Academy of Pediatrics. (www.aap.org).
- Consider taking cell salts (For more on *Cell Salts*, see *Chapter 3* on **page 39**).
- Eat lightly, focusing on foods that are bland and gentle on the stomach for a few days. Avoid foods that are raw, or high in acid, fat, and protein.
- Try drinking some miso soup or coconut water for electrolyte replacement.

WHEN TO CONTACT YOUR HEALTHCARE PROFESSIONAL

- severe diarrhea for longer than two days AND is not able to keep food or drink down
- dehydration as evidenced by the skin pinch test; pinch the skin either on the back of the hand or arm for a few seconds and then let go. If the skin returns to normal immediately the person is fine, but if it takes a moment the person may well be dehydrated
- diarrhea with fever that lasts longer than 24 to 48 hours
- bloody stools
- severe abdominal (stomach, belly) pain
- abdomen (stomach, belly) that looks swollen
- rash or jaundice (yellow color of skin and eyes)
- symptoms persist after several remedies

COMMON REMEDIES FOR DIARRHEA

	*Aloe	Arsenicum	Mercurius	*Podophyllum	Sulphur	*Veratrum
Onset	Inflammation of intestinal tract from medications. Food allergy reaction. Diarrhea of older people.	Food poisoning from anxiety and worry. After catching a chill. With stomach flu. Traveler's diarrhea.	Food poisoning.	Eating spoiled food. Teething.	After an acute disease. After alcohol. After skin eruptions being suppressed.	After anger. Anxiety with anticipation. After eating fruit.
Symptoms	Abdomen feels full, hot or burning. Drives person out of bed in the morning. Offensive burning flatus.	Profuse dark and foul smelling stool with a burning sensation around the anus. Painful cramping. Stools bloody and watery.	Burning, watery stool, sometimes blood stained. Offensive odor. Pinching pains in the belly. Chills.	Profuse, gushing and frothy, yellow diarrhea. Sweaty head. Cold skin.	May be hot and sweaty. Stools sometimes yellow and watery. Slimy and undigested food.	Copious and watery stool, often with projectile vomiting.
Mood	Weary, averse to mental or physical work.	Tired but restless. Chilly.	Exhausted.	Feels weak. Restless at night.	Unkempt and exhausted.	Fatigued.
Indications	Has to hurry to the bathroom immediately after eating or drinking. Before stool rumbling and gripping in lower abdomen with violent sudden urging. Involuntary stools.	Pain during diarrhea and discomfort afterwards. Vomiting may accompany. Lots of burning sensation. Thirsty for small sips.	Pain before, during or after stool. Frequent urge and never done feeling. Anus is raw from burning stool.	Gurgling sounds in the abdomen. Diarrhea shortly after eating. Cramps relieved by bending double and warmth.	Redness, itching and soreness of the anus. Thirsty for cold drinks. Offensive smelling stool.	Great weakness, shivering, cold sweats and cold skin. Person is on the verge of collapse. Very thirsty for ice cold drinks.
Worse	Early morning. Hot dry weather. After eating or drinking. Standing or walking.	Sight of food. Cold drinks. Cold weather.	Evening and night. Changes in temperature.	Mornings, 4-10 AM. After eating.	Early morning diarrhea that drives the person out of bed.	Warm foods.
Better	Cold water, cold weather, discharge of flatus and stool.	With head elevated. Heat. Warm drinks.	Rest.	Lying on stomach. Rubbing liver area.	In a warm room. At rest. External pressure. Sitting. Lying with head high.	Cold foods. Warmth.

Other remedies to consider for diarrhea include **Chamomilla, Calcarea carb, China, *Colocynthis, Gelsemium,** or **Pulsatilla.**

If there is a heavy loss of fluids, **China** may be needed if the person is weak, exhausted, and can't seem to get their energy back.

Dosing: If diarrhea is completely debilitating, constant and dehydrating, use ORANGE dosing. If the diarrhea is more manageable yet still present, use BLUE dosing. Observe and evaluate.

CONSTIPATION

Constipation is broadly defined as an unsatisfactory defecation characterized by infrequent stools, difficult stool passage, or both. Constipation can be caused by many things including a diet low in fiber, insufficient water intake, eating too much dairy, stress, overuse of laxatives, chemical medicines such as painkillers, and consistently resisting the urge to defecate.

ADDITIONAL SUPPORT FOR CONSTIPATION

- Drink six to eight glasses of water every day.
- Drink warm liquids, such as herbal tea or warm water with lemon, especially first thing in the morning to get peristalsis going.
- Add more fresh fruits and vegetables to your diet.
- Eat a few prunes daily and/or eat bran cereal. Add some ground flaxseed to your diet.
- Exercise—when you move your body, the muscles in your intestines are more active, too.
- Don't ignore the urge to stool—follow your body's signals.
- Consider taking a magnesium supplement daily.
- Consider taking a daily probiotic supplement to promote healthy gut flora.

COMMON REMEDIES FOR CONSTIPATION

	*Alumina	Bryonia	Calcarea carb	Lycopodium	Nux vomica	Sepia	Silicea
Symptoms	No urge to pass stool or a painful urge long before stool is passed.	Large, hard, dry stools. Difficult to expel.	Feels better when constipated.	Stool is hard and difficult to expel. Incomplete feeling. May alternate with diarrhea or a hard stool may end in soft or loose texture.	Frequent desire for stool. Stool never feels completely evacuated. May have heartburn or headache.	Stools hard, sometimes small, difficult to pass. Cold hands and feet.	Much straining. Sometimes no urge to pass stool.
Mood	Sluggish.	Ill-tempered and grumpy.	Lethargic.	Irritable but may not want to be left alone. Sensitive and easily annoyed.	Irritable. Effects of prolonged stress or partying.	Weary, irritable.	Anxious, yielding and nervous.
Indications	Constipation of newborns or during pregnancy or in old age. Stool and rectum very dry, may need to use fingers to assist evacuation. Dryness of all mucous membranes.	Difficult passing stool from lack of muscle tone. Very thirsty with a dry mouth.	Sour smelling stools. Craves eggs, ice cream and sweets. May crave indigestible things like chalk or dirt.	Abdomen feels distended. Pains come and go suddenly. Often chilled, but may want the room cool. Craves sweets. May be helpful for traveler's constipation.	Has a laxative habit. Overindulged in food, drugs or drink. Needs to loosen clothes around the waist. Has a lot of business stress.	Severe bearing down feeling with pelvic pains extending to rectum with an ineffectual urge to pass stool. Sometimes just before or after menses.	Rectum stings. Bashful stool (slips back into the rectum).
Worse	Waking in the morning or the afternoon. Eating potatoes. Heat. Warm room.	Morning. Eating. Motion. Touch. Warm drinks.	Hot food. Milk.	4-8 PM. Warmth but may want warm drinks. Eating even small amounts of food.	Morning, after eating. Cold. Narcotics, spices, stimulants. Open air.	When travelling. When pregnant.	Morning, during menses, cold, lying down.
Better	Open air, evening, damp weather.	Eating. Firm pressure. Rest. Open air. Cool room.	Ice cold drinks.	After burping or flatulence. Uncovering. Motion.	Evening. Strong pressure. Warmth. A nap.	Exercise.	Warmth. Warm foods. Wet and humid weather.

Other remedies to consider: **Natrum mur** and **Sulphur**.

Dosing: Use the BLUE dosing method. Observe and evaluate.

HEMORRHOIDS

Hemorrhoids, also known as piles, are swollen veins in the anus and lower rectum, similar to varicose veins. They are very common, nearly three out of four adults will have experienced hemorrhoids from time to time. Sometimes they don't cause symptoms but at other times they cause itching, discomfort, and bleeding.

Hemorrhoidal symptoms usually depend on the location. Internal hemorrhoids are located inside the rectum. Usually these can't be seen or felt, and they rarely cause discomfort. Straining or irritation when passing stool can damage a hemorrhoid's tissue and cause it to bleed. Occasionally, straining can push an internal hemorrhoid through the anal opening. This is known as a protruding or prolapsed hemorrhoid and can cause pain and irritation. External hemorrhoids are under the skin around the anus. When irritated, external hemorrhoids can itch or bleed. Thrombosed hemorrhoid is a condition where blood pools in an external hemorrhoid and forms a clot (thrombus) that can result in severe pain, swelling, inflammation, and a hard lump near the anus.

IT'S AN EMERGENCY WHEN

- There is a large amount of rectal bleeding, lightheadedness, dizziness or faintness.

Common Causes of Hemorrhoids

The veins around the anus tend to stretch under pressure and may bulge or swell. Swollen veins (hemorrhoids) can develop from increased pressure in the lower rectum due to:

- straining during bowel movements
- sitting for long periods of time on the toilet
- chronic diarrhea
- chronic constipation
- obesity
- pregnancy
- anal intercourse
- low-fiber diet

Symptoms can include

- painless bleeding during bowel movements — the person might notice small amounts of bright red blood on the toilet tissue or in the toilet
- itching or irritation in the anal region
- pain or discomfort
- swelling around the anus
- a lump near the anus, which may be sensitive or painful (may be a thrombosed hemorrhoid)

ADDITIONAL SUPPORT FOR HEMORRHOIDS

- Drink plenty of water.
- Eat a high fiber diet including plenty of fresh fruits and vegetables.
- Apply witch hazel pads or "Bottoms Up Balm" by Wise Woman's Herbals to the affected area.
- Don't strain or hold the breath while trying to pass stool as this creates greater pressure in the veins in the lower rectum.
- Move bowels as soon as there is an urge. If a person waits to pass a bowel movement and the urge goes away, the stool could become dry and be harder to pass.
- Exercise. Add movement to your days to help prevent constipation and to reduce pressure on veins, which can occur with long periods of standing or sitting. Exercise can also help lose excess weight that may be contributing to the hemorrhoids.
- Avoid long periods of sitting. Sitting too long, especially on the toilet, can increase the pressure on the veins in the anus.

WHEN TO CONTACT YOUR HEALTHCARE PROFESSIONAL

- The person experiences bleeding during bowel movements. While it is the most common sign of hemorrhoids, your healthcare provider can do a physical examination and perform other tests to confirm hemorrhoids and rule out more serious conditions or diseases.
- The person knows they have hemorrhoids and they cause pain, bleed frequently or excessively, or don't improve with home remedies.
- The person has rectal bleeding. Don't assume rectal bleeding is due to hemorrhoids, especially if you are over 40 years old.
- If you have bleeding along with a marked change in bowel habits or if your stools change in color or consistency.

HEMORRHOID
(vascular structures in the anal canal)

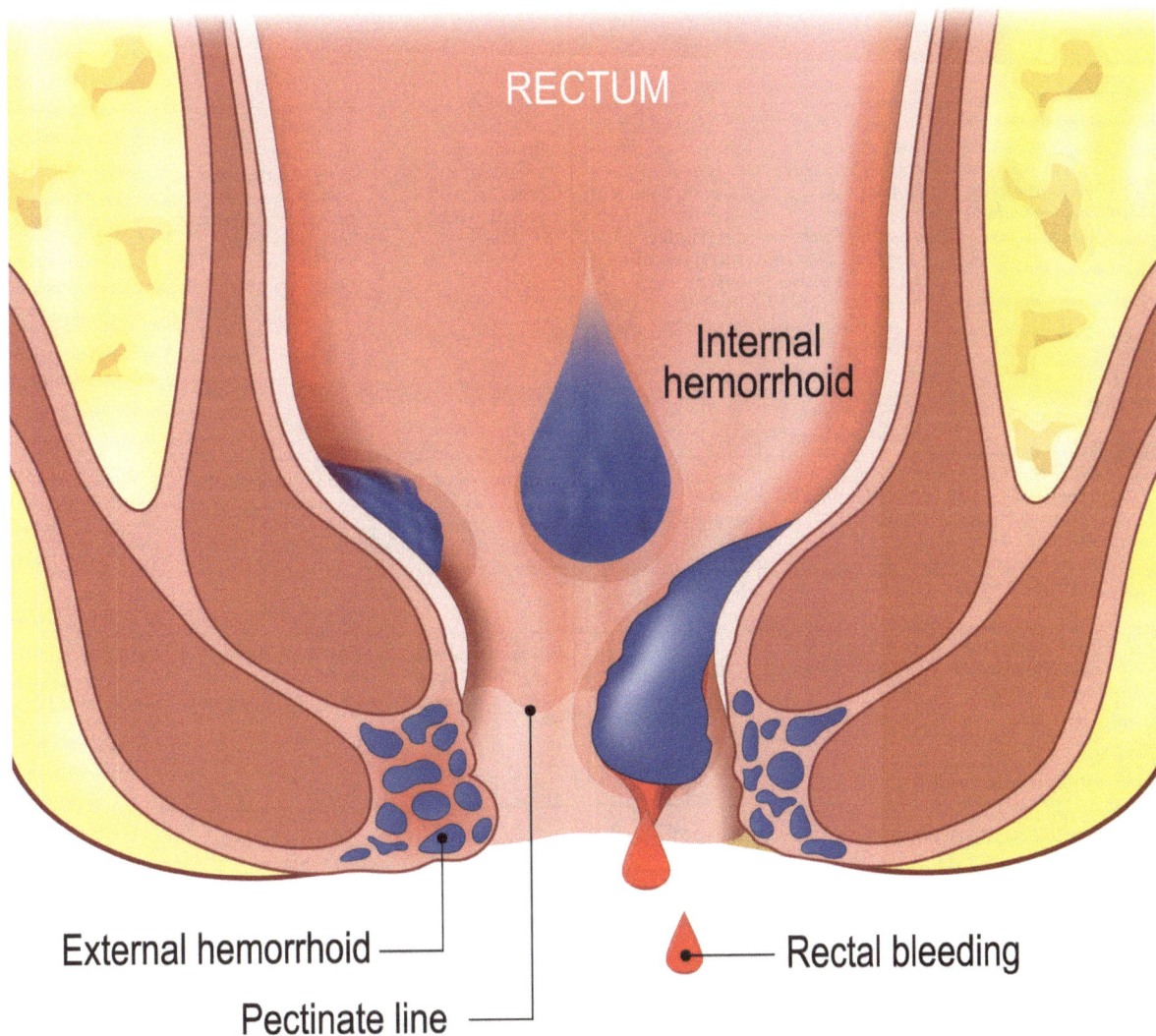

RECTUM

Internal hemorrhoid

External hemorrhoid

Pectinate line

Rectal bleeding

COMMON REMEDIES FOR HEMORRHOIDS

	*Aesculus	*Hamamelis	Lycopodium	Nux vomica	Sepia	Sulphur
Symptoms	Large, painful, bluish purple, protruding hemorrhoids.	Hemorrhoids that protrude, pulsate, bleed and itch.	Inflamed, achy, painful hemorrhoids when touched and may bleed.	Hemorrhoids from constipation.	Hemorrhoids. Can commonly show up during and/or after pregnancy. Hot and burning with swelling of the anus when hemorrhoids don't protrude. Itching of rectum and anus.	External and internal hemorrhoids. Great bunches, sore, raw, burning, tender, with bleeding and smarting with liquid stool.
Mood	Heavy or obese people with active minds and vivid imaginations that become lazy and inactive, loathing life.	Expects others to show respect for his opinions. Haughty. Conscientious about small matters.	Lack of self confidence. Feels weak and inadequate. Presents self as different from how they feel inside. Boasts, haughty, dictatorial, controls those they can. Timid and submissive to superiors. They may be generally mild tempered but bossy and domineering at home.	Irritable, sensitive, competitive, zealous, nervous and excitable. Typically angry and impatient.	Worn out, irritability often directed to spouse or family.	Mechanical thinking, inquiring mind, philosophical, reclusive, extroverted, practical idealist.
Indications	Aggravated by straining during bowel movement or standing for long periods of time.	Varicose veins may appear on the abdomen and legs along with ankle swelling after being on the feet all day. Varicose veins are especially worse with heat and may impair the ability to walk. If pregnant, may have nosebleeds.	Stools are large, hard and difficult to pass with a burning sensation afterwards. They are bloated and gassy after eating. They crave sweets, are hungry but quickly full.	Constipation with constant ineffectual urging. Constipation may alternate with diarrhea.	Abdomen feels bloated and full. Ineffectual urges and straining with bowel movements. May be a heavy, sagging or dragging down feeling in the pelvis.	Constant bearing down towards the anus. Sensation after stool as if stool was not evacuated. May bleed dark blood with violent bearing down pains from lumbar region to the anus. Itching and burning.
Worse	4 PM. Morning upon waking. Any motion, lying or stooping. After stool, urination or washing in water.	Pressure around the anus. Warm, moist air.	Pressure of clothes. Warm room. Lying in bed. Eating. Milk. Warm applications. 4-8 PM.	Early morning, cold, open air, coffee, alcohol, drugs, overeating, slightest noise, odors, touch.	During pregnancy, around menses, when travelling, when chilled.	Suppressions. Bathing. Milk. Becoming heated. Overexertion. In bed. Atmospheric changes. 11AM and at night.
Better	Cool, open air, bathing, bleeding, kneeling, continued exertion. Summer. Walking makes all symptoms better.	Rest. Lying quietly. Motion. Exertion in general.	Warm drinks or food. Cold applications. Motion. Burping. Urination. After midnight.	When allowed to finish the task at hand. Naps, resting, after dinner.	Being alone, hot applications, heat of the sun, exercise.	Open air. Motion. Drawing up the limbs. Sweating. Applying pressure to the painful part.

Other remedies to consider for hemorrhoids include: ***Aloe, *Collinsonia** and ***Nitric acid.**
Dosing: Use the BLUE dosing method. Observe and evaluate.

Note: It is not recommended to self-treat hemorrhoids longer than one week without any improvement. Seek the help of a professional homeopath or healthcare provider if symptoms persist or are severe.

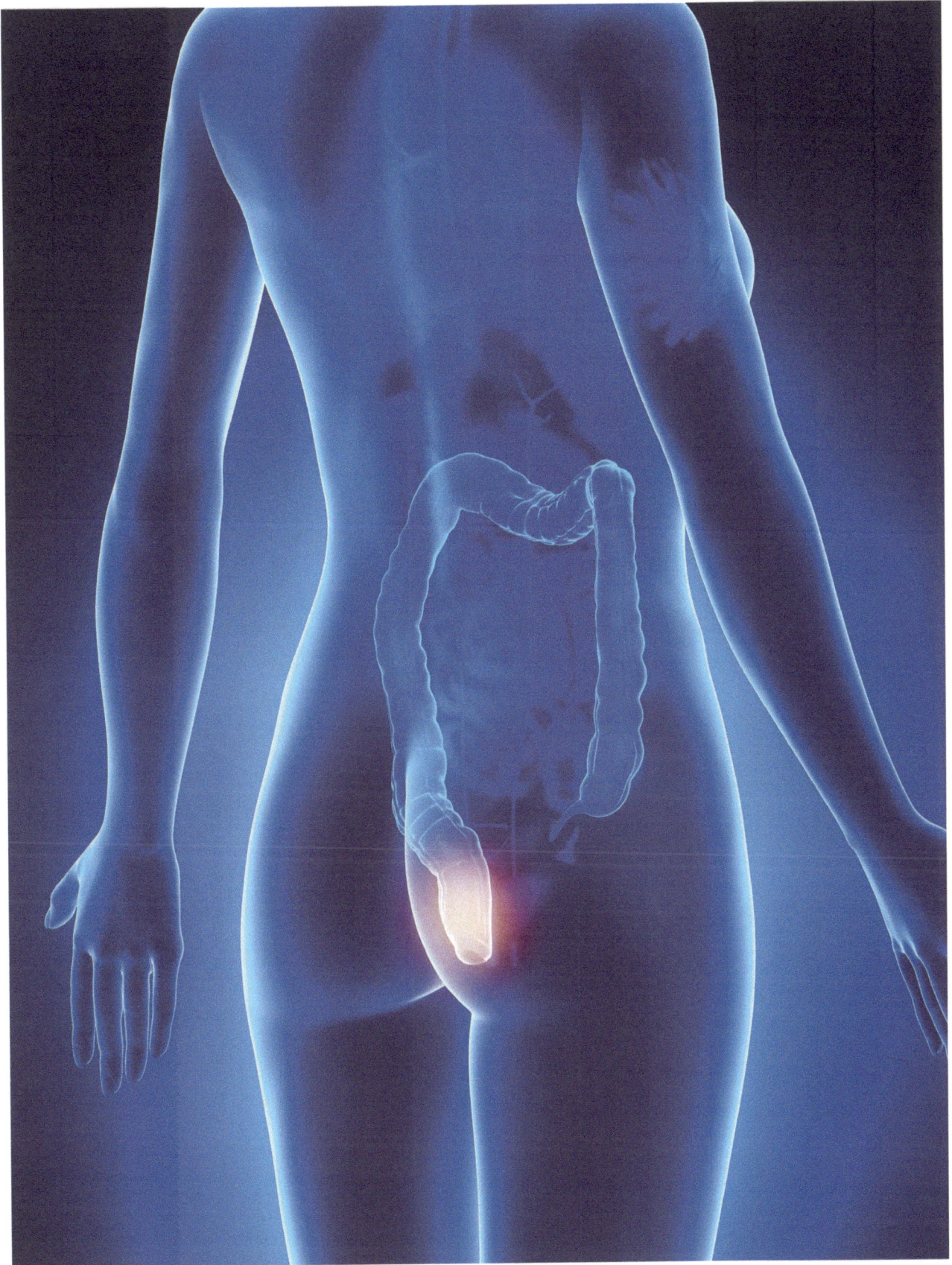

? WHAT'S THE FIRST REMEDY YOU THINK OF WHEN...

1. A person with burning diarrhea feels chilled.

2. A noisy stomach results in gushing stools.

3. A person has vomiting and diarrhea, with extreme chilliness, and includes a desire for cold drinks and food.

4. A person is dehydrated, cranky and is having trouble passing large stools.

5. An employee is impatient and feeling overworked and has to take frequent trips to the bathroom, but feels as if the stools are never fully evacuated.

6. A student, lacking grit, feels anxious over final exams and is experiencing "shy" stools.

7. A grocery cashier has bruised swelling around their anus.

8. A child who dislikes tight clothing around the waist from a bloated belly, craves sweets and is bossy.

9. A girl who hates to leave home, sits at her desk with legs drawn to the chest, and wears pads to deal with anal bleeding.

10. A traveler has painful and constant diarrhea after drinking contaminated water.

Answer key on page 324.

CHAPTER 13
Urinary Issues

Maintaining one's urinary health is very important for overall well-being and plays a crucial role in our body's functioning. Healthy urination:

- **Allows for the elimination of waste products, toxins and excess fluids.**
- **Prevents the build-up of waste materials in the kidneys, reducing the risk of kidney stones, infections, and other kidney-related disorders.**
- **Prevents excessive fluid retention, which can lead to conditions like edema (swelling), high blood pressure, and cardiovascular problems.**
- **Assists in the detoxification process by eliminating toxins, excess salts, and medications or their byproducts.**
- **Prevents urinary tract infections (UTIs) by flushing out bacteria and potential irritants from the urinary tract.**
- **Reduces the risk of conditions like cystitis and vaginitis.**

Knowing about some common homeopathic remedies can help regain a healthy urinary balance when discomforts arises.

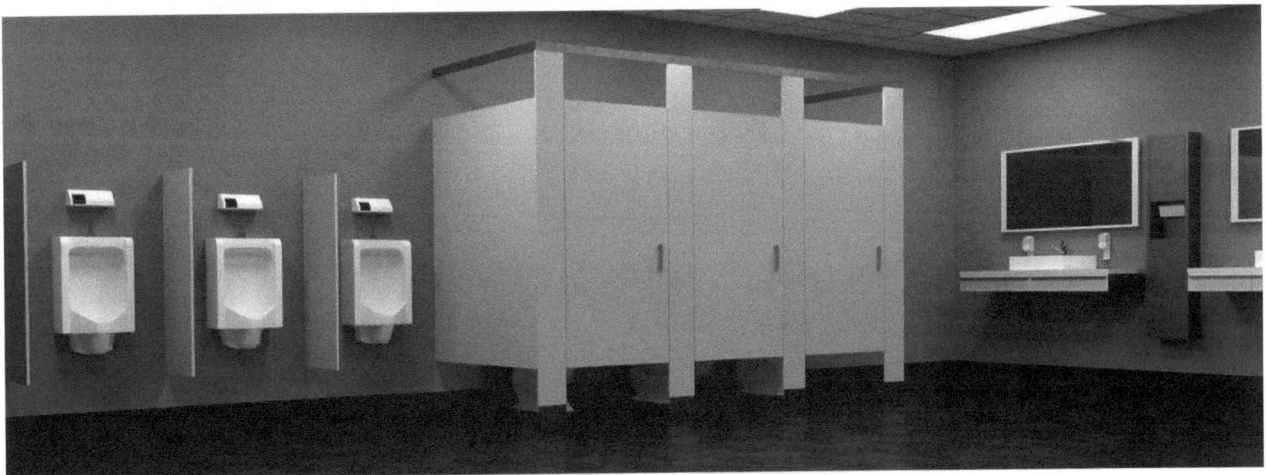

Urinary Tract Infections

When a urinary tract infection (UTI) is in the bladder, it's called cystitis. The bladder can normally hold up to two cups of urine and usually empties on average four to six times a day. The urinary tract can become irritated when there is local infection or other issues that prevent the bladder from emptying properly. Symptoms can include frequent urging for urination, leaking of urine, or painful urination. Homeopathy is a useful ally for urinary symptoms and can help to restore balance.

ADDITIONAL SUPPORT FOR URINARY TRACT INFECTIONS

There are several ways to support a healthy urinary tract, repair problems, and prevent their recurrence:
- Drink plenty of water. Water will be metabolized more efficiently if it contains a little fruit like a lemon slice or a bit of melon, a grain of sea salt, or a small spoonful of apple cider vinegar. Other drinks such as tulsi tea and ginger tea (without sugar added) have all been shown to improve urinary health.
- Temporarily eliminate (or severely reduce) coffee, black or green tea, alcohol , chocolate and seltzers as they can continue to "piss off" the infected bladder.
- Consider taking a D-Mannose supplement daily. It interferes with the ability of bacteria to attach to the wall of the bladder or urethra, relieving symptoms of irritation. It comes in powder or capsule form. Follow directions on the product label.
- Consider taking a cranberry supplement to discourage bacterial growth in the urinary tract. They are available at health food stores or pharmacies. Follow the directions on the product label. Or use unsweetened cranberry juice or take the extract and add it to water.
- Consider taking marshmallow root tincture or capsules several times a day to calm the immediate bladder discomfort.
- Include prebiotics and probiotic supplements or include kefir, yogurt, sauerkraut, kimchi, and/or naturally fermented pickles to your diet. All help the immune system to work more effectively.
- Void the bladder immediately after sexual intercourse.

WHEN TO CONTACT YOUR HEALTHCARE PROFESSIONAL

- If experiencing unusual frequent urination without indicators of infection (pain, heat, odor) for evaluation of other conditions.
- If experiencing continuing uncomfortable urinary symptoms soon after pregnancy/delivery.
- If urination continues to be frequent or painful.
- If there is pus in your urine.
- If symptoms do not improve with the suggested homeopathic remedies.

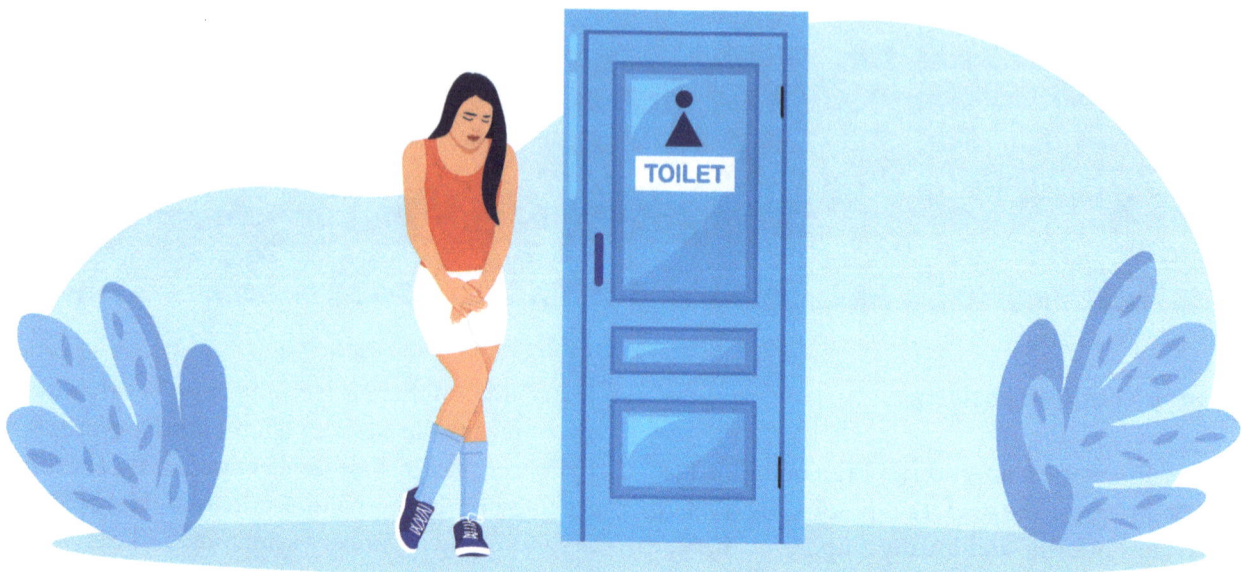

COMMON REMEDIES FOR URINARY TRACT INFECTIONS

	Apis	Cantharis	*Causticum	Pulsatilla	*Sarsaparilla	Sepia
Onset	Ailments from fright, rage, bad news, anger.	Quick onset symptoms that tend to progress rapidly.	After childbirth. When circumstances require a delay in urinating.	Feeling forsaken. Retention of urine after childbirth.	From vexation. Some experts recommend this as the most common choice for cystitis.	After sexual activity (known as "honeymoon cystitis"), pelvic examination, operation, labor, episode of marked or suppressed anger, humiliation or violation.
Sensation and Appearance	Difficulty passing urine, incomplete. Hot urine passed drop by drop burning the skin. Strong color and odor. Swelling of genitals.	Urgency, frequency, intense burning. Urine passes in drops. Inflammation can cause feelings of arousal. Violent burning pain, razor-like or scalding.	Frequent urging. Involuntary dribbling during coughing or sneezing. Difficulty voiding urine if retained too long.	Spasms of bladder after urination. Urine in dribbles, involuntary urination with walking, sneezing, coughing or laughing. May be weepy and want consolation. Burning in urethra during and after urination.	Frequent urging. May have a spasm at the close of urination - cries out with pain. Urine scanty, sandy and sometimes bloody.	Frequent urging, though urination may be constricted, passing slowly. Pain is felt during and after urination with burning in the urethra.
Worse	Warmth of any kind.	Before and after urination. Seeing running water. Coffee. Any movement.	Becoming cold. After childbirth.	Lying down, especially on the back, causes desire to urinate.	At end of urination. While sitting. Before menstrual period. Motion.	After sex. During urination. After urination. Walking, riding. Cold.
Better	Cold applications, even ice.	Rest, laying down. Warmth.	Warm applications. Cold drinks.	Cold applications. Open air.	Urinating when standing.	Lying curled up on the side. Rest. Heat.

Other remedies to consider: ***Berberis, Mercurius, Nux vomica.**
Dosing: Use the BLUE Method. Observe and evaluate.

For more specific information about women's UTIs, see **Chapter 15—Female Issues** *starting on* **page 162**.

Yeast Infections

Both women and men can get yeast infections. In women, the vagina is a remarkable combination of tender and strong tissues, providing a channel for menstrual flow and intimacy, and is able to expand to allow for childbirth. Like other areas of the body that are open to the environment, these tissues interact with a variety of microbes. Collectively, they make up the microflora that forms an internal environment. Just like the microbes that live in the gut, mouth, or sinuses, some are helpful and others not. When the not helpful ones overpopulate these tissues, they create irritation and cause the symptoms of yeast infection that include itching, burning, irritation, and discharge. One of the most common microbes is candida, a form of yeast. The result is commonly called a "yeast infection."

In men, yeast infections are common because candida—the fungus that causes yeast infections—is normally present on skin, especially moist skin. When some contributing factor—such as having sexual intercourse with a partner who has a vaginal yeast infection or prolonged heat and moisture in the area—can result in an infection.

For specific remedy suggestions, see **Yeast Infections** *in* **Chapter 14—Male Issues** *on* **page 152** *and/or* **Chapter 15—Female Issues** *on* **page 163**.

URETHRITIS for Men

See **Chapter 14—Male Issues** *on* **page 150**.

BEDWETTING (ENURESIS)

Bedwetting is also known as nocturnal enuresis and though it is sometimes seen in adults, it is more commonly found in children, hence the focus on children here. It can be a significant source of embarrassment and make traveling or sleepovers very challenging.

Physical causes include:

- genetic factors (it tends to run in families)
- difficulties waking up from sleep
- slower than normal development of the central nervous system— which reduces the child's ability to stop the bladder from emptying at night
- hormonal factors (for example, decreased anti-diuretic hormone—this hormone reduces the amount of urine made by the kidneys)
- urinary tract infections
- abnormalities in the urethral valves in boys or in the ureter in girls or boys
- abnormalities in the spinal cord

Bedwetting can lead to additional problems because of the guilt and embarrassment a child feels. Some feel that a child should take responsibility for bedwetting, which could mean having the child help with the laundry and re-making the bed. However, parents should refrain from making the child feel guilty about something he or she can't control. Because bedwetting is a very emotionally stressful problem for older children, psychological counseling may be in order. It may help a child to know that the exact cause of bedwetting is unknown.

If bedwetting tends to run in a family, it is important that a parent share that they also wetted the bed as a child. It also helps the child know that they can get "better" faster if the child, the family, the doctor, and/or the psychologist all work together. A few dry nights can work wonders to help the child feel better.

♥ ADDITIONAL SUPPORT FOR BEDWETTING

If a medical professional has eliminated physiological symptoms as a cause, the following measures can help in addition to homeopathic remedies:
- Change the diet, eliminating caffeinated drinks, dairy products, anything with artificial sweeteners, citrus fruits, and/or any juices that cause an increased passing of urine, also known as a diuretic effect.
- Begin bladder training exercises to help the child withstand longer periods of time between trips to the bathroom.
- Limit how much the child drinks by avoiding liquids two hours before bedtime.
- Use a moisture sensing alarm to wake the child when the child begins to wet the bed. This type of training gets the child into the habit of waking up in the night to go to the bathroom.
- Employ motivational therapy to take away guilty feelings and give emotional support and positive reinforcement to the child and parents.

WHEN TO CONTACT YOUR HEALTHCARE PROFESSIONAL

- Parents suspect any of the mentioned physical conditions exists; a urologist should be consulted.
- Parents suspect this is having a detrimental effect on their child; a psychologist should be consulted.
- There is any possibility of inappropriate sexual touching in the child's life.
- You are an adult and are experiencing enuresis.
- The well indicated homeopathic remedies are not eliminating the bedwetting.

COMMON REMEDIES FOR BEDWETTING

	Arsenicum	*Causticum	*Kreosotum	Lycopodium	Pulsatilla	Sepia
Symptoms	Bedwetting in nervous, anxious, restless and fastidious children. Often very chilly and irritable. Usually wets the bed between 1-2 AM.	Useful in children who wet the bed, especially in first sleep. Often the urine passes so easily that the child is unaware of it. Can also leak urine on laughing or coughing.	Urine flows during first deep sleep, from which the child is roused with difficulty. Wakes with urging, but cannot hold the urine or dreams is urinating and wets the bed.	Involuntary urination during sleep. Passes enormous quantities of clear urine. Difficult to see color of urine on sheets. Can also have red sand in urine (in which case a urine sample should be tested for infection). Typically craves sweets, likes hot drinks. Tendency to feel worse from 4-8 PM and is irritable on waking.	For children who are gentle, sensitive, weepy and want affection. Might sleep on their back with arms above head or on their abdomen. Wants open windows or fan when sleeping.	Involuntary urination as soon as the child goes to sleep at night. Child is often indifferent, does not like sympathy and often wants to be alone. Possible history of sexual abuse.

Special Dosing Instructions: Give the chosen remedy half an hour before bedtime for up to one week. If there is no change, re-evaluate and try another remedy. If still no change, consult a healthcare provider or professional homeopath.

WHAT'S THE FIRST REMEDY YOU THINK OF WHEN...

1. There is difficulty passing urine that burns the skin when coming out drop by drop.
2. The person gets a urinary tract infection called "Honeymoon Cystitis," a first time sexual experience, with pain both before urination and after.
3. Your child wets the bed in the middle of the night and is often anxious and irritable.
4. When there is a large quantity of clear urine involuntarily passed during the night and often accompanied by a craving of sweets.
5. The person involuntarily urinates during sleep.
6. Your child is typically sensitive, weepy and gentle and is experiencing issues with bedwetting.
7. Urgent, frequent and intense burning happens during urination.
8. The person is weepy with their urinary tract infection symptoms.
9. Urinary tract infections feel better with warm applications and cold drinks.
10. You want to think of the most common choice for a urinary tract infection.

Answer Key on page 324.

CHAPTER 14
Male Issues

Men's health encompasses a range of issues that affect the well-being of men physically, mentally, and emotionally. While it's crucial to remember that individual experiences may vary, some of the more common men's health issues are discussed in this chapter with suggestions for how to deal with them homeopathically.

PROSTATITIS

Prostatitis is swelling and inflammation of the prostate gland, a walnut-sized gland situated directly below the bladder in men. The prostate gland produces fluid (semen) that nourishes and transports sperm. Prostatitis often causes painful or difficult urination. Other symptoms include pain in the groin, pelvic area, or genitals and sometimes flu-like symptoms.

Prostatitis affects men of all ages but tends to be more common in men 50 or younger. If prostatitis is caused by a bacterial infection, it can usually be treated with antibiotics. Homeopathy can also help. Depending on the cause, prostatitis can come on gradually or suddenly. It might improve quickly, either on its own or with treatment. Some types of prostatitis last for months or keep recurring (chronic prostatitis).

The many possible causes of prostatitis include a bacterial infection, pelvic floor dysfunction, urethral infection, prostate stones, sexually transmitted diseases, trauma or injury. It accounts for nearly two million visits per year to outpatient urology practices in the United States. Approximately 10 to 12 percent of all men experience prostatitis symptoms and is the most common prostate problem in men under the age of 50. Prostatitis can be an acute illness or a chronic condition.

Symptoms include:

- pain or burning sensation when urinating
- difficulty urinating, such as dribbling or hesitant urination
- frequent urination, particularly at night
- urgent need to urinate
- cloudy urine
- blood in the urine
- pain in the abdomen, groin, or lower back
- pain in the area between the scrotum and rectum
- pain or discomfort of the penis or testicles
- painful ejaculation
- flu-like signs and symptoms (with bacterial prostatitis)

♡ SUPPORTIVE MEASURES FOR PROSTATITIS

- Soak in a warm bath (sitz bath) or use a heating pad.
- Limit or avoid alcohol, caffeine, and spicy or acidic foods, which can irritate your bladder.
- Avoid activities that can irritate the prostate, such as prolonged sitting or bicycling.
- Drink plenty of caffeine-free beverages. This will cause the person to urinate more and help flush bacteria from the bladder.

WHEN TO CONTACT YOUR HEALTHCARE PROFESSIONAL

- The person has pelvic pain, difficult or painful urination, or painful ejaculation. If left untreated, some types of prostatitis can cause worsening infection or other health problems.
- When well-chosen homeopathic remedies aren't working.

COMMON REMEDIES FOR PROSTATITIS

	*Baryta carb	Calcarea carb	*Conium	Silicea	*Thuja
Symptoms	Benign enlargement of prostate.	Benign enlargement of prostate.	Benign enlargement and hardness of prostate.	Enlarged prostate.	Enlarged prostate.
Mood	Immature, timid, childish, lack of self-confidence. Neat and often perfectly dressed. Suspicious, laughing immoderately, dependent in relationships.	Capable, hardworking, over-responsible. Conscientious. Weakness of will. Intelligent, but slow comprehension.	Materialistic, practical, business-minded. Strong attachment to partner and material items. Fixed ideas. Gradual estrangement from family. Emotions become weak and paralyzed.	Lascivious thoughts, keenly sensitive to noise or pain. Every hurt annoys. Faint-hearted, anxious, concerned with everything being in its place. Internal restlessness. Timidity about appearing in public.	Fixed ideas. Perceives he is divided into two parts. Indifference to the opposite sex. Anger from contradictions. Anxiety about salvation. Aversion to company. Avoids the sight of people.
Indications	Swollen glands. Genitals feel numb. Urging to urinate, can't retain urine, frequent night urination, dark brown urine. Diminished sexual desire and premature impotency.	Scrotal swelling, burning in urethra and ineffectual desire to urinate, sour smelling urine at night, frequent urination at night.	Great difficulty in voiding urine. Urine flows and stops again, intermittent. Prostatic fluid emitted when straining for stool and with every emotion.	Prostate gland enlarged, without pain, but irregularly hardened. One point being hard, another soft. Prostatic fluid emitted when straining for stool.	Flow of prostatic fluid during difficult stool. Irresistible inclination to masturbate even during sleep, nightly painful erection causing sleeplessness. Forked urine stream.

Other remedies to consider include ***Ferrum phos**, ***Digitalis**, and **Pulsatilla**.

Dosing: Use the BLUE Method. Observe and evaluate.

URETHRITIS

Urethritis is inflammation of the urethra, the tube that carries urine from the bladder to outside the body. Pain with urination is the main symptom of urethritis. Most episodes of urethritis are caused by infection by bacteria that enter the urethra from the skin around the urethra's opening. Though this section is geared toward men, many of these remedies are useful for women's symptoms as well.

Symptoms include:

- feeling the frequent or urgent need to urinate

- burning during urination

- difficulty starting urination

- pus or whitish, mucus discharge from penis

- burning or itching around opening of the penis

- itching, pain, or discomfort when a person is not urinating

- pain during sex

- discharge from the urethral opening

- blood in the semen or urine

ADDITIONAL SUPPORT FOR URETHRITIS

- Have the affected person's partner checked for bacteria too which may require treatment. Both the person and their partner should be checked three months after last symptoms to ensure the treatment cleared the bacteria and no reinfection is happening.

WHEN TO CONTACT YOUR HEALTHCARE PROFESSIONAL

- Before beginning homeopathic treatment, the person should see a healthcare provider to determine if they have an STD (sexually transmitted disease) or other condition that requires medical attention.

COMMON REMEDIES FOR URETHRITIS

	Argentum nit	Cantharis	Mercurius	*Sarsaparilla	Staphysagria	Sulphur
Symptoms	Sensation of swelling in urethra.	Intolerable spasms before, during and after urination with violent burning and cutting in the neck of the bladder.	Extremely swollen penis and testis. Red urethral orifice. Swollen and hot glans penis.	For burning at conclusion of urination.	Comes on after sexual intercourse. Urging and pain after urinating.	Stitches in penis. Involuntary emissions with burning in the urethra.
Indications	Sensation as if there is a splinter. Urethra swollen with a feeling as if the last drops remain behind. Increased gonorrhea, erections, pain and burning sensations. Bloody urine and fever. Retention of urine. Urine stream is divided.	Heaviness in bladder, feels sore on slightest motion. Violent paroxysms of cutting and burning in whole renal region and painful urging to urinate. Bloody urine, emissions in drops. Intense burning in urethra before and after urinating. Cutting and contracting from ureters down to penis. Intolerable urging to urinate. Urine scalds and is passed drop by drop with a constant desire to urinate.	Thick greenish and/or bloody discharge. Intense urethral burning. Stabbing pain from urethra to bladder. Perspires after urinating, which is passed only in drops causing much pain. Painful stinging in left testicle.	Frequent urging to urinate with little passing. Burning in urethra. Excruciating pain at the conclusion of urination. Blood in urine which helps pain abate. Obstinate constipation.	Prostatic troubles. Frequent urination, burning in urethra when not urinating. Frequent call to urinate, though little dark-colored urine is discharged. Smarting and burning at the orifice of the urethra, when not urinating.	Itching in genitals when going to bed. Seminal discharge too quick after an erection. Icy cold sensation of genitals. Discharge of prostatic fluid after urination and stool.

Dosing: Use the BLUE Method. Observe and evaluate.

YEAST INFECTIONS

See also **Yeast Infections** *in* **Chapter 13—Urinary Issues** *on* **page 145**.

Men can experience yeast infections although they are more common in women. In men, yeast infections are common because candida—the fungus that causes yeast infections—is normally present on skin, especially moist skin. When some contributing factor—such as having sexual intercourse with a partner who has a vaginal yeast infection or prolonged heat and moisture in the area—can result in an infection.

The main causes can include:

- taking antibiotics for a long time

- having sexual relations with someone who has a yeast infection

- being diabetic

- being overweight

- having a weak immune system

- having trouble cleaning oneself

- sensitivity to soaps, perfumes, dyes, and chemicals.

- steroid use.

For men, some indicators of a yeast infection include:

- swelling around the tip of the penis and foreskin

- trouble pulling back the foreskin (if uncircumcised)

- discharge that looks like cottage cheese and might have a bread-like or unpleasant smell

- itching or burning on the tip of the penis or foreskin

- a moist feeling on the tip of the penis

- sores or white patches of skin

- a hard time getting or keeping an erection

ADDITIONAL SUPPORT FOR YEAST INFECTIONS IN MEN

- Take a good probiotic several times a day during and a few weeks after the infection.
- Cleaning and drying your penis well, including pulling back the foreskin to wash and dry the skin beneath it.
- Managing your diabetes if you have it.
- Losing weight if obese.
- Avoiding any soaps or other chemicals that cause irritation.

WHEN TO CONTACT YOUR HEALTHCARE PROFESSIONAL

- If there is intense discomfort or a strong, foul odor.
- If the person has a high fever, chills, upset stomach, and headache with the infection.
- If the person has a hard time peeing or keeping control of the urine stream.
- If the person gets frequent yeast infections.
- If the condition is not helped by homeopathic remedies.
- If you suspect that you may have contracted a Sexually Transmitted Disease (STD).

The top three remedies to consider are:

- **Nux vomica**: There is a cottage cheese-like discharge from the penis or that sits under the foreskin (if uncircumcised). If no discharge, there can be a moist sensation on the tip of the penis accompanied by discomfort or a burning type of pain. The symptoms are worse from alcohol, coffee and stress. It can be difficult to get or keep an erection.

- **Rhus tox:** For swelling around the tip and under foreskin of the penis (if uncircumcised). There can be itching or a burning sensation. There can be sore or white patches on the skin. The swelling and pain can be relieved by bathing in warm water. It can be worse from sitting for a long time. The discomfort is worse from cold and dampness.

- **Sulphur:** There is a creamy white discharge that is itchy. The foreskin, of uncircumcised males, can be stiff and difficult to pull back. There can be difficulty getting an erection. There is a feeling of weak sexual power. Symptoms are worse from bathing, resting, milk and sweets. Symptoms are relieved by motion and dry heat.

Dosing: Use the **BLUE** Method.
Observe and evaluate.

PREMATURE EJACULATION

Premature ejaculation is when ejaculation happens sooner than a man or his partner would like during sex. Occasional premature ejaculation is also known as rapid ejaculation, premature climax, or early ejaculation. In the U.S., about one in five men 18 to 59 years old have problems with premature ejaculation and it is one of the most common sexual complaints. There is no medical time limit that defines ejaculation as "premature," but typically ejaculation within two to three minutes from beginning intercourse is regarded as premature.

Symptoms include:

- ejaculation that routinely occurs with little sexual stimulation and with little control

- decreased sexual pleasure because of poor control over ejaculation

- feelings of guilt, embarrassment, or frustration

Though the actual cause of premature ejaculation is not completely known, premature ejaculation is more often caused by a psychological stressor such as anxiety or depression. Though much less common, it can also have a physical cause such as an injury, infection, or hormonal problem.

ADDITIONAL SUPPORT FOR PREMATURE EJACULATION

- Premature ejaculation can be helped with behavior modification and counseling to help with emotional issues or stressors that may be contributing to it.

WHEN TO CONTACT YOUR HEALTHCARE PROFESSIONAL

- In addition to these remedy suggestions, it is strongly advised to consult with a healthcare practitioner to make sure there isn't any underlying health issue.

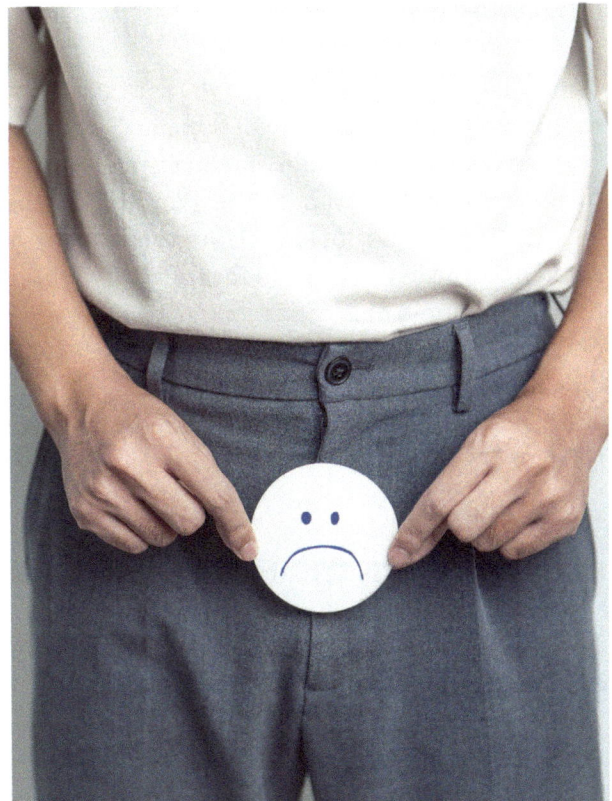

COMMON REMEDIES FOR PREMATURE EJACULATION

	Calcarea carb	*Graphites	*Natrum carb	Nux vomica	Phosphorus
Symptoms	Premature ejaculation with increased desire.	Strong and painful erections with too early or no ejaculation, feeble enjoyment during sex.	Too strong or too weak erections with quick ejaculation.	Premature ejaculation. Inability to be in the company of those desired without emission.	Premature ejaculation. Strong desire with feeble erection.
Mood	Capable, hardworking, over-responsible, conscientious. Desires to be magnetized. Weakness of will. Intelligent, but slow comprehension.	Difficult to make choices/anxiety about decisions made. Obstinate, discontented, changeable moods, irritability about trifles.	Premature ejaculation, flaccidity during sex. Inability to be in the company of those desired without emission.	Very irritable, insensitive to all impressions. Competitive. Zealous, nervous and excitable. Angry and impatient.	Strong sexual desire. Easily vexed and fears when thinking about unpleasant things. Deep desire to be magnetized. Anxiety with thunderstorms.
Indications	Increased desire or erections incomplete. Ejaculation is too quick.	Lascivious feeling in the genitals, uncontrollable sexual excitement. Seminal emissions at night with flaccid penis that wake him, but no voluptuous feelings. Sensation of great weakness in genitals, from previous sexual abuse or overall dislike of sex. After sex, coldness of legs, exhaustion, or heat of the body and sweat.	Prolonged, painful erections without desire. Head of penis easily becomes sore from constant inflammation and swelling. Nightly emissions with or without an erection.	Sexual desire, but lacking an erection. Heat, stitching and drawing up sensation in testicles. Easily excited desire, especially in morning in bed. Painful erections midday after a nap. Dry heat with dry mouth without thirst after sex.	Impotence after excessive excitement or frequent masturbation. Erections absent. Irresistible desire with premature ejaculation. Involuntary emissions, lascivious dreams, frequent emissions at night, even after sex.

Dosing: Use the BLUE Method. Observe and evaluate.

HEMORRHOIDS

Hemorrhoids are swollen veins in the anus and lower rectum, similar to varicose veins. Hemorrhoids may be located inside the rectum (internal hemorrhoids), or they may develop under the skin around the anus (external hemorrhoids). Hemorrhoids are very common. Nearly three out of four adults will have hemorrhoids from time to time. Sometimes they don't cause symptoms but at other times they cause itching, discomfort, and bleeding.

Read more about Hemorrhoids in Chapter 12—Stool Issues on page 138.

ERECTILE DYSFUNCTION

Erectile dysfunction (ED) is the inability to get or keep an erection firm enough to have sexual intercourse. Occasional ED is fairly common. Many men experience it during times of stress. ED is often a side effect of smoking and/or pharmaceutical use. Frequent ED can be a sign of health problems that need treatment. It can also be a sign of emotional or relationship difficulties that may need to be addressed.

Because erectile dysfunction is a complex issue, consider consulting a professional homeopath.

MUSCLE SPRAINS

See Blows and Contusions/Bruises in Chapter 4—First Aid on page 49 and Sprains, Strains and Overexertion of Ligaments and Tendons in Chapter 17—Muscle, Joints and Bones on page 185.

JOCK ITCH

See Fungal Infections in Chapter 18—Skin on page 214.

DANDRUFF

See Chapter 5—Head on page 76.

BLOWS TO THE TESTICLES

Receiving a blow to the testicles is one of the most painful experiences for a male. Thankfully, the pain, soreness and nausea gradually subside within a few hours.

ADDITIONAL SUPPORT FOR BLOWS TO THE TESTICLES

- Lie down, rest, and apply cold compresses to the groin area.
- Wear supportive underwear which can help to lessen the pain.
- Avoid any strenuous activity or lifting and take it easy for a few days.

WHEN TO CONTACT YOUR HEALTHCARE PROFESSIONAL

- The pain is not subsiding, at all, after an hour and is continuing to be extreme.
- There is swelling or bruising of the scrotum or a puncture of the scrotum or testicle.
- The nausea is not subsiding and vomiting ensues.
- A fever develops.

Remedies to consider: Give one dose of **Arnica** immediately. 15 minutes after giving **Arnica**, give a dose of **Staphysagria** and continue on an as-needed basis up to every 15 minutes for four doses. If the pain subsides after an hour, use additional remedies only if there is a return of pain or swelling.

DECREASED LIBIDO (SEXUAL DESIRE)

It's common to lose interest in sex from time to time, and libido levels vary through life. It's also normal for your interest not to match your partner's at times. However, low libido for a long period of time may cause concern for some people. It can sometimes be an indicator of an underlying health condition.

Because decreased libido is a complex issue, consider consulting a professional homeopath.

LOW SPERM COUNT

The symptoms of a low sperm count are not apparent and can only be checked via sperm count testing by a healthcare provider. If the person is having trouble conceiving, it is advisable to see their healthcare practitioner. Also, consider consulting with a professional homeopath.

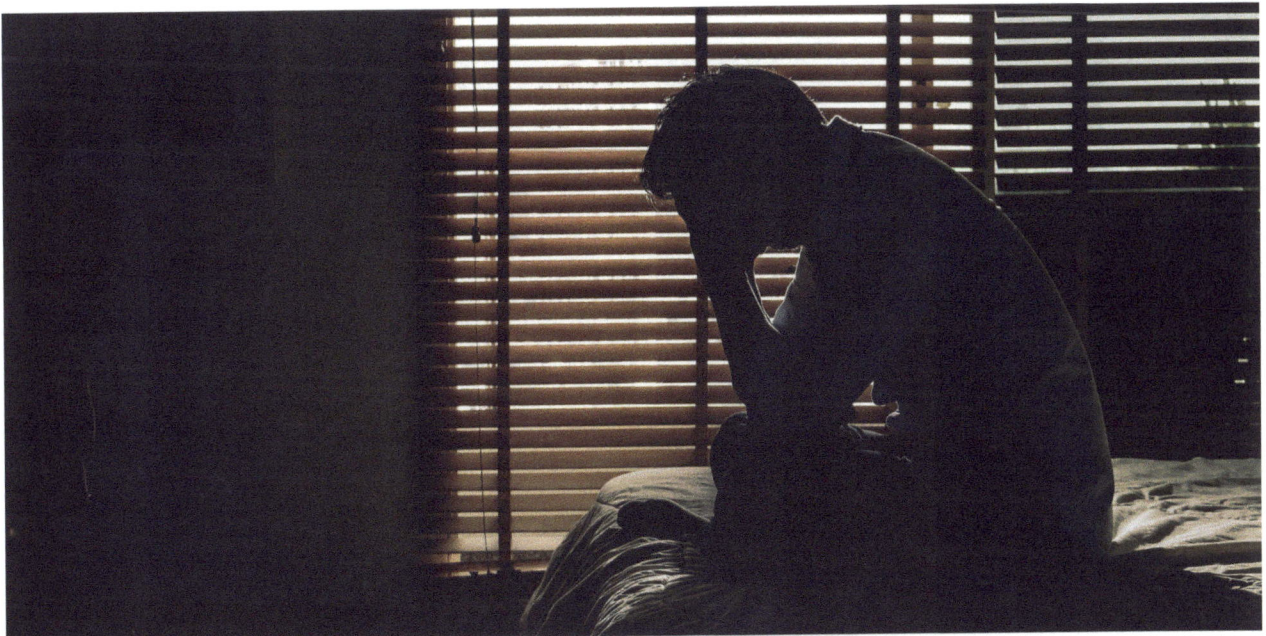

? WHAT'S THE FIRST REMEDY YOU THINK OF WHEN...

1. Dry hair or skin is violently itchy at night. The itchy spots can bleed and feel hot after itching.

2. There is an erection that is lacking despite sexual desire or there is premature ejaculation when sexually aroused.

3. There is benign enlargement of the prostate and the genitals feel numb with a difficulty in retaining urine.

4. There are intolerable spasms before, during and after urination along with violent burning. The urine is released drop by drop.

5. Hemorrhoids that are large, painful and protruding are aggravated by straining during bowel movements.

6. The scalp oozes honey-like sticky yellow discharge. The itching is aggravated by heat. The skin is often crusty with scales.

7. Enlargement of the prostate, without any pain, has an irregular shape. There can be anxiety and restlessness accompanying this condition.

8. There are achy, painful hemorrhoids that may bleed with stool that is large, hard and difficult to pass.

9. There is soreness around the tip of the penis and some sore white patches on the skin that cause pain.

10. Urethritis comes on after sexual relations with burning in the urethra when not urinating.

11. Having strong sexual desire produces a feeble erection or having irresistible desire with premature ejaculation.

12. There is a period of great stress accompanied by a cottage cheese-like discharge from the penis.

Answer Key on page 324.

CHAPTER 15
Female Issues

Women experience unique health considerations and challenges throughout their lives. From adolescence to menopause and beyond, females navigate a myriad of biological, hormonal, and societal factors that influence their overall health. Addressing women's health issues involves understanding the complex events of a woman's life including menstruation, urinary and vaginal infections, pregnancy issues and menopause, interpersonal relations and sexual health. This chapter will share some of the specific issues females experience at different stages of their lives and some homeopathic remedies that can help with them.

MENSTRUATION ISSUES

Menstruation, also called menses, is a monthly event for females, starting at about 12 years old and continuing until she reaches menopause, typically in her 50s. The uterus goes through changes each month, setting up ovulation (the monthly creation of an egg in the ovary) while the inner lining of the uterus thickens in preparation for potential pregnancy. When there is no pregnancy, the lining of the uterus discharges with a flow of blood and tissue that exits through the vagina.

A typical female now averages about 450 menstrual periods in her life, for a total of about 3500 days of flow. A menstrual period typically releases up to half a cup of blood over a three- to five-day period, recurring every 28-30 days. For many women, these periods appear regularly without difficulty, but a variety of difficulties can occur and homeopathy can help when they do. Each woman will have her own pattern of menstrual symptoms. Through matching that pattern to a homeopathic remedy, she can support all aspects of her menstruation.

Where some difficulties can arise:

- **Premenstrual Syndrome (also called PMS)**: As many as three out of four women report some type of discomfort in the 7-10 days before their menstrual period, including but not limited to fatigue, emotional moodiness, headaches, bloating, backache, constipation or diarrhea, food cravings and/or sleep disturbances. About 5% of women —primarily in their 30's—are likely to experience intense and disruptive symptoms preventing them from carrying out normal daily and work activities in the days before or during her period.

- **Irregular Periods**: A usual menstrual cycle—calculated from the first day to the next first day of the period—is an average of 28 days with the range being between 21-35 days, or up to 45 days in teens who are still developing a menstrual rhythm. Up to 25% of women report that their cycles are irregular, too short, too long, or inconsistent in their occurrence. The menstrual cycle can be affected by stress, medications, body weight, and interactions with other menstruating women. Menstrual synchrony was coined in 1971 by Martha McClintock, a University of Chicago psychologist, who had observed during her undergraduate days that close friends living in the same dorm tended to get their periods at the same time.

- **Painful Periods**: Painful periods are a common complaint affecting more than eight out of 10 women at some time in their lives. About 43% of women report pain with periods some of the time and another 41% of women experience pain with every period. Interestingly, menstrual periods are statistically heavier, longer, and more painful during cold winter months. Menstrual pain can appear before, during, or even after the actual flow. Other symptoms such as constipation or diarrhea may also appear. Women who have recently had an intrauterine device (IUD) placed for contraception may have a few periods with increased pain as they adapt to its presence. Although they don't get periods from hormonal IUDs, the ovary still cycles regularly, indicated by premenstrual cyclical breast tenderness.

• **Heavy Periods**: Excessive menstrual bleeding is experienced by one in five women. The menstrual flow is so heavy that they are not able to maintain usual activities because there is so much blood loss. Excessive flow soaks through one or more heavy sanitary pads or tampons per hour, for multiple hours. It is common for these women to use double protection to prevent accidents (using both a tampon or cup and a pad to prevent leaking). Women who bleed heavily or for longer than a week are at risk of anemia, a lack of iron and the related symptoms of fatigue and weariness.

• **Missing Periods**: Some women may miss their period(s) completely from not ovulating regularly (commonly called poly cystic ovarian syndrome or PCOS). They may menstruate only at every second or third cycle or perhaps only a few times per year. Women with very low body fat, such as athletes or women with eating disorders, may find that their cycle stops until a greater body weight can be maintained. Some women find that their menstrual cycles do not re-establish after they have used a contraceptive that stops the periods for a time.

ADDITIONAL SUPPORT FOR MENSTRUATION ISSUES

Good self-care can help improve one's menstrual health and and minimize symptoms:
• Be mindful of one's diet: Coffee, alcohol, and tobacco can aggravate symptoms and are best avoided. Increase intake of water while staying away from salty foods, even though they may be craved, as excess salt can dehydrate a woman which increases uterine cramping. Eating regular meals of lean protein can reduce cravings in the days leading up to and during the period. Add extra fiber to reduce bloating and support digestion.
• Heat can be a nice friend: Hot showers, heating pads, and hot drinks often ease menstrual pain. Hot baths with a handful of Epsom salts can also bring relief.
• Exercise is known to reduce the stress that may cause menstrual pain. Physical activity helps your blood circulation and the release of "feel-good hormones" called endorphins. The combination of exercise and heat together can be more effective than common over-the-counter pain tablets such as acetaminophen or ibuprofen.
• Sleep! Create a regular nighttime schedule around the menstrual period. Sleeping on either side is a way to reduce pressure on the abdominal muscles. Pulling knees up to the chest can also bring additional comfort and warmth.

WHEN TO CONTACT YOUR HEALTHCARE PROFESSIONAL

• Persistent menstrual irregularity or severe pain can be a symptom of more complicated ailments, such as polycystic ovaries or endometriosis.
• Periods that do not resume after contraception removal may suggest an ongoing effect on the hormonal system from the birth control method used.
• Women who experience heavy bleeding or normal bleeding over a longer time should check with their health care practitioner to ensure that they are not anemic.

The remedies on the following chart can help with the array of symptoms related to one's menstruation issues. Each woman's particular way of feeling menstrual pain is important in helping to select the best matching remedy. For example, menstrual pain may be felt in the abdomen or back, left or right side, down the legs, or around the belly button, before or during the flow—all specifics identifying a unique pattern for each woman.

COMMON REMEDIES FOR MENSTRUATION ISSUES

	Belladonna	Gelsemium	Nux vomica	Pulsatilla	Sepia
Onset	Pain worse before period starts. Headaches before onset. Sudden and violent onset.	Periods are late and scanty, preceded by a congestive headache, vomiting, dark red face.	Periods always arrive too early, always irregular.	Irregular. Sensation of band around throat just before menses.	Menses too late or too early, too scanty or too profuse.
Symptoms	Skin hot and flushed. Bright red blood with clots. Bearing down sensation in uterus when sitting bent forward. Cramping in tail bone area before menses. HEAVY flow.	Uterus feels as if squeezed by a hand. Cramping extends to back and hips.	Pain in sacrum and urging to pass stool. Cramps spread over whole body. Nausea in the morning with chilliness. Pain extends deep into the pelvis before menses.	Bearing down sensation worse lying down. Clotted blood. Intermittent or scanty flow. Changeable menses. Nausea and vomiting. Chilliness.	Menses appears in the morning. Sometimes other symptoms include toothache, headache, nose bleed and limb pain. HEAVY flow.
Mood	Excitable. Sudden flares of anger.	Weakness on all levels. Anticipatory anxiety. Reacts strongly to fright, bad news, or excitement.	Irritable. Impatient. Easily offended. Never feels finished (e.g., work, stool, urinating).	Sadness and weeping before menses. Nervous and excitable during menses. Restless and sleepless at night. Wants affection and consolation.	Sadness and weeping often without knowing why. Indifference to loved ones.
Indications	Violent bearing down sensation in low back and thighs. Worse lying down, better standing and sitting erect. Menses offensive and feels hot.	Thirstless. Scanty flow. Sore throat or difficulty talking.	Prolonged periods, blood is dark or black. Feels like she will faint in a warm room. Cramping causes her to double up and cry. Must stay in bed. Pain extends into umbilicus and stomach causing strong nausea. Menses can return at full moon.	Chilliness before and during menses with yawning and stretching. Periods do not resume after stopping contraceptive use.	Bearing down sensation, worse standing. Indicated after child stops nursing and still no menstruation in mother. Itching eruptions on chin, cheeks, and temples before scanty menses. Uterine prolapse.
Worse	Sitting bent forward. Walking. Early morning. Head is sensitive to drafts. Jarring movement. Being touched. Company.	Motion. Walking.	Cold. Dry and windy weather. Early morning (unrefreshed, irritable, depressed, pains worse).	Before menses. When discharge is most profuse there is the most pain. Catching cold.	Before, during, and after menses. Coition. Acne, worse before menses.
Better	Pains ameliorated by pressure. Lying on abdomen. Sitting erect. Cold applications. Eating before menses. Rocking back and forth. Expelling clots.	Sharp pain better with hot applications. Profuse urination.	Heat.	Consolation. Warmth.	Hot applications. Warm bed. Being alone.

Dosing: Use the BLUE Method. Observe and evaluate.

MENSTRUAL CRAMPS — DYSMENORRHEA

Dysmenorrhea, also known as menstrual cramping, produces muscular contractions of the uterus due to fluctuating hormonal levels. The pains can be mild or intense, shooting, radiating to other parts of the body, or just on one side and can occur before, during, or at the end of the period.

In severe cases, dysmenorrhea symptoms can include headache, dizziness, nausea, vomiting, diarrhea, back pain and fatigue. Any of these symptoms can start prior to the onset of menstruation and can continue during and after the cycle is complete. Dysmenorrhea can interfere with school, sports, and other daily activities.

When trying to find a good remedy, take a menstrual history.

Ask the following questions:

- At what age did the periods start (also known as menarche)?

- How long does menstrual bleeding last?

- Is bleeding light or heavy? What's the color of the blood clots?

- What is the interval between periods? (This is measured from the first day of one period to the first day of the following period).

Here are symptoms to look for:

- Where are the cramps? Ask her to point where they are.

- Do the cramps move? From left to right? Front to back? Down the legs?

- How long do the cramps last?

- Is there a time of day they feel worse? Morning, afternoon, night? All day?

- What makes the cramps feel better or worse?

- Do the cramps change into something else?

- Do the symptoms impact school or work?

- Are other symptoms present that accompany the cramping pains? Nausea, vomiting, diarrhea, back pain, etc.

WHEN TO CONTACT YOUR HEALTHCARE PROFESSIONAL

- If there is abnormal uterine bleeding, anemia and iron deficiency, scoliosis, and/or depression.
- If there is severe cramping from the onset or if severe cramping continues.
- If there is severe cramping month after month with no relief.

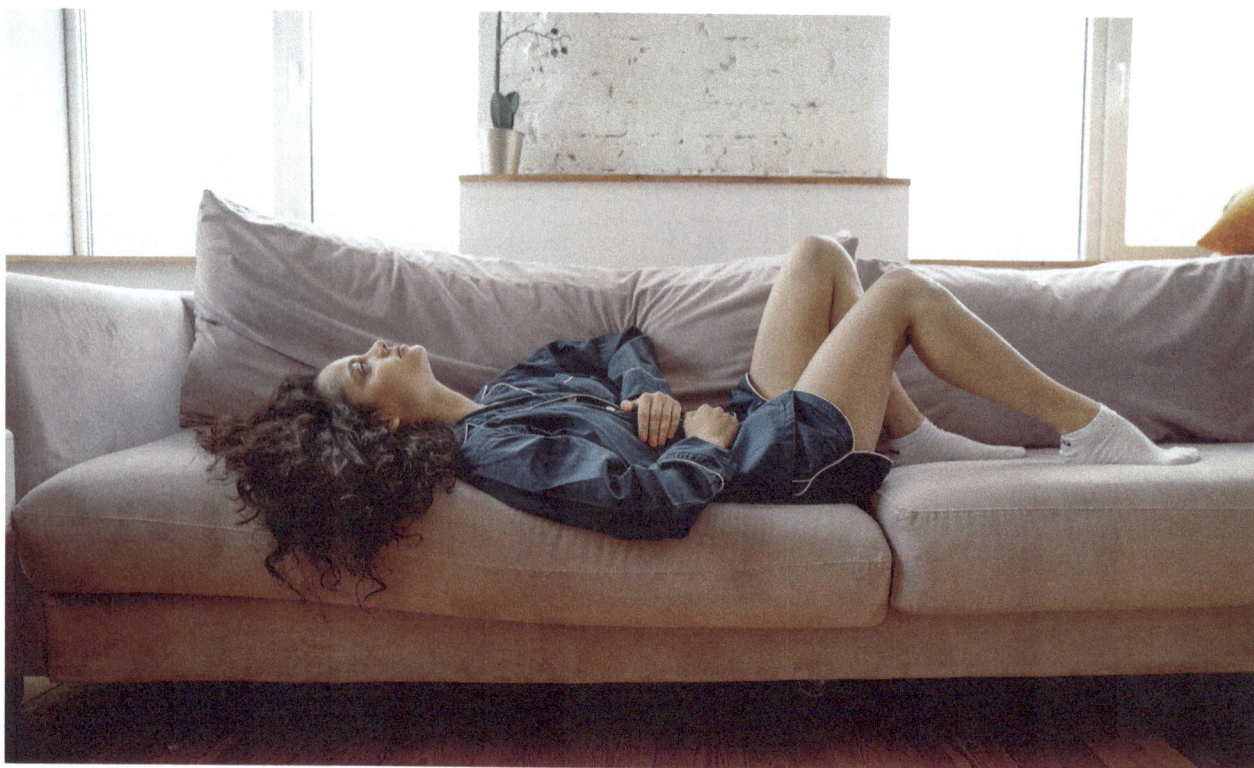

COMMON REMEDIES FOR DYSMENORRHEA

	Belladonna	*Colocynthis	Magnesium phos	Nux vomica	Pulsatilla	Sepia
Onset	Pain worse before period starts.	Pains worse before the flow starts.	Pain worse before period starts or at start of menses.	Periods always arrive too early, always irregular.	Irregular. Sensation of band around throat just before menses.	Menses too late or too early, too scanty or too profuse.
Symptoms	Skin hot and flushed. Bright red blood. Bearing down sensation in uterus when sitting bent forward. Cramping in tail bone before menses.	Pain boring into and bearing-down in the ovarian area, coming in waves. Usually heavy flow. Wants to be doubled up and press something hard into pelvic area like a chair. Intense pain may cause vomiting.	Crampy pains, darting, like lightning, shooting. Pains over entire pelvis, sharp pains in both ovaries and small of back, can feel womb contract and force out blood.	Pain in sacrum with urge to pass stool. Cramps spread over the whole body. Nausea in the morning with chilliness. Pain extends deep into the pelvis before menses.	Bearing down sensation, worse lying down. Clotted, intermittent, changeable menses. Scanty periods, nausea, vomiting, chilliness.	Menses comes in the morning. Sometimes toothache, headache, nose bleed, and limb pain accompany.
Mood	Excitable. Sudden flares of temper.	Pains brought on by intense anger. Feelings easily hurt. May become angered when asked questions.	Lamenting about pain. Inability to think clearly.	Irritable. Impatient. Mean. Easily offended. Never feels finished (work, stool, urinating).	Sadness and weeping before menses. During menses nervous and excitable. At night restless and sleepless. Wants affection and consolation.	Sadness and weeping often without knowing why. Indifference to loved ones.
Indications	Violent bearing down which is worse lying down, better standing and sitting erect. Menses very offensive and feels hot.	Restless, easily offended, extremely irritable, irritated by the pains, indignant.	Intermittent pain precedes flow and/ or at start of menses. Period flow could come too early.	Prolonged periods, blood black, feels as if will faint in warm room. Cramping causes her to double up and cry, must stay in bed. Pain extends into umbilicus and stomach causing strong nausea. Menses can return at full moon.	Chilliness before and during menses with yawning and stretching.	Bearing down feeling. Indicated after child stops nursing and still no menstruation. Itchy eruptions on chin, cheeks, and temples before scanty menses.
Worse	Sitting bent, walking. Early morning. Being jarred, touched, company.	Anger, feeling indignant, drafts, getting chilled, evening, nighttime, eating, and drinking.	Right side. After coition (sexual relations).	Cold. Dry and windy weather. Early morning (unrefreshed, irritable, depressed, pains worse).	Before menses. Pain is greatest when discharge is most profuse.	Before, during, and after menses. Coition. Acne. Standing. Before menses.
Better	Pressure. Lying on abdomen. Sitting erect. Cold applications. Eating before menses. Rocking back and forth.	Beginning of flow, pressure, heat, lying doubled up or on painful side, rest, gentle motion, a bowel movement, and passing gas.	Heat. Flow of period. Warm drinks. Bending double.	Heat.	Heavy pressure, open air, gentle motion.	Hot applications. Warm bed.

Dosing: Use the **BLUE** Method. Observe and evaluate.

Urinary Tract Infections

Though Urinary Tract Infections (UTI) are discussed in **Chapter 13** starting on **page 143,** women tend to get more of them because of sexual relations, bathroom habits, menopause, perfumed products and more, hence the need to include this additional information. Up to 60% of women worldwide experience urinary tract symptoms at least once during their lifetime.

Urinary tract infections can often result in symptoms such as pain and/or burning before, during or after urinating, increased urgency and frequency of going to the bathroom, and cloudy or unusually smelly urine. The average woman urinates six to eight times a day. If there is a local infection, excessive withholding, long-term use of some prescription medications or other issue that prevents the bladder from emptying properly, UTI symptoms can occur. Homeopathy is a useful ally for urinary symptoms and can help to restore balance.

♡ ADDITIONAL SUPPORT FOR URINARY TRACT INFECTIONS

There are good ways to support a healthy urinary tract, repair problems, and prevent their recurrence:
- Drink plenty of water, double than what you normally drink when having symptoms. Water will be metabolized more efficiently if it contains a little fruit like a lemon slice or a bit of melon, a grain of sea salt, or a small spoonful of apple cider vinegar. Other drinks such as tulsi tea and ginger tea (without sugar added) have all been shown to improve urinary health.
- Temporarily eliminate (or severely reduce) coffee, black or green tea, alcohol , chocolate and seltzers as they can continue to "piss off" an infected bladder.
- Take a D-Mannose supplement. It comes in powder or capsule form. It interferes with the ability of bacteria to attach to the wall of the bladder or urethra, relieving symptoms of irritation. Follow directions on the product label.
- Take a cranberry supplement to discourage bacterial growth in the urinary tract. Follow the directions on the product label. Drink diluted cranberry juice (full strength has a lot of unnecessary sugar) by adding a few splashes of cranberry juice to water or drink unsweetened cranberry juice full strength. You can also add cranberry extract to water.
- Include more probiotics in the diet: either as a nutritional supplement several times a day during an infection and/or consuming more probiotic-rich foods including kefir, yogurt, sauerkraut, kimchi, and naturally-fermented pickles to help boost the beneficial bacteria.

💡 OTHER IDEAS FOR PREVENTING URINARY TRACT INFECTIONS

- Always wiping your bottom from front to back after urinating to avoid bacteria on the genitals.
- Emptying your bladder as soon as possible, especially after having sexual relations.
- Avoid using anything perfumed or containing dyes, i.e., bubble bath, soap, or powder around your genitals.
- Taking a shower instead of a bath.
- Urinate as soon as you feel the urge, don't hold it in.
- Avoid using a diaphragm for contraception—find an alternative.
- Wearing underwear made from cotton (instead of synthetic material such as nylon) and not wearing tight pants.

WHEN TO CONTACT YOUR HEALTHCARE PROFESSIONAL

- If there is back pain with the urinary issues.
- If there is a high fever with chills with the urinary issues.
- If experiencing nausea and vomiting with urinary issues.
- If you see blood in the urine.
- If you have more than two per year.

COMMON REMEDIES FOR URINARY TRACT INFECTIONS

	Apis	Cantharis	*Causticum	Pulsatilla	*Sarsaparilla	Staphysagria
Onset	Ailments from fright, rage, bad news, anger.	Quick onset symptoms tend to progress rapidly.	After childbirth. When circumstances require a delay in urinating.	Feeling forsaken. Retention of urine after childbirth.	From vexation. Some experts recommend this as the most common choice for cystitis.	After sexual activity (known as honeymoon cystitis), pelvic examination, operation, labor, episode of marked anger, humiliation or violation.
Sensation and Appearance	Difficulty passing urine, incomplete. Hot urine passed drop by drop, burning the skin. Strong color and odor. Swelling of genitals.	Urgency, frequency, intense burning. Urine passes in drops. Inflammation can cause feelings of arousal. Violent burning pain, razor-like or scalding.	Frequent urging. Involuntary dribbling during coughing or sneezing. Difficulty voiding urine if retained too long.	Spasms of bladder after urination. Urine in dribbles, involuntary urination with walking, sneezing, coughing, or laughing. May be weepy and want consolation. Burning in urethra during and after urination.	Frequent urging. May have a spasm at the close of urination—cries out with pain. Urine scanty, sandy and sometimes bloody.	Frequent urging, though urination may be constricted, passing slowly. Pain is felt during and after urination with burning in the urethra.
Worse	Warmth of any kind.	Start of and after urination. Any movement. Seeing running water. Coffee.	Becoming cold. After childbirth.	Lying down, especially on the back, causes desire to urinate.	Sitting can bring on slight dribbling of urine. Before menstrual period.	After sex. During urination. Burning after urination. Walking, riding. Cold.
Better	Cold applications, even ice.	Rest, laying down. Warmth.	Warm applications. Cold drinks.	Cold applications. Open air.	Urinating when standing.	Lying curled up on the side. Rest. Heat.

Dosing: Use the **BLUE** Method. Observe and evaluate.

Yeast Infection

*Also see **Yeast Infections** in **Chapter 13—Urinary Issues** on **page 145**.*

Yeast infections are a form of vaginitis. Women tend to get more of them than men for many reasons including sexual intercourse, bathroom issues, perfumed products, over consumption of sugar, tampon use, contraceptives and more. It includes bothersome symptoms including intense vaginal itching, burning, irritation, and discharge. The cause is usually a change in the balance of vaginal bacteria. If you have a yeast infection, be aware that your partner may have one also. Therefore, your partner should consider treatment as well. The body contains millions of microbes which are tiny living things unseen by the naked eye. The vagina contains microbes, similar to those that live in the gut, mouth, or sinuses. When the microbes that live in these places become overrun by unfriendly bacteria, infections occur. One of the most common microflora imbalances found in the vaginal area is called candida, a form of yeast. When candida overruns a healthy microbiome, the result is often a "yeast infection."

Interesting to note that vaginal candida does not generally occur without estrogen so young girls who haven't menstruated yet and older menopausal women typically do not get vaginitis.

It's important to be aware of some of the factors that can increase the tendency for yeast infections:

- antibiotics, birth control pills, and certain steroids

- high sugar and/or alcohol intake

- a weakened immune system

- unmanaged diabetes

- sexually transmitted diseases

- obesity

- contraceptives

- frequent use of antibiotics

- pregnancy

- stress

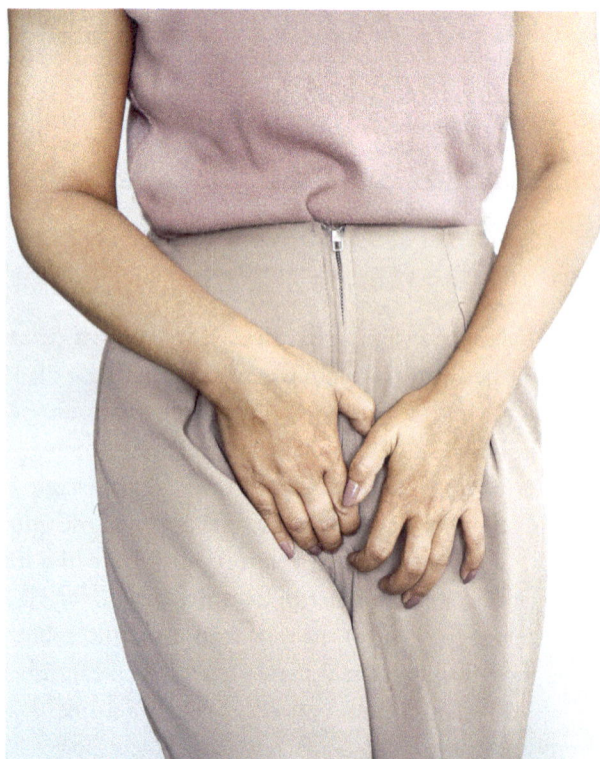

For women, some indicators of a yeast infection include:

- itching and irritation in the vagina and vulva

- a burning or itching sensation, especially during intercourse or while urinating

- thick, white, and possibly odorous vaginal discharge with a cottage cheese appearance

- redness and swelling of the vulva

- watery vaginal discharge

- history of other candida infections

ADDITIONAL SUPPORT FOR YEAST INFECTIONS (For Women)

- Take a good probiotic several times a day during and a few weeks after the infection.
- Include more probiotic rich foods in your diet including kefir, yogurt, sauerkraut, kimchi, and naturally-fermented pickles to help boost the beneficial bacteria.
- Candida (yeast) feeds on sugar and yeast so it's recommended to reduce or eliminate both in your diet for a few weeks. If you're prone to getting frequent yeast infections, review your diet and continue to reduce or eliminate them both.
- Avoid wearing any thong underwear and any other underwear with synthetic fabric against the vaginal opening; cotton is best.
- Change out of a wet bathing suit, stretchy workout clothes, or yoga pants after exercising.
- Make your own douche rinse with a quart of lukewarm water and add two tablespoons of apple cider vinegar OR a probiotic capsule. Avoid over-the-counter douches, as they contain strong chemicals that affect the vaginal tissues, including irritating perfumes and dyes.
- Use condoms without spermicides, at least until normal balance has returned. Contraceptive spermicidal condoms, spermicidal creams, or gels can disrupt tender tissues.
- During menstrual flow, only use sanitary pads.

For Extra Support: Help the vaginal tissues repair the microflora imbalance by using these options for up to a week at a time, discontinuing when symptoms have improved.

- One option is to swab the vaginal interior with a tablespoon of plain yogurt (unsweetened, unflavored, with active cultures) at room temperature each morning and evening for up to a week. This is a natural probiotic that supports healthy microbial balance.
- Another option is to insert a small tampon that has been coated with **calendula oil** (be sure to use OIL, not a tincture, which contains alcohol that can burn tissues) before bed at night and remove it in the morning. **Calendula** inhibits the reproduction of troublesome microbes, helping to clear the problem. These supports are also useful if a woman is taking antibiotics for any reason.

WHEN TO CONTACT YOUR HEALTHCARE PROFESSIONAL

- If there is intense discomfort or a strong, foul odor.
- If the person has a high fever, chills, upset stomach, and headache with the infection.
- If the person has a hard time urinating.
- If the person gets frequent yeast infections.
- If the condition is not helped by homeopathic remedies.

COMMON REMEDIES FOR YEAST INFECTIONS (Female)

	*Borax	Calcarea carb	Pulsatilla	Sepia	Sulphur	*Thuja
Onset	Appears midway between menstrual periods.	Before menstrual period. Menses too early and profuse.	During pregnancy or with menstrual period. Puberty or perimenopause.	Perimenopausal. Pain on or after intercourse.	Combination of warm moisture, high sugar intake, and/or stress.	From one menstrual period to the next.
Sensation	Burning pains. Feels like warm water running out.	Itching and burning.	May be itching, but usually there is very minimal irritation. Bland discharge that turns acrid. Painless.	Irritation and burning, sensation of swollen tissue. Vagina may feel dry, even with discharge. Sensation of weakness in uterus with bearing down feeling.	Voluptuous itching with burning. Aggravated by warmth and bathing.	Itching. Very sensitive vagina that prevents sex.
Appearance	Egg-white colored discharge. Inflamed, swollen, burning labia.	Milky or white-yellow discharge.	Discharge thick, creamy or milky. Yellowish color.	Yellowish-green or milky discharge. Corrosive and burning.	Red, hot, swollen tissue.	Profuse, thick, greenish discharge.
Odor	Unremarkable.	May have odor like yeast.	Not usually any strong odor.	Has a very unpleasant odor.	Offensive smelling, may be like rotten eggs.	Possibly pungent, sour, sweetish.

Dosing: Use the BLUE Method. Observe and evaluate.

PREGNANCY AND BEYOND

Safe, gentle homeopathy has been the choice of pregnant women worldwide for more than 200 years. It is fantastically effective for keeping moms and babies healthy and for relieving or averting common problems before, during, and after childbirth.

> ### What is a Doula?
>
> *Some new mothers engage the services of a doula. Doulas can perform different roles, depending on your needs:*
> - *Labor or birth doulas provide continuous care during labor.*
> - *Antepartum doulas support women who are put on bed rest to prevent preterm labor. They help with household tasks and childcare.*
> - *Postpartum doulas support the new mom during the first few weeks after birth. They help with care and feeding of the baby and household tasks.*

MORNING SICKNESS

Most women experience some degree of morning sickness during the first trimester of pregnancy due to hormonal changes and/or poor nutritional choices. Morning sickness, despite its name, can be experienced at any time of day. The symptoms of morning sickness are nausea with or without vomiting.

ADDITIONAL SUPPORT FOR MORNING SICKNESS

- Try eating a dry cracker before getting out of bed.
- Avoid rich, high-fat foods.
- Eat small, frequent high protein and fat meals to keep blood sugar stable.
- If the nausea is worse when hungry, eat frequently but in small amounts.
- Make some homemade limeade: water, salt, sugar and fresh lime juice with the lime rind is the best way to hydrate.

WHEN TO CONTACT YOUR HEALTHCARE PROFESSIONAL

- For some women, morning sickness can be severe and can lead to dehydration. If she has been unable to keep down any fluids and hasn't urinated for eight hours, seek medical attention.

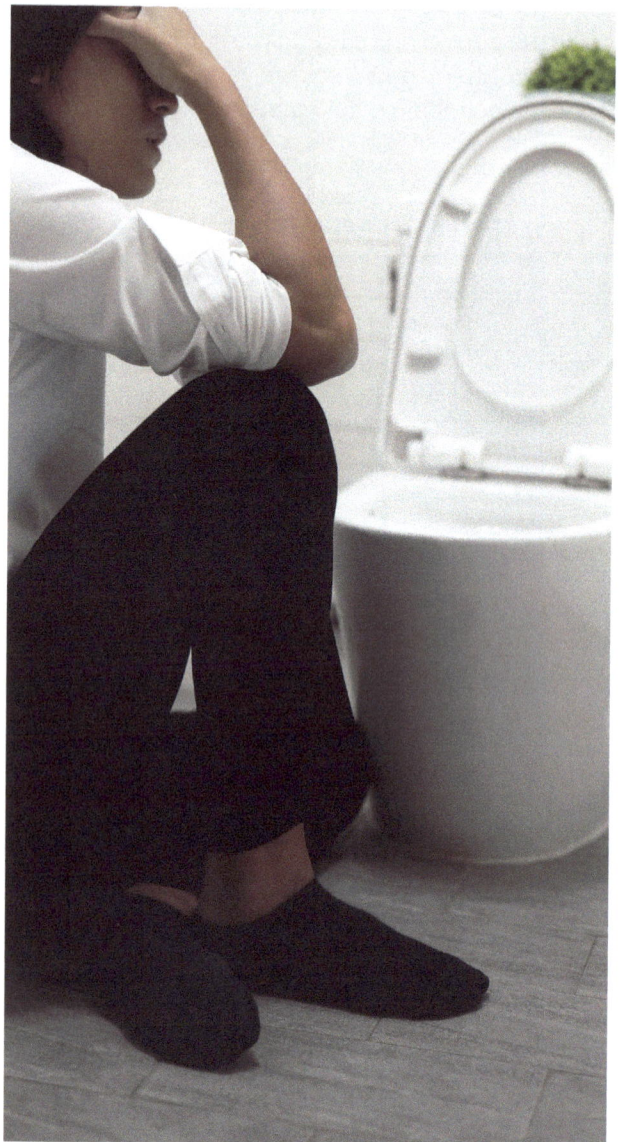

COMMON REMEDIES FOR MORNING SICKNESS

	*Colchicum	Ipecac	Nux vomica	Pulsatilla	Sepia
Onset	First trimester.	First trimester.	First trimester.	First trimester.	First trimester.
Symptoms	Nausea and retching which can last all day.	Severe, constant nausea which is not relieved by vomiting.	Strong nausea especially on waking.	Nausea.	A sinking feeling in the stomach that makes her feel faint.
Mood	Sad, irritable, fretful.	Dejected, whiny.	Irritable.	Weepy with changeable moods.	Indifferent to loved ones. Irritable or moody.
Indications	Very sensitive to food. Wants carbonated drinks. Can have painful abdominal distention from gas.	Salivates profusely and may have to spit frequently. Can experience a feeling of the stomach hanging loosely. Can be accompanied by headache.	Unable to vomit. Great hunger. Over-sensitive to noise and light.	May also complain of headaches above the eyes.	Craves vinegar and pickles, as well as sweets. Has a sensation of heaviness or sagging in the pelvis.
Worse	Smelling or even the thought of food, especially eggs or fish. Stretching out the legs. Motion.	Smell or thought of food.	Feels worse after eating, with indigestion and cramping.	Warm, stuffy room. Rich, sweet, or fatty food.	Smell and thought of food.
Better	Lying with knees drawn up.	Open air. Drinking.	Being in a dark, quiet space.	Walking slowly in the open air.	Eating may relieve, but only temporarily. Better for exercise.

Important note: The remedy **Ipecac** is homeopathically prepared and is NOT interchangeable with the common drugstore *Ipecac* used to induce vomiting.

Special Dosing Instructions: If symptoms are only in the morning, take a dose of the chosen remedy before getting out of bed. Do this for three days and then repeat only if symptoms return. If symptoms are throughout the day and more severe, such as vomiting, take a dose every two to four hours, depending on the severity. Observe and evaluate.

HEARTBURN

Heartburn is one of the most common complaints of pregnant women. This is because hormonal changes relax the esophagus, allowing acid to back up, and the growing baby pressing against the stomach.

ADDITIONAL SUPPORT FOR HEARTBURN IN PREGNANCY

- Avoid or eliminate these foods: citrus, spicy, fatty (especially fried or greasy) foods, caffeine, and carbonated drinks
- Eat some yogurt or have some milk with honey.
- Sleep with head and shoulders elevated.
- Ginger tea can be helpful if it is drunk before or during a meal, rather than when heartburn actually occurs.
- Try drinking a glass of water or have a cup of licorice tea as they can also help when heartburn occurs.

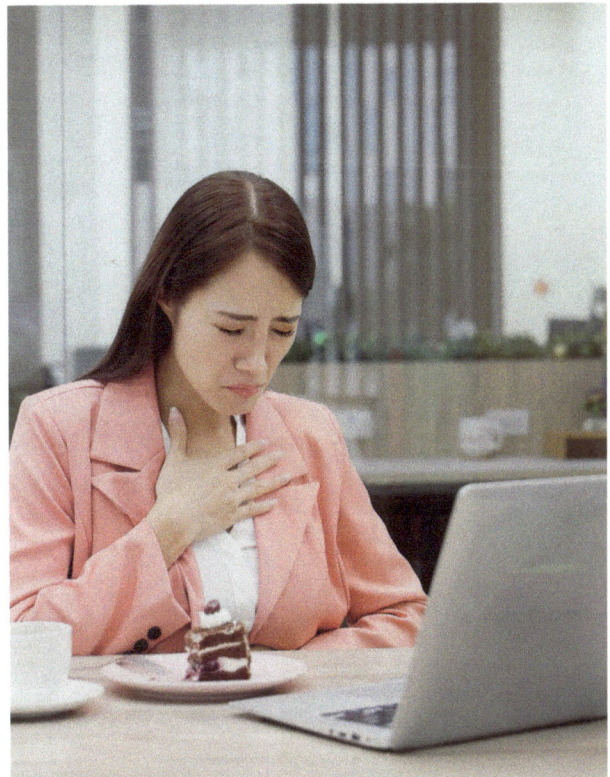

Two most common remedies for heartburn during pregnancy include:

- **Pulsatilla**: Heartburn comes on at different times of the day and after eating various kinds of foods (especially rich, greasy ones). Burps have a sour, bitter taste. The stomach and abdomen feel empty, with gurgling and rumbling in the evening, and pressing pains. The woman feels better in the fresh air (See *Morning Sickness* chart on the previous page).

- **Carbo veg**: Bitter, sour, rancid burping along with nausea and a very bloated abdomen are typical; burping gives temporary relief. She may feel worse after rich, high-fat food. She craves fresh air and wants the windows open and fans turned on. She feels physically exhausted and mentally sluggish, but when she lies down the indigestion is worse. She tends to have cold hands and feet and varicose veins.

Dosing: Use the BLUE Method.
Observe and evaluate.

*Read more about **Heartburn** in **Chapter 11—Stomach** on **page 127**.*

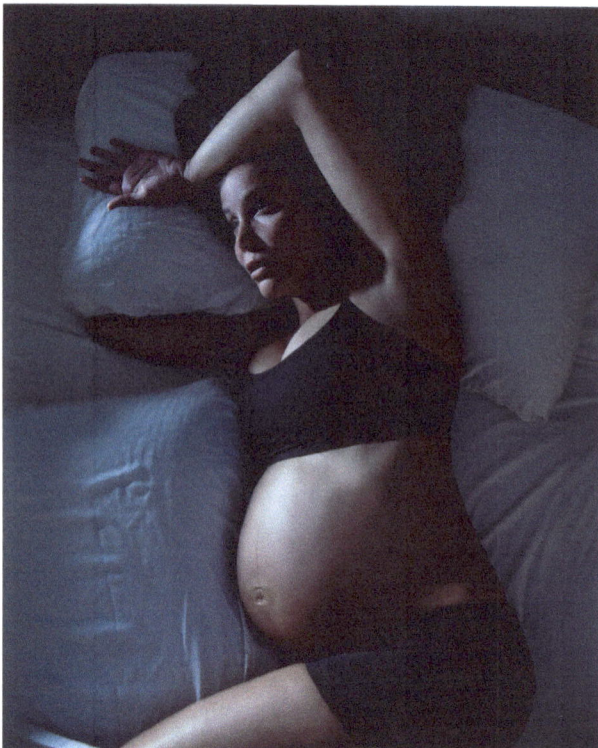

HEMORRHOIDS AND CONSTIPATION

Hormonal changes that relax the muscles of the pelvis in preparation for labor can slow down digestion, while the growing uterus puts pressure on other organs and veins. This can make an expectant mother prone to constipation and hemorrhoids.

*See more and compare remedies about **Constipation and Hemorrhoids** in **Chapter 12—Stool Issues** starting on **page 137**.*

BACKACHE AND LIGAMENT PAIN

*See **Chapter 16—Back and Neck** on **page 177**.*

INSOMNIA in Pregnancy

During the early stages of pregnancy, changing hormone levels may contribute to insomnia. During the last trimester, discomfort from the growing baby, increased urination, and anticipation of the birth may keep an expectant mother awake at night.

- ***Coffea**: The woman can't sleep because she's excited and euphoric—or she's uptight and extremely sensitive to the slightest pain. All her senses are very acute, and she wakes at the slightest sound. Her mind is overactive, and her dreams are vivid. She is anxious, energetic, and very tired at the same time—much like someone who drank too much coffee.

- **Aconite**: The mother to-be is having a lot of fears, the biggest being that she will die in labor. She is restless in sleep with vivid, frightening dreams.

Special Dosing: Take the chosen remedy one hour before bedtime and also on waking in the night if needed. If no response after three days, re-evaluate and give a new remedy.

*Read about more options for **Insomnia** in **Chapter 19—Mind and Emotions** on **page 230**.*

A NOTE ABOUT LABOR

The first stage of labor starts with sustained and progressive contractions. The baby is in the uterus, and the cervix is being dilated. The second stage of labor starts when the baby begins the journey into the vagina and ends with birth. The third stage of labor starts when the baby has been born and ends with the expulsion of the placenta.

Homeopathy can be helpful during any of the three stages, especially if the stage does not progress as expected; however, one option is to seek the services of a professional homeopath or a midwife with experience in using homeopathy to be present at this time. Either will know best how to match a laboring woman's specific and fast-changing symptoms to the broader patterns in various remedies.

HEALING AFTER THE BIRTH

Homeopathy works beautifully to speed healing and relieve pain after birth.

COMMON REMEDIES FOR HEALING AFTER BIRTH

	Arnica	*Bellis per	Calendula	Hypericum	*Phytolacca	Staphysagria
Onset	Take as soon as possible after the birth.	Use if Arnica has not helped.	For cuts or incisions incurred from childbirth.	Pain that may follow an episiotomy, a forceps or vacuum delivery, or an epidural or other IV injection.	When breast feeding.	Pain from deep surgical incisions after Cesarean sections or episiotomies.
Symptoms	Feeling bruised all over or bleeding excessively. Violent afterpains.	Deep aching pain and bruised soreness in the pelvis.	Infected wounds and inflamed areas of skin.	Shooting pains. Pain in the tailbone or perineum.	Painful, inflamed, red breasts. Lumps in the breasts. Cracked nipples. May have fever and flu-like symptoms.	Severe pain and sensitivity of the genital organs.
Mood	There may be physical and mental shock. Fears touch.	Impulse to move. Thinking is difficult.	Extremely nervous and easily frightened.	May be sad, restless, or nervous.	May feel depressed and discouraged.	May have feelings of anger, shame, or humiliation from the experience of birth.
Indications	Nervous. Cannot bear pain. Whole body is oversensitive.	Following a Cesarean section, forceps delivery, or similar trauma.	Inflamed areas. For sore, cracked nipples or perineum.	Pain along the path of a nerve.	Mastitis. When child nurses, pain radiates from nipple all over body.	Pain at the surgical site.
Worse	Least touch. Motion.	Hot bath and warmth of bed. Before storms. Cold bathing.	Moving.	Cold and touch.	Cold and dampness.	Loss of fluids.
Better	Lying down.	Continued motion. After eating.	Lying still.	Bending back. Rubbing.	Warmth and rest.	After breakfast. Warmth. Rest at night.

Note: Topical **Calendula cream** or **ointment** can also be applied on clean incisions, available at most health food stores. Avoid the gel version as it may sting.

Dosing: Use the **BLUE** Method. Observe and evaluate.

BREASTFEEDING

Mothers have much to do in caring for their babies; making and delivering healthy milk for them is an important part for those that choose to breastfeed. Consuming a minimum of 1800 calories per day along with adequate water intake will allow the building blocks of nutritious milk. While it is not a requirement, many women choose to continue to take their prenatal vitamins during this time to ensure adequate nutrition.

It is quite normal for a newborn baby to eat every two to three hours around the clock and to spend about seven hours per day eating, whether at the breast or from a bottle. Accepting this as normal will hopefully help with the family's expectations. Breastfeeding mothers need frequent liquid intake in order to keep a healthy supply. Both mother and baby should have some nourishment during each feeding time! You can ask a family member to help by stocking a water bottle and a container of fruit and nut mix on a table by a favorite feeding chair to make this easy.

Making milk takes energy; energy requires rest. New mothers often feel the need to use baby's sleeping times to get things done. At least for the first several weeks, it will help for mom to rest whenever the baby sleeps. Mothers can ask for help in re-prioritizing, limiting visitors, allowing for a daily 'to do list' of eat, sleep, drink, bathe, and take care of the baby.

While all goes well much of the time, the problems that come up can often benefit from help with homeopathy. In the early days of breastfeeding, the nipples can become irritated or cracked. The milk supply may be excessive or too little. Plugged milk ducts can progress into mastitis, an infection in the breast. The breast may become tender, swollen, or hot. There may be a reddened area on the skin. Mastitis can become an issue when a woman is overextended, e.g., lots of visitors and activities or on the initial return to work. Risk factors are extra energy expenditures, a longer time between feedings or pumping, and less attention to hydration. Mastitis needs to be addressed at first indication of symptoms; if unresolved, mastitis can sometimes progress toward the formation of a breast abscess. Homeopathy can be included as part of the plan to help smooth a bumpy road toward healthy breast feeding.

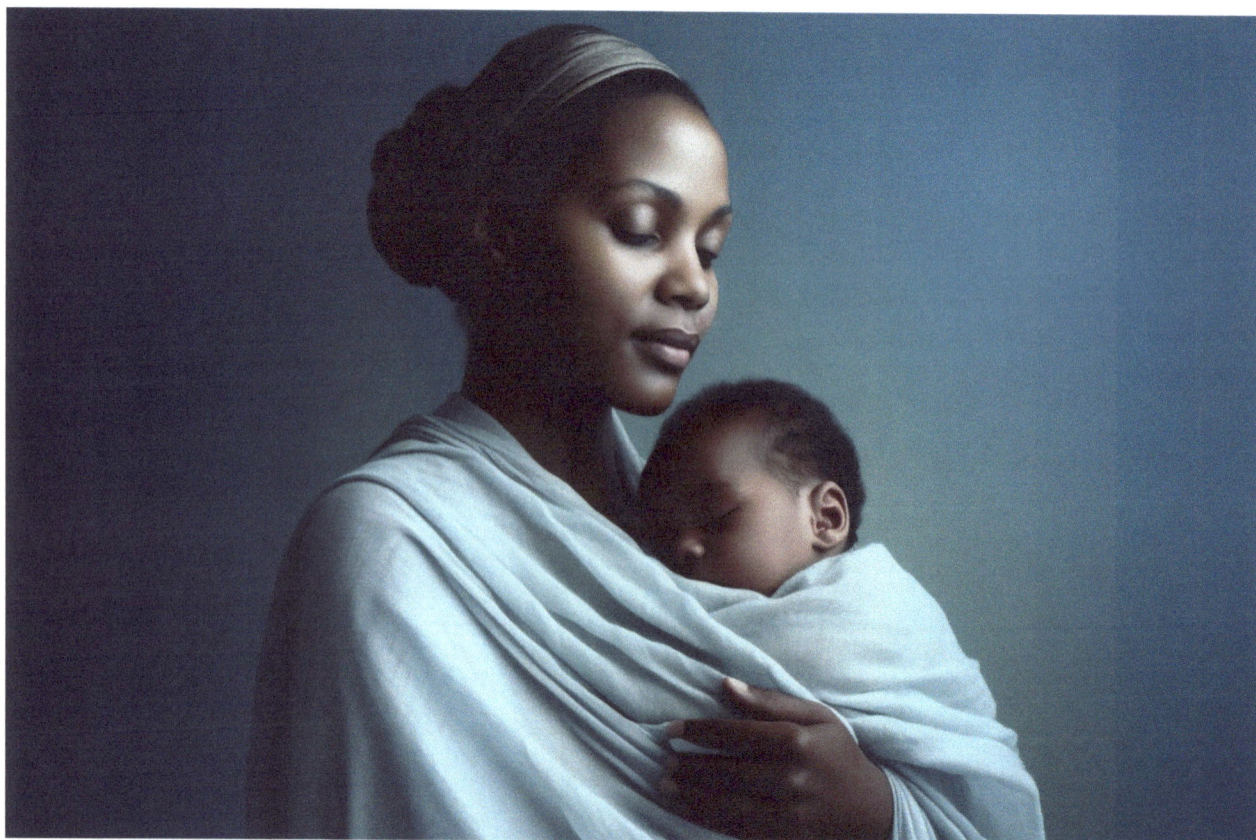

IT'S AN EMERGENCY WHEN

- There is pus and blood in the breast milk.
- There are red streaks on the breasts.

ADDITIONAL SUPPORT FOR BREASTFEEDING

There are several supportive measures that women can use to support healthy breasts and ample milk supply:

- The mom and baby need to get together as a 'nursing couple', which is easier for some and more difficult for others. Take advantage of any offered support by your doctor's office, hospital, delivery center programs, lactation consultant, or postpartum doula to help guide the process. Excellent support can be offered by a local La Leche League chapter. Get help early if there are problems.
- Help each breast to empty by changing the baby's position from one feeding to the next so all areas of the breast are drained. Allow the baby to fully empty one breast before switching to the other.
- Help the nipples to maintain healthy tissue by allowing them to air dry when possible and rubbing a small amount of breast milk onto nipples that are sore, chafed, or cracked. Repeat with each feeding. It is normal for the nipples to be uncomfortable when the baby latches in the first few days of breastfeeding; this feeling will pass. If it is necessary to stop feeding, avoid pulling away abruptly. Instead, first place a finger gently inside the baby's mouth to break the suction with the nipple.
- Any flu-like or 'coming down with something' sensations in a woman who is breastfeeding should be suspected to have mastitis until proven otherwise. This is especially true for women who have recently returned to work. This feeling should be taken seriously with 24 hours of rest, plenty of fluids, and frequent breastfeeding on both breasts. **Ferrum phos 6X** cell salt taken four times per day can help restore balance. If other specific symptoms are present, the remedy chart can help to identify the best remedy choice.
- If a plugged duct forms, massage the breast from the area behind any lump or sore area, moving toward the nipple. Apply heat (hot water bottle/warm compress). Remember that the milk is still safe for the baby to drink. Breastfeed at least every two hours to keep milk flowing and prevent the breast from being overfull.
- Every mother can benefit from reminding herself often that no matter what is happening today, there is sweetness to be treasured in those moments of holding, feeding, and bonding with the baby.

WHEN TO CONTACT YOUR HEALTHCARE PROFESSIONAL, MIDWIFE OR PROFESSIONAL HOMEOPATH

- There are symptoms of mastitis in both breasts, lasting more than 24 hours.

COMMON REMEDIES FOR BREASTFEEDING

	Arnica	Belladonna	Bryonia	*Phytolacca	Pulsatilla
Characteristics	Soreness in the breasts and nipples in the first days of nursing.	Heat, throbbing and redness in plugged duct or mastitis. May follow Bryonia.	Initial feeling of flu or coming down with something may suggest mastitis. Low milk supply.	Breasts overly full, excessive milk supply. Plugged duct. Mastitis.	Useful for helping dry up milk from the breasts during weaning.
Indications	Sensation of tenderness and bruising in the nipples.	Redness in a spot, streak, or region on surface of breast. Aching or burning pain. Heat in breast. Breast may be hard and overfull. Generally feverish. Face may be flushed.	Aching pain in breast. Early stage of mastitis may feel like flu coming on, with aching in joints and muscles. Breast may not yet appear swollen or have lump. Thirsty.	Sore or cracked nipples with fissures. Lump in the breast. Breasts hard, swollen, tender.	Sore or cracked nipples. Mother may weep every time baby is put to the breast.
Worse	Baby's initial latching onto nipple.	Bumping or jarring to the breast, as from stepping. Sensitive to light, sound.	Motion. Consolation.	When child nurses, mother nearly goes into spasms of pain that extend down the back and limbs and all over body.	When baby latches to the breast, pain extends from nipple through breast to the entire body.
Better	Uncovering nipples in open air. Cool compress.	Lightly wrapped up.	Remaining still.	Supporting the breasts. Applying pressure with the hand.	Cold application.

Dosing: Use the **BLUE** Method. Observe and evaluate. The trio of remedies **Bryonia, Belladonna** and ***Phytolacca** can also be taken in alternation with each other. Always observe and re-evaluate if there is no response after several doses.

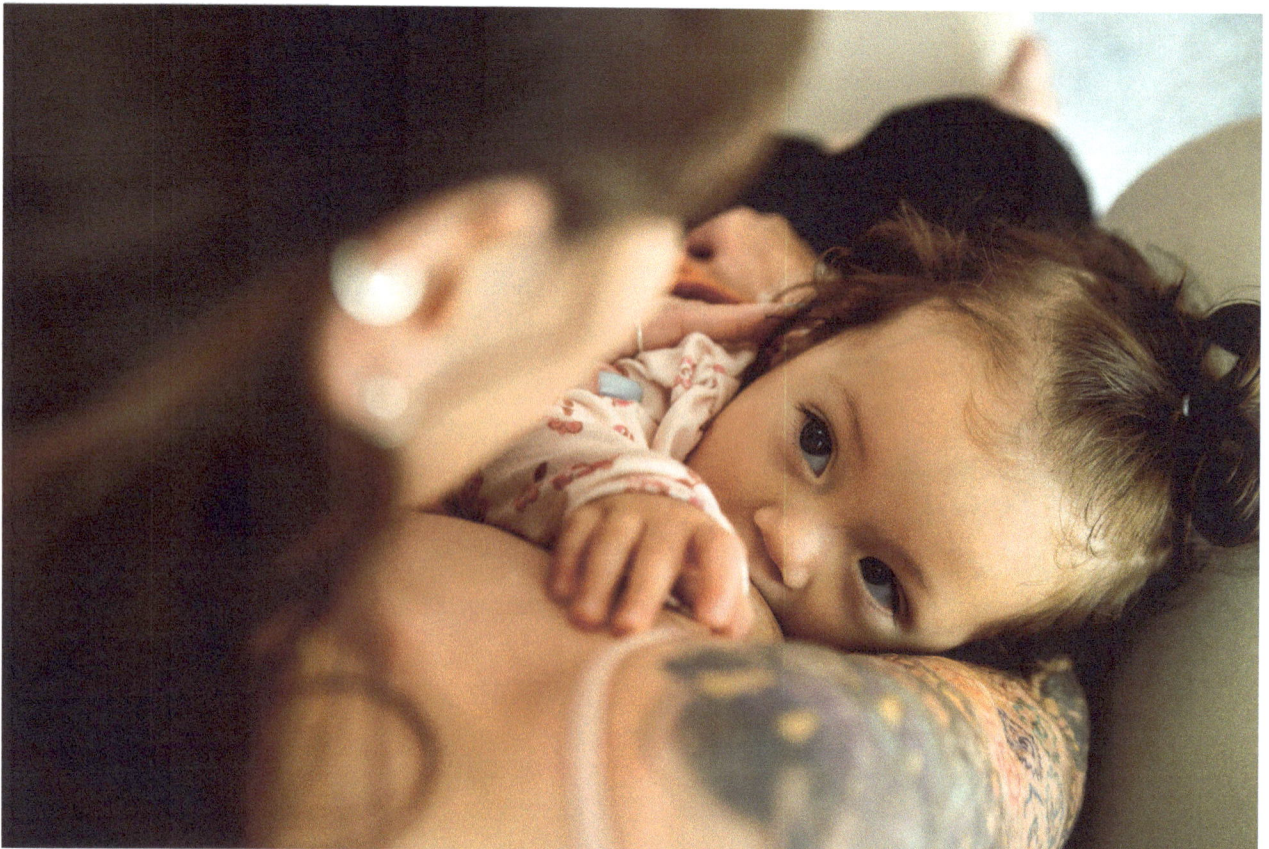

MENOPAUSE

A natural part of each woman's life is the ending of the menstrual periods, a time known as menopause, when biology changes gears. The average age for this is midway through the 51st year. While many women make the transition smoothly, others find this passage to be quite challenging. Research indicates that more than 75% of women have mild to severe symptoms. Additionally, women who have had a hysterectomy may experience menopausal symptoms.

The approaching months or years to this change is a time called perimenopause. Menstrual periods can become irregular or unusually heavy. Hot flashes, night sweats, difficulty sleeping, vaginal dryness, mood swings, irritability, and foggy thinking can also cause problems as hormonal levels change.

After the menstrual periods have stopped for a full year, then the woman is considered to be in menopause. In health, her body reaches a new and stable hormonal balance without troublesome symptoms. When the hormones are not able to reach a new equilibrium, previously mentioned symptoms can continue for years. Homeopathy has been helping women with symptoms of this transition for more than 200 years.

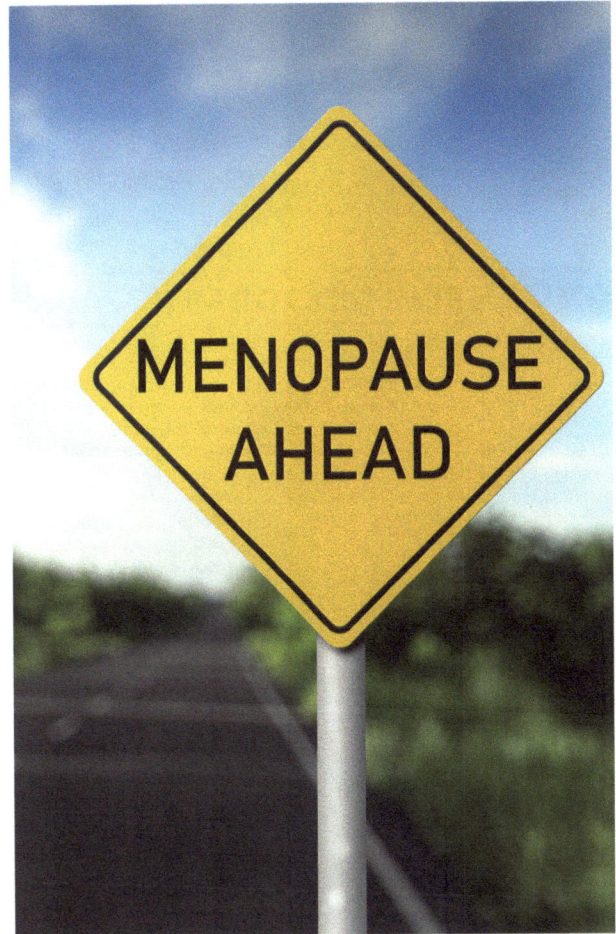

♡ ADDITIONAL SUPPORT FOR MENOPAUSE

- Exercise: Multiple research studies have shown that women who exercise (walk, dance, or other aerobic activity) for 60 minutes three times weekly had improved sleep and mood, better vitality, fewer hot flashes, and less sweat.
- Optimize body weight: Increased body fat impacts the hormonal balance. Research shows that women with higher body fat have more hot flashes, poorer quality sleep, and increased night sweats. Those who lost even 10% of their body weight and 5% reduction in body fat reported markedly improved symptoms.
- Avoid common dietary triggers: Coffee, alcohol, tobacco use, and spicy food can increase hot flashes and sleep disturbances.
- **Bach Flower Rescue Remedy®**: This is a combination of Dr. Bach's flower essences that is available in spray, pastilles, and drops. It can be used multiple times daily to relieve the intensity of irritability, mood swings, anxiety, and lack of clarity. There is also a **Bach Flower Rescue Sleep®** formula that can be used at night to improve sleep.
- Dress in layers: Wearing light clothes in layers that are easy to adjust with heat or sweat will ease discomfort.
- Iron rich diet: For women with frequent or heavy perimenopausal menstrual flow, be sure to have adequate iron in the diet to prevent anemia. **Ferrum phos 6X** cell salts taken three to four times daily on any day of menstrual flow can support healthy iron metabolism.

WHEN TO CONTACT YOUR HEALTHCARE PROFESSIONAL

- There is repeated or frequent heavy menstrual flooding.
- There is any bleeding one year after menopause.

COMMON REMEDIES FOR MENOPAUSE

	Lachesis	Nux vomica	Pulsatilla	Sepia	Sulphur
Characteristics	Intense irritability before menstrual flow. Temperature instability in general, with hot flashes. Long-lasting impacts. "Never well since menopause."	General irritability. Very irregular and early periods, heavy menstrual periods and intermittent spotting. Headaches. Digestive disturbances may accompany.	Emotional symptoms predominate. Weepy and moody. Early menopause. Changeable symptoms.	Irritability. Sensation of heaviness in the pelvis as if everything would fall out.	Flushes of heat followed by sweat as the heat is relieved. Generally feels too hot, needs to open windows, puts feet out of covers.
Symptoms	Menstrual flooding. Headaches that begin around menopause. Hot flashes appear suddenly with mottled appearance on skin. Insomnia with overactive mind. Sweat feels hot in daytime, cold at night.	Perimenopausal irregular bleeding and spotting. Hot flashes with heavy sweat. Headaches pressing on the crown of head.	Anxiety felt just before or during a hot flash. Menstrual periods irregular, late, with clotting.	Menstrual irregularity, heavy periods. Hot flashes with hot sweat and feeling of anxiety or weakness. Hair falling out at menopause.	Hot flashes with redness of the skin, insomnia, night sweats. Heat with a sensation of burning in the face, palms, feet, vagina. General sense of heat, with cold feet. Perspiration has a strong odor.
Mood	Extremes of emotion before menstrual periods: rage, depression, jealousy. Often very talkative.	Irritable and impatient. Insomnia from busy thoughts on waking in early morning hours.	Weepy, mood swings. Desires reassurance and comfort from companions.	Irritability or dissatisfaction, often directed toward spouse or family.	Indifferent to loved ones.
Worse	Before the menstrual flow begins. After sleep or on waking. From tight clothing, especially around the throat and waist. More left-sided symptoms.	Cold, open air.	Warm room. From heat and sun. Hot flashes, especially at night. Varicose veins.	Cold.	Exposure to heat. Heat of bed once it becomes warm.
Better	After menstrual flow is established. Cold drinks.	With loosening tight clothing. Heat (such as heating pad on abdomen).	Walking outdoors. Fresh air from open window. Cooling influences. Consolation and reassurance.	Vigorous movement, dancing, and exercise.	Open air.

Dosing: Use the BLUE Method. Observe and evaluate.

BLOWS TO THE BREASTS

Blows to the breasts in either women or men can damage the ducts, lymph nodes, mammary glands (in women), or fatty tissue. A severe blow can have long-lasting and serious consequences, including pain and swelling. Always give a remedy, especially ***Bellis per**, if there has been any blunt force trauma.

WHEN TO CONTACT YOUR HEALTHCARE PROFESSIONAL

- The person had a severe blow to the breast; this includes being hit with a hard ball or hitting the breast on a steering wheel in a car accident.

Remedies to consider:

- **Arnica:** Give this remedy at once. If the blow was severe, call your homeopath immediately. Then, always follow with ***Bellis per.**

- ***Bellis per:** Pains are achy, squeezing, and throbbing. Give this remedy every two hours on the first day, then give three times a day if soreness or pain returns or persists. Re-evaluate if there is no response. Repeat only if symptoms return. **Note:** Give this remedy at least six hours before bed because it can disrupt sleep. However, it is best to give the remedy, if needed, rather than be concerned about sleep.

- **Staphysagria:** Give this remedy if the blow was the result of anger or physical abuse.

Dosing: Use the **BLUE** Method. Observe and evaluate.

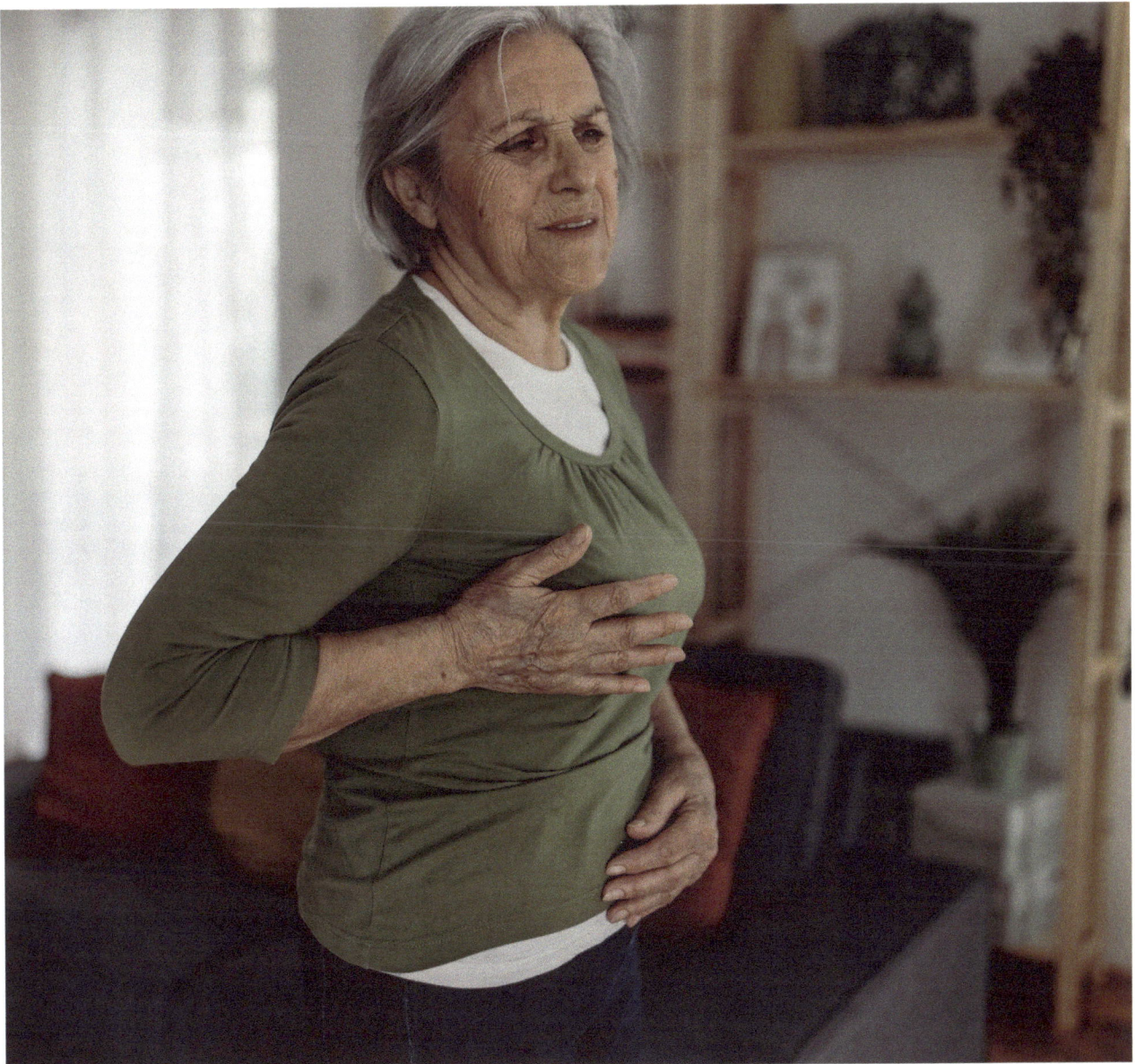

? WHAT'S THE FIRST REMEDY YOU THINK OF WHEN...

1. A person has heavy frequent periods.
2. A girl is experiencing very painful menstrual cramps.
3. A woman is experiencing sweaty hot flashes with irregular bleeding cycles and spotting.
4. Breastfeeding causes a fluish feeling, with a seemingly low milk supply and aching pain in the breasts.
5. Severe pain and swelling of the genital organs after childbirth is accompanied by feelings of shame or anger.
6. Experiences of nausea and weepiness along with changeable moods occur during the first trimester of pregnancy.
7. Lower back and ligament pain extends down the leg during the last month of pregnancy.
8. A need to rebalance menstruation, that comes too early or too late, is too scanty or too profuse.
9. The woman has frequent urination urging with a spasm at the end of urination after anger.
10. There is voluptuous vaginal itching with a swelling of the labia and a feeling of heat.
11. Intense burning pains are accompanied by urine passing in drops.
12. Pain occurs on intercourse and there is irritation and burning with the vagina feeling dry despite having a discharge
13. A case of "honeymoon cystitis" happens after sexual activity during your post-wedding trip.
14. The pain needs to be relieved after an episiotomy.

Answer key on page 324.

CHAPTER 16
Back and Neck

In today's fast-paced world, it's not uncommon for people to experience back or neck problems at some point in their lives. The human spine, comprising numerous delicate vertebrae, intricate muscles, and supportive ligaments, is tasked with providing structural support and facilitating a wide range of movements. However, factors such as poor posture, sedentary lifestyles, heavy lifting, repetitive motions, stress, and age-related changes can place undue strain on the spine, leading to discomfort, pain, and potential injuries. Fortunately, there are remedies that can reduce the discomfort while keeping one healthy in the long run.

BACKACHES AND LIGAMENT PAIN

Backaches and ligament pain can have a major impact on your quality of life. It can occur for a multitude of reasons including but certainly not limited to poor posture, an accident, over-exertion/over-exercising, sitting at a desk all day, or even just stress.

ADDITIONAL SUPPORT FOR BACKACHE AND LIGAMENT PAIN

- Apply cold pack to the injured area—10 minutes on, 20 minutes off, several times a day for the first few days.
- Apply heat if the pain had been there longer than 48 hours. Better to use cold in the first 48 hours.
- Find gentle ways/exercises to strengthen your abdominal muscles that then help support your back.
- Check the age of your mattress as older one's can break down and not provide the support needed for good back health.
- Lie flat on your back with knees bent at a 90 degree angle and legs propped up and supported on the seat of a couch or chair allowing gravity to hold your back. Stay for 5-10 minutes (or more) if comfortable.
- Use good body mechanics when sitting, standing and lifting. Avoid twisting movements and over-lifting. Look online to get ideas for ways to lift more safely.
- Consider taking cell salts ***Calc phos 6X** and ***Calc flour 6X** twice daily for up to two months to strengthen a weak back.
- Wear comfortable, low-heeled shoes.

WHEN TO CONTACT YOUR HEALTHCARE PROFESSIONAL

- If you have pain that interferes with sleep.
- If you have injured your lower back several times before.
- If you have severe pain and cannot walk more than a few steps.
- If you have numbness in the area of injury or down your leg.

The first remedy to consider is **Arnica. Arnica** is especially helpful when the body feels injured in some way, feels sore and/or bruised. See chart for additional considerations.

COMMON REMEDIES FOR BACKACHE AND LIGAMENT PAIN

	Belladonna	*Bellis per	Bryonia	*Kali carb	Sepia
Onset	Pain comes on fast and disappears just as quickly.	The last months of pregnancy. Deep tissue trauma, repetitive strain and sprains. After surgery.	Arthritic pains or sudden injuries/fractures.	From injury or exertion. Can be sudden.	Overwork. Exhaustion.
Symptoms	Pain in sacrum. Cutting pain from hip to hip. Burning, throbbing, stiff and swollen.	Pain in the groin extending down the legs, e.g., sciatica. Like **Arnica** injury, but deeper with more swelling and bruising.	Stitching, sharp, cutting pains. Stiffness in the back and neck.	Bruised, dragging feeling with sudden sharp pains up and down the back, buttocks, and thighs. Pain in the hip joint is common.	Back feels tired with an aching, dragging pain in the lower back. Aching, dull pains. Sudden stitches as if struck by a hammer.
Mood	Restless.	Impulse to move.	Grumpy, irritable with the pain.	Irritable, touchy, and domineering.	Weepy, indifferent to work. May be depressed and chilly.
Indications	May have a flushed, red face with dilated pupils, and be thirsty for lemonade.	Old back strains. Becoming chilled when hot. Ill-effects of getting overheated.	Any motion causes pain. Inflammation of joints and bursa.	Weak back feeling. Must lie down or lean on something. Must walk stooped over. Very sensitive to changes in weather, cold, and drafts and wants to be warm, but not overheated.	Weak, tired low back. Aching. Sensation of heaviness or bearing down in the pelvis as if everything might fall out.
Worse	Any touch, especially sudden jarring movements. Bending head backward.	Touch. Left side. Hot or cold bathing. Warmth of bed.	Motion, touch, becoming hot, in cold wet weather, morning on waking.	Standing, sitting erect, bending back. Gentle touch.	Sitting, standing, cold wet weather, before, during or right after menses. Left side.
Better	Laying semi-erect. Warmth.	After eating. Continued motion.	Absolute stillness, rest, lying on painful side, cool air.	Hard pressure over the painful area. Lying down.	Exercise. Pressure. Warmth of the bed and hot applications. After sleep.

Dosing: Use the BLUE method. Observe and evaluate.

WHIPLASH

Whiplash is a neck injury that occurs when your head is forcefully and quickly thrown backward and then forward. This motion can injure bones in the spine, discs between the bones, ligaments, muscles, nerves, or other tissues of the neck, and may tear blood vessels.

Symptoms of whiplash include neck pain, stiffness, and headaches. Most people with whiplash recover within a few weeks with good remedy choices and targeted exercises. However, some people have chronic neck pain and other long-lasting complications.

Signs and symptoms of whiplash usually—but not always—develop within 24 hours of the injury and may include:

- neck pain and stiffness

- worsening of pain with neck movement

- loss of range of motion in the neck

- headaches, most often starting at the base of the skull

- tenderness or pain in the shoulder, upper back, or arms

- tingling or numbness in the arms

- fatigue

- dizziness

Some people also have:

- blurred vision

- ringing in the ears (tinnitus)

- sleep disturbances

- irritability

- difficulty concentrating

- memory problems

- depression

A whiplash injury may result from:

- Auto accidents. Rear-end collisions are a major cause of whiplash, or sudden stops.

- Physical abuse or assault. Whiplash can occur if you are punched or shaken. It's one of the injuries seen in shaken baby syndrome.

- Contact sports. Football tackles and other sports-related collisions can sometimes cause whiplash.

- Risk factors: Having had whiplash before, older age, and/or existing low back or neck pain.

IT'S AN EMERGENCY WHEN

- You suspect broken bones or tissue damage that can cause or worsen symptoms.

ADDITIONAL SUPPORT FOR WHIPLASH

- Rest the neck.
- Do gentle exercises as possible.
- Get chiropractic or osteopathic care (if not too invasive).
- Go for physical therapy.

WHEN TO CONTACT YOUR HEALTHCARE PROFESSIONAL

- You have any neck pain or other whiplash symptoms after a car accident, sports injury, or other traumatic injury.

Remedies to consider:

The first remedy to consider after any accident is **Arnica**. This is one of the times giving a 200c potency would be possible, if you have it, especially if the person claims nothing is wrong with them. After a few doses of **Arnica** (either 30c or 200c) then consider the options below as needed.

- **Belladonna:** Sudden back pain, herniated discs with great aggravation from motion or jarring.

- **Bryonia:** If the person has extreme back or neck pain and does not want to move or be moved.

- ***Calcarea phos:** Cervical pain and stiffness. Vertigo, worse from wind or draft. Worse from exertion and/or swallowing.

- **Gelsemium:** Aching and stiffness in neck which may extend to forehead. Chills running up and down the spine. Numbness and weakness of limbs.

- **Rhus tox:** When the pain decreases to help heal the soft tissue injury and promote mobility.

Dosing: Use the **BLUE** method.
Observe and evaluate.

BLOWS TO THE BACK

Getting a blow to the back is never an expected event. You can get hit by many things like a ball when playing sports, in a car accident or by an accidental fall onto the back.

IT'S AN EMERGENCY WHEN

- If there is severe pain or tenderness in the kidney area, on the back on either side of the spine just below the ribcage.
- If there is any blood in the urine after a blow to the back.
- If the person has suffered a severe fall or received a hard blow on their back.

ADDITIONAL SUPPORT FOR A BLOW TO THE BACK

- Consider seeking the care of a craniosacral osteopath, cranial sacral therapist, a massage therapist, acupuncturist, or chiropractor if symptoms linger.

Some remedies to consider:

- **Arnica:** Give this remedy immediately if the person has had the wind knocked out of them in a fall. This will help with shock and release spasms in the diaphragm, which tenses upon impact. Repeat if the tenseness returns. The pain produces a sore and bruised feeling; they feel beaten-up. This remedy will also help if a person falls on their back awkwardly, causing a twist. Start with the ORANGE dosing method, then consider BLUE if the person is in less pain. Observe and evaluate.

- **Hypericum:** Give this remedy for trauma to the spine. The pains are intense, violent, and shooting upwards from the point of impact. The pains appear suddenly and then disappear gradually. The area is very tender and sore. There may be tingling, twitching, trembling, or numbness. The back feels weak. Use the ORANGE dosing method. Observe and evaluate.

- **Nux vomica:** This remedy will relieve intense muscle spasms where there is also great sensitivity to pain. Bruised or sharp pains, feels as if broken. Must sit up in order to turn over. Pain radiates to hips. Use the ORANGE dosing method. Observe and evaluate.

TORTICOLLIS

Torticollis, also known as wryneck, is a twisting of the neck that causes the head to rotate and tilt at an odd angle. It can be caused by a trauma, such as when a baby is being born its head can get twisted, or to a related inflammatory syndrome. The symptoms are painful spasms of the neck with an opposite tilting of the head. Stiffness can be intense, limiting any neck movement.

Indicated remedies include:

- **Aconite:** when the cause is exposure to extreme and sudden cold such as a chilly wind or the person catches a chill after sweating outside and not drying off quickly.

- **Rhus tox:** to be given after **Aconite**, if it was needed, and when the neck at first feels pain upon first movement but feels better after continued motion.

Rotator Cuff Tendonitis

Rotator cuff tendonitis, also called supraspinatus tendonitis, is an injury to one's shoulder area. It can be caused by repetitive motions of the arm girdle such as those executed by a baseball pitcher, a lap swimmer, gardener or landscaper, or frequent arm exerciser. It can also be caused by repeatedly lifting heavy things. There can be sharp electrical pain with a locking sensation as if the muscles and tendons are too short, especially if the arm is taken out away from the body. It is worse from pressure and stiffness can be present because of spasm of the muscles.

ADDITIONAL SUPPORT FOR ROTATOR CUFF TENDONITIS

- Ice the area for 20 minutes every two hours to bring down the inflammation until the pain is reduced or use heat after the first 48 hours.
- Consider seeking the care of a craniosacral osteopath, cranial sacral therapist, a massage therapist, a physical therapist, an acupuncturist, or chiropractor if symptoms linger.

WHEN TO CONTACT YOUR HEALTHCARE PROFESSIONAL

- If you suspect a complete rupture or tear of the rotator cuff muscles that is resulting in total loss of movement.

COMMON REMEDIES FOR ROTATOR CUFF TENDONITIS

	Arnica	*Causticum	Rhus tox	Ruta	*Sanguinaria
Onset	From mechanical injury due to repetitive strain on the shoulder girdle.	From carrying something heavy.	Spraining or straining a single part, muscle or tendon. Overlifting, particularly stretching high up to reach things.	Sprains. Overexertion. Carrying heavy weight.	After exposure to cold.
Symptoms	Sore as if bruised. May be a tingling sensation down the arm. Cold fingertips.	Sensation as if muscles and tendons are too short. Awakened from sleep due to discomfort.	Rigidity, stiffness, numbness and pain as if sprained or a muscle or tendon was torn from its attachment.	Bruised, lame, sore, aching, sensation all over, as after a fall or blow. Feels sprained. Stiffness.	Frozen shoulder. Cannot lift the arm but can swing it back and forth. Cramping up of arms during sleep.
Mood	Fears being touched.	Anxious, sad mood.	Restless with the pains.	Weak and restless.	Feeling of helplessness because of a sensation of being paralyzed.
Indications	Limited movement of the upper arm after overuse.	Sharp stitches in the top of the shoulder. More left-sided.	May have arthritis in the shoulder causing chronic wear and tear on the shoulder. Pressure feeling on shoulders like a heavy weight.	Often a puffy appearance along with pain and stiffness caused by fluid in the joint.	Right sided rheumatism of shoulder.
Worse	Anything pressing on the area.	Change of weather especially to cold, windy weather. Night. Any exertion.	Cold, damp weather. Beginning to move. Rest. Before storms.	Lying down. Tosses and turns in bed. Cold.	Jarring. Motion. Touch. Raising arm. Turning in bed at night.
Better	Cold applications. Supporting the arm. Hanging arm down.	Gentle supported movement of the upper arm. Damp wet weather.	Hot applications and bathing. Gentle continued movement.	Lying on back. Supporting and resting the arm.	Passive, supported movement. Lying on back.

Dosing: Use the BLUE method. Observe and evaluate.

SCIATICA

Sciatica refers to pain, weakness, numbness, or tingling in the leg. It is caused by injury to or pressure on the sciatic nerve located in the spine. The pain occurs when there is a herniated disc, or rupture, or an overgrowth of bone, sometimes called bone spurs, that form on the spinal bones. Typically there are intervals of low back pain that are worse bending forwards or backwards, or after sitting for a long time causing stiffness in the back. It can be aggravated by sneezing and walking OR can be better from walking even though the person feels heaviness and weakness in the lower back. As the situation progresses, the pains can worsen and radiate down the leg with decreased sensation in the leg and foot. The affected leg may be colder or hotter than normal.

ADDITIONAL SUPPORT FOR SCIATICA

- Try applying cold packs to the back and/or alternate with warm packs.
- Learn some targeted stretches for the specific area the pain is in.
- Consider seeking the care of a craniosacral osteopath, cranial sacral therapist, a massage therapist, physical therapist, acupuncturist, or chiropractor if symptoms linger.

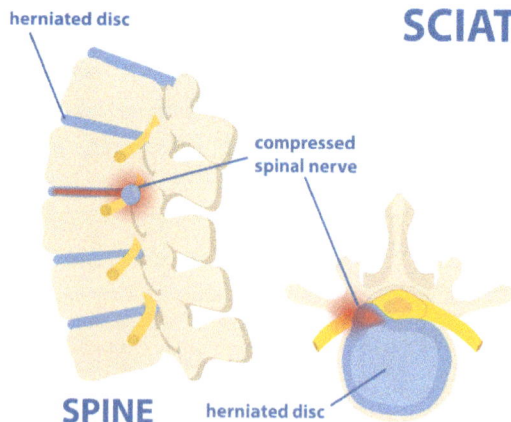

SCIATICA

SPINE

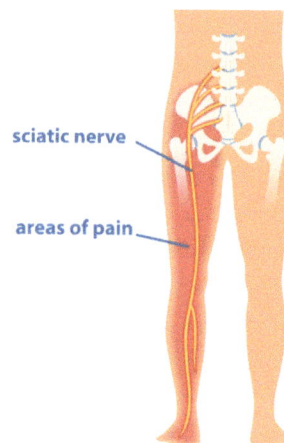

WHEN TO CONTACT YOUR HEALTHCARE PROFESSIONAL

- If the pain becomes intolerable and/or movement isn't possible.

Some common remedies for Sciatica include:

- **Bryonia:** For sciatica due to a herniated disc or from lifting a heavy object. The person is in extreme pain. They don't want to be bothered by anyone and they are irritable.

- **Colocynthis:** When sciatica comes on with muscle cramps in the lower back extending to the hip.

- **Hypericum:** This is a 'go to' remedy for any trauma to the nerves. It has a particular affinity for areas rich in nerves such as the coccyx.

Dosing: Start with the ORANGE dosing method, then consider BLUE if the person is in less pain. Observe and evaluate.

BLOWS TO THE TAILBONE

The tailbone, also known as the coccyx bone, is an area rich in nerves. A blow to the tailbone is commonly caused by either falling down on ice or cement pavement, or on the sharp edge of something like rocks. The blow can send a shock wave all the way up to the head and negatively affect the bowels, uterus, sacrum, sciatic nerve, bladder, or lower-back area. In the mid-back area, the lungs, heart, and digestive processes can also be negatively affected. The shock can even trigger excess mucus production in the sinuses, above the bridge of the nose. The person may have sharp electrical pains and are worse from sitting on a hard surface. The area is quite tender to the touch and may feel or look black and blue.

ADDITIONAL SUPPORT FOR A BLOW TO THE TAILBONE

- Apply an ice pack wrapped in a towel to the painful area for twenty minutes, repeat three times a day for first few days.
- Purchase a blow-up donut for the person to sit on. This will relieve pressure on the tailbone and make them more comfortable.
- An injury to the tailbone can have long-term consequences. It is best to see a craniosacral osteopath as soon as possible.
- Consider seeking the care of a craniosacral osteopath, cranial sacral therapist, a massage therapist, acupuncturist, or chiropractor if symptoms linger.

WHEN TO CONTACT YOUR HEALTHCARE PROFESSIONAL

- If the pain becomes intolerable and/or movement isn't possible.

First remedies to consider:

- **Arnica:** Give this remedy immediately for shock to the spine.

- **Hypericum:** This remedy acts as a tonic for injured nerves. It is for pain in nerve-rich areas such as the tailbone. The area is very tender and sore. They feel pressure, and the pains are intense, violent, and shooting upwards. The pains appear suddenly and then disappear gradually. There may be tingling, twitching, trembling, or numbness.

Special Dosing Instructions: **Alternate these two remedies every 15 minutes** until the person becomes more comfortable. Then continue with **Hypericum** only, on an as-needed basis.

ADDITIONAL REMEDIES TO CONSIDER FOR COCCYX PAIN OR INJURY

	Bryonia	*Bellis per	*Causticum	Rhus tox	Ruta	Silicea
Onset	A sudden blow or fall.	A blow to the coccyx.	After a fall or blow. Condition comes on slowly.	Arthritis can trigger it.	Injury to the attachments of the ligaments of the sacrum.	Injury to the coccyx when there is an existing condition and the spine has been weakened such as with osteoporosis.
Symptoms	Painful stiffness. Back feels worse with any movement.	Deep bruised pain.	Back muscles feel constricted and contracted, as if they are too short.	Pain feels as if the back is broken. Pain in the deeper muscles in the area.	Feels bruised, sore to the touch.	Back feels weak. Legs may tremble and can hardly walk.
Mood	Wants to be left alone and be quiet. Grumpy.	Anxious, may scream with the pains.	Thinking about what happened makes them feel worse.	Restlessness of the body. Desire to move.	Irritable and anxious.	Anxious, may cry out with the pains.
Indications	Resists movement.	Acts like **Arnica** for deep soft tissues.	Complaints of tightness and stiffness, which ascend up the back to the neck.	Pain is aggravated at the beginning of movement, but better with continued movement.	Indicated for sprains.	In the elderly or frail. Can also be triggered by drafts.
Worse	Any movement.	Sitting. When having a bowel movement.	Cold, damp weather.	Lying in bed, resting or sitting still.	In the morning before getting out of bed.	Lying on the painful part. Feet becoming cold.
Better	Resting, no movement. Pressure applied to or lying on the painful part. Hot applications.	Cold applications. Supporting the painful area.	Continued gentle motion.	Bending backwards. Gentle walking. Warm applications.	When pressure is applied.	With rest. Cold compresses.

Other remedies to consider: ***Kali bich** and ***Carbo animalis**.
Dosing: Use the BLUE method. Observe and evaluate.

? **WHAT'S THE FIRST REMEDY YOU THINK OF WHEN...**

1. The person is experiencing shooting pains after an injury.

2. A remedy is needed immediately after any physical trauma.

3. There is blood in the urine after a blow to the back, you give this remedy on the way to the hospital.

4. A heavily pregnant woman complains of backache.

5. The back pain has the quality of feeling heavy, tired and dragging.

6. The person has been in a car accident and now has aching and stiffness in the neck which radiates all the way round to the forehead.

7. The person is in extreme pain and cannot bear to be moved. This could be a fracture. Do not move the person, call for an ambulance and give this remedy in the meantime.

8. A teenager comes in with restricted movement and stiffness in the shoulder. She says it happened after swimming. It loosens up as she gently moves it.

9. You instruct the person with an inflammatory condition: apply an ice pack wrapped in a towel to the painful area for twenty minutes, repeat three times a day and give this remedy.

10. An older person with osteoporosis falls on her tailbone. She has already had an x-ray and doesn't have a fracture, but she is complaining of sharp stitching pains and is having trouble walking.

11. There is a history of a herniated disc. The person has bouts of back pain which come on suddenly and go away suddenly. They are much worse from walking and riding in a car.

Answer key on page 324.

CHAPTER 17
Muscle, Joints, and Bones

Muscles, joints, and bones form the foundation of our body's structure and movement, playing a vital role in our overall well-being. These interconnected systems provide support, stability, and mobility, enabling us to perform daily activities and engage in physical pursuits. Healthy muscles ensure proper movement and posture, joints allow for smooth articulation and flexibility, and bones provide structural support and protect vital organs. Conditions like arthritis, fractures, muscle imbalances, and joint disorders can cause discomfort, pain, and functional limitations. By learning the remedies in this chapter, you will be better equipped to relieve these conditions.

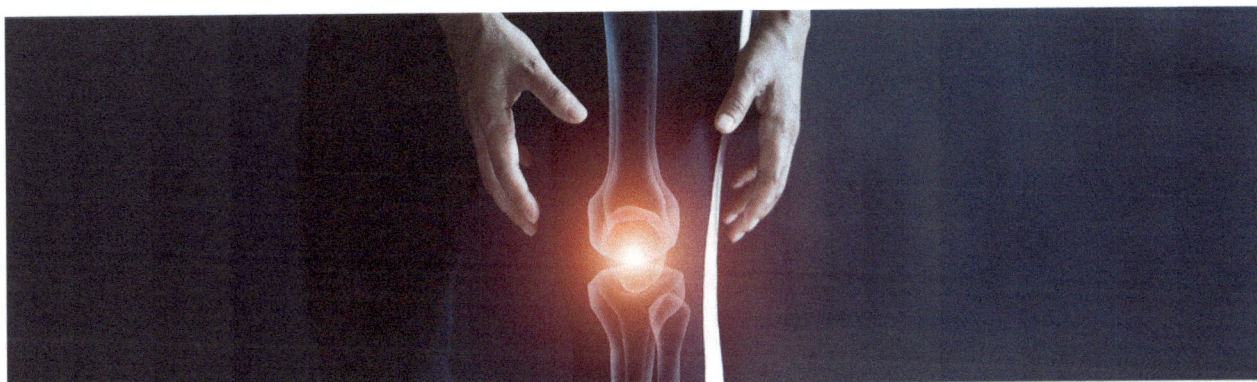

SPRAINS, STRAINS AND OVEREXERTION OF LIGAMENTS AND TENDONS

Just about everyone is familiar with the discomfort of a sprain or strain. Anyone who has enjoyed a day of gardening, winter sports or who has shoveled heavy snow knows the discomfort and even exhaustion brought on by overexertion.

Ligaments are strong, fibrous bands of tissue that connect bones and provide stability to joints, while tendons connect muscles to bones, enabling movement.

Sprains occur when ligaments are stretched or torn due to sudden twisting or trauma, often resulting in pain, swelling, and joint instability.

Strains, on the other hand, involve the stretching or tearing of muscles or tendons and can cause localized pain, muscle weakness, and limited range of motion. This can be caused by trauma, overexertion or overstretching a muscle or a tendon beyond its normal range.

Overuse injuries, such as tendonitis, develop gradually from repetitive motion or excessive stress on tendons and can lead to chronic pain, inflammation, and reduced functionality. These kinds of injuries cause pain when normal pressure is applied, produce swelling, and cause loss of range of motion.

Important Note: This section addresses sprains and deep strains of ankles, knees, hips, wrists, elbows, shoulders, and backs. If there is severe pain and no response to remedies, an x-ray may be needed to rule out dislocation, a deep tear, or a bone fracture.

ADDITIONAL SUPPORT FOR SPRAINS, STRAINS AND OVEREXERTION OF LIGAMENTS AND TENDONS

- Applying an ice pack over a thin cloth placed on the affected area for 20 minutes at a time, with an hour between applications, during the first 24 hours. This will help to reduce swelling.
- Continue icing as needed to reduce swelling. Some sprains will feel better if heat is applied after the first 24 hours, but ice is best to keep the swelling down. Wrists, ankles, knees, and elbows can be supported by wrapping them firmly with an Ace™ bandage. Give the sprain plenty of rest. Do not let the person run or play sports after the injury until you are sure that the healing is complete.
- Reduce your activity to avoid overexertion. Find others who can help with your physical work until you are feeling strong again.
- To relieve pain and encourage healing, protect the injured area with a brace or splint if necessary.
- Consider wrapping the injured area with an elastic bandage in order to decrease swelling.
- Keep the affected part(s) elevated.
- Encourage rest, avoiding activities that cause pain until the injury has resolved.
- **Rhus tox cream** and/or **Ruta cream** may be applied to dry skin in addition to the internal dose of the appropriate homeopathic remedy.

WHEN TO CONTACT YOUR HEALTHCARE PROFESSIONAL

- The person is prone to having accidents, their clumsiness results in frequently hurting themselves, or they are always dropping things.
- You suspect a bone might be broken.
- The injury is accompanied by a fever.
- The person has a popping sound with the injury or cannot walk or use the limb at all.
- There is significant swelling or pain that does not improve with homeopathic treatment.

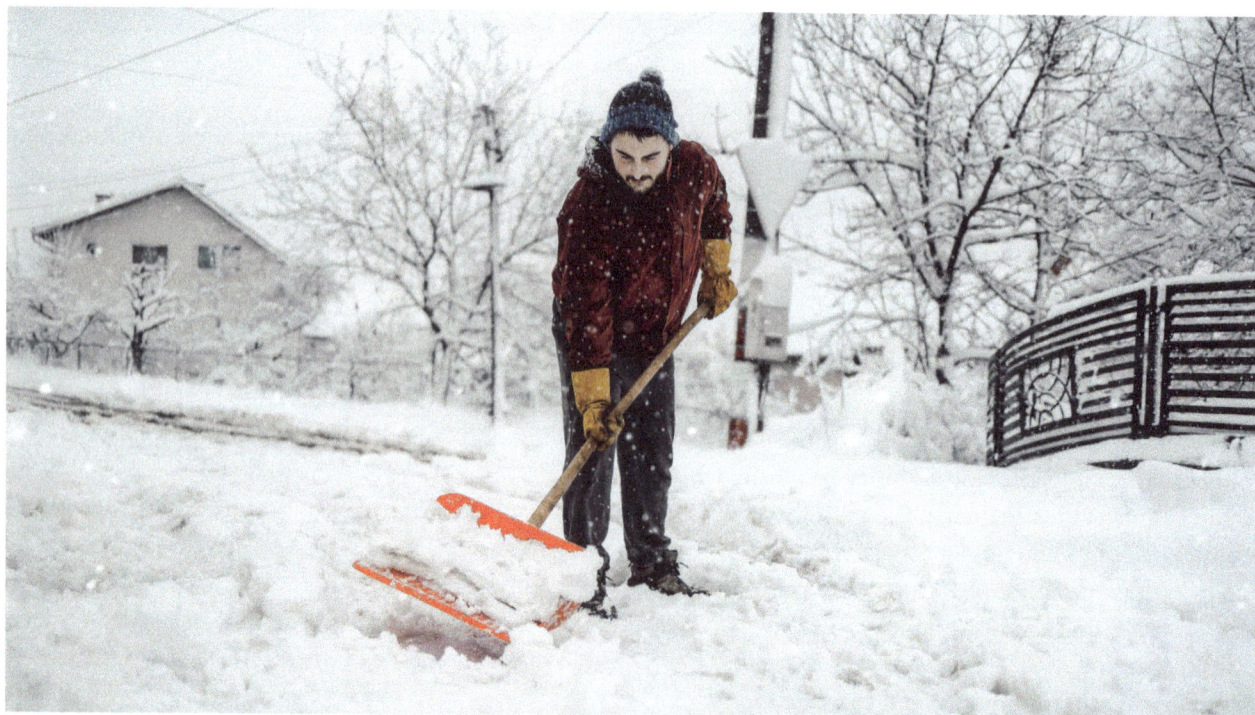

COMMON REMEDIES FOR SPRAINS, STRAINS AND OVEREXERTION—part 1

	Arnica	*Bellis per	Bryonia	Hypericum
Onset	The first remedy to give for sprains and strains. Relieves pain, bruising, and swelling associated with overexertion from sports or activities such as shoveling snow.	Useful for injuries to the trunk, deep tissues and organs. After blows or falls.	Helps with deep exhaustion. Any movement is painful. Ailments from lifting, sciatica, and disc problems. Slow onset of symptoms.	Relieves sharp, shooting nerve pains, especially if the tailbone or any part of the spine is injured in a fall or accident. Also for concussion and whiplash.
Symptoms	Stitching pains in the heart. Feeble, irregular pulse. Concussion. Muscles feel sore, bruised and beat up. Injury can feel cold.	Feelings of muscle soreness, stiffness, lameness as if sprained, or coldness developing in the injured area. Much swelling and bruising around a joint. Resembles **Arnica**, but its action goes deeper.	Muscle stiffness with shooting pains from the back through chest that make breathing difficult (also consider for pleurisy). Pains are tearing and stitching.	Pains travel up and down the spine and limbs. Walking, bending, or any movement of the neck or limbs cause intolerable, radiating pains.
Mood	Fears, approach of helpers and being touched. Insists they are fine.	Excitable. Impulse to move.	Annoyed. Grumpy like a bear and does not want to be disturbed.	Restlessness, can't concentrate.
Indications	Shock and trauma, such as a fall on ice. Insists nothing is wrong. May be given after overexertion or overstretching to prevent soreness or strain from developing later on. Injuries to muscle tissue, bone or blood vessels.	Hip pain, sprains, rheumatism, tendonitis, with swelling. May be used if **Arnica** has not helped enough. Injury to soft tissue, especially of breast and abdomen, bruises or deep tissue injury. Useful for deep trauma with achy, squeezing, and throbbing pains.	Painful inflammation of connective tissue, stiffness of joints. Dryness. For a twisted or strained knee, and for sprains where there is much inflammation, swelling, redness, and heat around a joint.	Burning and tingling sensations. Injuries to nerve rich areas.
Worse	Continued movement, being touched or jarred, alcohol (may crave alcohol to relieve pain), tobacco smoke. After sleep.	Touch, becoming chilled when overheated. Left side. Hot bath. Immobility.	Early morning, even slightest movement, light touch to the back, pressure, noise, coughing, deep breathing overheating, cold drafts, bright light.	Cold and damp, stuffy rooms, touch, pressure and motion.
Better	Cold applications, stillness, rest, privacy. Lying with head low, or lying out-stretched.	Pressure, gentle rubbing. Continued motion and localized cold packs.	Rest, quiet, low light, pressure, heat, or lying on the painful side. Firm bandaging. Hot applications after first 24- 48 hours depending on the degree of swelling.	Lying on face, bending backwards, rubbing and quiet.

Dosing: Use the BLUE method. Observe and evaluate.

COMMON REMEDIES FOR SPRAINS, STRAINS AND OVEREXERTION—part 2

	Magnesium phos	Rhus tox	Ruta
Onset	Anti-spasmodic remedy for painful muscle cramps, spasms, convulsion, and paralysis.	Used if aching, stiff joints with stitching pains, numbness and prickling, especially when lifting, straining or twisting while lifting a heavy load.	Relieves strained, sore ligaments and tendons, bruised bones, and sciatica.
Symptoms	Sciatica. Sharp, radiating, shooting, shifting muscle and nerve pains that are improved by warmth and pressure.	Dislocations, sciatica, tearing pains in lower back that cause restlessness. Pain on first movement, but pain subsides with continued movement.	Tearing pains in lower back that cause restlessness. Sore bruised feeling. Deeply aching pains that can be quite intense. Sensations of heaviness and weariness. Affected area can be quite lame. May crave iced drinks.
Mood	Irritable, fearful.	Restlessness, especially at night. Wants to move.	Restless, quarrelsome. Intense lethargy, weakness, despair, fretfulness, weepiness.
Indications	Injuries to connective tissue, periosteum, muscles and tendons, especially flexor tendons of the ankles and wrists.	Dislocations, and slipped vertebrae. Injury to connective tissue around joints tendons. Sprains, strains and overlifting. Pains are tearing, shooting, and stitching. Injured part is stiff and gets worse if kept still for too long. Area is weak and trembles after exertion.	Injuries to bones and periosteum, with pains as if bones are broken. Dislocations, slipped vertebrae, lameness. Back weakness & stitching pains. Inflammation of cartilage, joints, tendons and the protective sheath. Strains and sprains of ankles, hips, lower back, neck, wrists, and elbows (including tennis elbow).
Worse	Light touch, cold air, drafts, and movement.	Cold damp air, wet weather. Night. Stooping, sitting or lying down. Beginning motion, after rest, after midnight. From ice and cold drinks.	When sitting, resting, especially at night in bed, and during first movements. Overexertion. Cold damp, wet weather. Ascending and descending steps.
Better	Warmth, pressure, bending over, rest, and massage.	Lying on hard surface, hard pressure, changing position, stretching, warm applications. Gentle rubbing, continued motion, limbering up, stretching, flexing. Hot bath.	Lying on back. Warmth, rubbing, scratching and movement. Gentle pressure.

Dosing: Use the BLUE method. Observe and evaluate.

Also consider:

- ***Calcarea phos:** This remedy is useful for lumbago (pain in the muscles and joints of the lower back) from over lifting, bone bruises, aggravation of old or slow healing fractures or injuries that lead to soreness in the bones, especially if the area feels cold or numb and improves with warmth. The muscles near the injury may ache or stiffen. Worse for cold and damp, better for rest and dry warmth.

- ***Strontium Carb:** This remedy is helpful when legs feel weak and the muscles cramp or twitch. Also recommended for deep, tearing and burning bone pain. Also, for sprains in ankles, knees, hips, wrists, shoulders, neck and back. Worse from exertion, being uncovered or drafts and better for quiet, wrapping up and warmth. Indicated when **Rhus tox** or **Ruta** have been tried.

ARTHRITIS

Arthritis is a general term that refers to a group of more than 100 inflammatory joint diseases. Arthritis can affect people of all ages, genders, and backgrounds, and it is a leading cause of disability worldwide.

The most prevalent form of arthritis is osteoarthritis which occurs when the protective cartilage that cushions the ends of bones wears down over time. It commonly affects the joints in the hands, knees, hips, and spine, causing pain, stiffness, and reduced range of motion. Other forms of arthritis include rheumatoid arthritis, psoriatic arthritis, ankylosing spondylitis, gout, lupus-related arthritis, and juvenile idiopathic arthritis, among others. Each type has its own distinct characteristics and may affect different joints or organs.

Since homeopathic remedies treat a person's individual symptoms, not diagnoses, there might well be a remedy or two listed here that can help with the symptoms.

Common symptoms of arthritis include:

- joint pain

- swelling and inflammation

- stiffness, especially in the morning or after periods of inactivity

- reduced range of motion

- fatigue

- warmth or redness around affected joints

Some possible factors for experiencing arthritis include:

- a person's increasing age

- the person's gender: Some types are more common in women (e.g., rheumatoid arthritis), while others affect men more (e.g., gout)

- genetics can play a role in certain types of arthritis

- excess weight can strain joints, particularly in the knees and hips

- sedentary lifestyle

- diet consisting of inflammatory foods

ADDITIONAL SUPPORT FOR ARTHRITIS

- Get moving daily—motion is the joint's lotion. Walk, swim, yoga, tai chi and other gentle movements can help the joints keep lubricated.
- Avoid inflammatory foods—sugar, alcohol, a lot of red meat, white flour foods like pasta and white bread, fried foods, and sugar sweetened soda. Instead consider an anti-inflammatory mediterranean-type diet which consists of fresh vegetables, fruits, healthy fats, fish and poultry, nuts and more.
- Avoid nightshades, at least for a two week period, if you think you may be sensitive to them—potatoes, tomatoes, eggplant, bell peppers, and spices like paprika and cayenne. If you feel better after the two weeks, then you know to continue avoiding them.
- Consider anti-inflammatory supplements that include Curcumin, Tumeric and/or Omega-3's.
- Apply heat or cold to the affected area if either makes you feel better.

WHEN TO CONTACT YOUR HEALTHCARE PROFESSIONAL

- If you continue to have a lot of pain making it difficult to function.
- If you're not sure what your joint pain is about and you are concerned.
- Arthritis can be considered a chronic condition which may warrant a visit to a professional homeopath.
- If none of the well-selected remedies help.

COMMON REMEDIES FOR ARTHRITIS

	Aconite	Apis	Belladonna	Bryonia	Ledum	Pulsatilla	Rhus tox
Onset	After a fright or shock. Sudden onset and very painful. Exposure to cold winds.	Can be any sort of joint inflammation and swelling. Can also be from suppressed measles.	Violent onset. Acute bursitis, synovitis, arthritis.	Injury, trauma, sprains, fractures. Also after getting chilled when hot in summer.	For rheumatism or gout.	Issue often starts during puberty or pregnancy or they have never been well since then.	Spraining or straining a single part, muscle or tendon. Overlifting, particularly stretching high up to reach things.
Symptoms	Intense unbearable pains. Tearing, cutting or bruised. Burning pains like boiling water. Tingling and numbness. Cracking of joints. Limbs feel lame.	Joints are burning, stinging, red and swollen.	Red, hot swollen joints. Spasms. Throbbing or pulsating pain. Stiffness, feels as if would break.	Affected joints are red, swollen and hot. Stiffness. Constipation.	Swelling of the feet that travels up to the knees, with unbearable pain when walking, as from a sprain or false step. Ball of the great toe swollen. Painful heels as if bruised.	Pain which shifts rapidly from place to place. Drawing, tensive pain in thighs and legs, with restlessness, sleeplessness and chilliness. Joints swollen, red. Legs feels heavy and weary.	Pains as if sprained. As if a muscle or tendon was torn from its attachment. As if bones were scraped with a knife. Affected part is sore to touch.
Mood	Restless and tired. Anxiousness. Easily startled. Hyperventilation possible.	Very restless and fidgety.	Fearful, excitable, moaning with pain.	Wants to be left alone and not be disturbed. Easily angered and irritated.	Seems dissatisfied and doesn't want company.	Mild, weepy, whiny, sweet. Changeable moods.	Extreme restlessness, with a desire for continuous change of position. Impatient and hurried.
Indications	Thirsty. High fever. Redness and swelling. Sticking, tearing pains with numbness. Red shiny inflamed joints. Possible fever.	Joint feels tense, stiff, puffy and hot. Thirstless.	Sensitive to touch. Can be accompanied by a headache or fever.	Extremely thirsty for large quantities of water, especially cold.	Stiffness of all joints. Can only move them after applying cold.	Chilly but seeks open air and doesn't want to cover up. Thirstless.	Sprains and strains. Bursitis, tendonitis. Stiffness, numbness and pain are experienced on first moving but better with walking or continued motion.
Worse	Strong emotions, getting chilled, lying on the affected side, night, pressure or touch.	From heat, slightest touch, after sleep and 4 PM.	Touch, motion, exertion.	Motion. Touch, becoming hot, 9 PM.	At night. From touch. Warmth of any kind. Walking. Motion.	Being in a warm stuffy room. Being in the sun. Resting. On beginning to move. Evening. At twilight.	Initial movement. Jarring. Damp rainy weather.
Better	Rest, sitting still, open air.	Gentle motion, cold applications, open air.	Pressure, warm wraps. Lying on painful side with head high.	Lying on the painful part. Applying pressure. Hot compress. Rest. Quiet.	Ice cold water applications even though they may be chilly. Cold bathing. Rest.	Cold applications. Gentle motion. Continued motion. Pressure. Rubbing.	Continuous motion. Hot applications. Hot bathing. Change of position. Warm dry weather.

Dosing: Use the BLUE method. Observe and evaluate.

Other remedies to consider: **Calcarea carb, *Causticum, *Dulcamara, *Kalmia, *Rhododendron, Ruta.**

CHARLEY HORSE

A charley horse is another name for a muscle spasm or muscle cramp. This can occur in any muscle, but they're most commonly found in the legs, particularly in the calf or hamstring (thigh).

Symptoms include involuntary, sometimes painful, and uncomfortable muscle contractions. If the contracting muscles don't relax for several seconds or more, the pain can be severe. Severe charley horses can result in muscle soreness that lasts anywhere from a few hours to a day. This is normal, so long as the pain isn't prolonged or recurring.

Many things can trigger a muscle cramp, including:

- dehydration

- poor blood circulation in the legs

- working calf muscles too hard while exercising

- not stretching enough

- being active in hot temperatures

- muscle fatigue

- lack of nutrition, especially magnesium and/or potassium deficiency

- a problem such as a spinal cord injury or pinched nerve in the neck or back

- muscle cramps can also occur as a side effect of some medications

To prevent cramps:

- Eat foods high in vitamins and magnesium and calcium.

- Stay well-hydrated.

- Stretch properly, regularly, and especially before and after exercise.

♡ SUPPORTIVE MEASURES FOR A CHARLEY HORSE

- **Traumeel®** (https://traumeel.com) can be taken internally or as an ointment applied externally. You can use the internal and topical simultaneously.
- Take **Mag phos 6X** cell salt for cramping four tablets, four times a day. Taper off as cramping subsides.
- Take extra magnesium, especially at bedtime with night time cramps, and stay hydrated.
- Eat a variety of organic fruits and vegetables which will provide additional nutritional support.

⚕ WHEN TO CONTACT YOUR HEALTHCARE PROFESSIONAL

- The cramps continue even after following the supportive measures.

COMMON REMEDIES OR CHARLEY HORSE

	Calcarea carb	*Causticum	*Colocynthis	*Cuprum met	Magnesium phos
Symptoms	Cramping of the thigh, calves, foot muscles, especially when stretching or straining, or when in bed at night.	Cramps in the calves and feet. Contracture of muscles and tendons.	Useful in cases of neuralgia and sciatica. Cramps in the thigh and calf. Pains are almost always better from pressure and often ameliorated by bending double and from heat.	For hand or leg cramps, particularly following loss of fluids that cause dehydration, after childbirth or from diarrhea.	Classic remedy for neuralgia and nerve pain. Cramps especially in the hands and fingers. e.g., writer's cramp. Sciatica, better heat and pressure, worse motion and cold, right sided.

Dosing: Use the **BLUE** method. Observe and evaluate.

SHIN SPLINTS

The term "shin splints" refers to pain along the shin bone (tibia)—the large bone in the front of your lower leg that runs from the knee to the ankle. Shin splints are common in runners, dancers, aerobic exercisers, and military recruits.

Medically known as medial tibial stress syndrome, shin splints often occur in athletes who have recently intensified or changed their training routines. The increased activity overworks the muscles, tendons, and bone tissue.

Most cases of shin splints can be treated with rest, ice, and other self-care measures. Wearing proper footwear and modifying your exercise routine can help prevent shin splints from recurring. Shin splints are commonly caused by repetitive stress on the shinbone and the connective tissues that attach your muscles to the bone often due to any motion that causes the knee to be stretched out over the toes, as in aerobics or yoga.

If you have shin splints, you might notice tenderness, soreness or pain along the inner side of your shinbone and mild swelling in your lower leg. At first, the pain might stop when you stop exercising. Eventually, however, the pain can be continuous and might progress to a stress reaction or stress fracture.

ADDITIONAL SUPPORT FOR SHIN SPLINTS

- To prevent shin splints, do not stretch the knee over the toes, e.g., running up hill, certain yoga poses.
- With shin splints, elevate the affected leg, ice the leg to reduce inflammation about four times daily, as tolerated.
- Wear compression stockings until you fully recover.
- Gently message the shins as tolerated.
- Consider a good quality fish oil, turmeric and/or curcumin supplements to reduce the inflammation.

WHEN TO CONTACT YOUR HEALTHCARE PROFESSIONAL

- There is no improvement after a week using additional supports and homeopathic remedies.

Remedies to consider for shin splints:

- **Rhus tox:** The pain may be aching, drawing, tearing, can also be shooting or cutting. The pain gets worse at night and with rest. There is a desire to move legs to get relief. Restless and stiff. Bruised feeling. Better warmth. Crossing the legs is worse.

- **Ruta:** The pain is present in the leg along the tibia bone. Feels sore as if beaten and extreme soreness is felt on touch. Pain can be worse from stretching, by exertion and on first motion. Better continued motion. Intense weariness and lameness. Better from pressure and rubbing. Despairing mood.

- ***Causticum:** The pain feels tearing, stitching or bruised in the lower leg with every movement. The legs are also sore to touch. Swelling in legs may also be present.

Dosing: If in acute, sudden pain, use the ORANGE dosing method. If shin splints are chronic, use the BLUE dosing method. Observe and evaluate.

STITCHES IN THE SIDE

Side stitches, sharp pains in the side, are muscle spasms of the diaphragm, and they occur occasionally during strenuous exercise. Most people experience stitches on their right side, immediately below the ribs, commonly after running or briskly walking. During exercise, your trunk muscles become tired and your back muscles over-engage to compensate, pressing on nerves felt in your abdomen, side, or shoulders. Although a side stitch is basically harmless, it can be quite painful and can cause aspiring athletes to stop in the midst of their competition.

ADDITIONAL SUPPORTS FOR STITCHES IN THE SIDE

- Stay hydrated.
- Stop eating at least two hours before you exercise.
- Remember to breathe properly while exercising.
- Pay attention to your posture when exercising.
- Avoid quick starts.
- Strengthen the abdominal muscles.

WHEN TO CONTACT YOUR HEALTHCARE PROFESSIONAL

- The pains don't resolve quickly upon ceasing your activity or with a chosen remedy.

COMMON REMEDIES FOR STITCHES IN THE SIDE

	Arsenicum	*Berberis	Bryonia	Sepia
Onset	Stitching pains in abdomen aggravated by motion or physical activity.	Sudden sharp, stitching pains in abdomen, aggravated by motion or physical activity.	Stomach pain aggravated by motion or physical activity. Thirst for large quantities of water, which may contribute to symptoms.	Sudden stitching pains typically on left side, aggravated by motion, running, etc.
Symptoms	Anxiety about health. Great restlessness. Chilly and aggravated by cold. Pains usually burning in nature. Thirst for small quantities often. More right-sided, but could be left-sided.	Sharp, sudden, radiating pain—neuralgic in nature—from one point to another. Left side or right to left. Great chilliness, or coldness of isolated spots. Perspires easily.	Averse to being disturbed, must be left alone and quiet. Aggravation from motion. Aggravation rising in the morning.	Stitching pain, one-sided (left).
Mood	Overwhelming sense of vulnerability and fear for health and well-being. Fastidious (desire to control environment). Anxious, proper, tense and worried. Tremendous restlessness. Anguish, worse when alone.	Obvious sudden stitches of pain, from exertion of the body.	Irritability.	Young children and teens are excitable and affectionate or are introverted. Adults may be irritable.
Indications	Stitching, burning pains on side, often doubled over.	Sudden sharp, stitching pains in abdomen or on sides.	Stitching pains in abdomen or on side.	Stitching pains, left side.
Worse	Cold. Exertion. Drinking. Physical exertion. Running. Night.	Least motion, jarring, stepping hard, rising from sitting. Fatigue. Urinating.	Motion. Rising from lying, stooping, exertion, coughing, a deep breath, sneezing, swallowing and motion of eyes. Drinking, while hot. Eating. Vexation. Touch. Getting cold. Lying on painless side. Ascending. Morning. During sleep. Closing eyes.	Alone, yet dreads being completely alone. Cold. Morning and evening. After first sleep. During and right after eating. Mental exertion. Afternoon. 5 PM. Before thunderstorms.
Better	Warmth. Motion. Walking about. Sitting erect. Having company.	Rest, motion.	Rest, and when quiet. Pressure on painful part. Cold air, food and water. Being quiet. Cloudy, damp days. Drawing knees up. Heat to inflamed parts. Dark room. Eructations (belching).	Violent motion (e.g., running, walking fast, power yoga). Dancing. Warmth. Cold drinks. When busy. Loosening clothes. Open air.

Dosing: Use the BLUE method. Observe and evaluate.

TENNIS ELBOW

Tennis elbow is caused by repetitive motions of the forearm muscle, such as in playing tennis. Overuse of the forearm muscle can cause microscopic tears in the tendon causing inflammation and pain.

Symptoms can include:

- severe pain in upper arm, especially when trying to play tennis or other sport using your elbow to swing

- inability to squeeze a tennis ball

- severe pain near the elbow, which may affect bones and joints of the arm

WHEN TO CONTACT YOUR HEALTHCARE PROFESSIONAL

- Pain is not greatly alleviated in 48 hours or becomes chronic.

Remedies to consider:

- **Bryonia:** Stitching pains, worse with motion, desire to keep the arm still. Better with rest, pressure, lying on the painful side, perspiration and/or wet weather. Worse from motion, heat, and in the morning upon rising.

- **Ruta:** Aversion to motion, yet relieved by it. Better from motion, warmth, and in the daytime. Worse from overexertion, cold and/or pressure on an edge.

- **Rhus tox:** Stiffness and pain are relieved by movement. Perspiration is prominent. Better from continued motion of affected parts, moving affected parts, rubbing, heat (local or general), warm drinks, change of position, stretching limbs, and/or lying on something hard. Worse when first beginning to move, from rest, overexertion, after midnight, before storms, getting wet (especially by perspiring), cold air, chill or draft when hot or sweaty, uncovering.

Dosing: Use the BLUE method. Observe and evaluate.

GROWING PAINS

Growing pains result from a growth spurt in growing children. These pains can localize in the legs but could be felt in the shins, ankles, and knees.

Remedies to consider:

- ***Calcarea phos:** Used for big growth spurts where the child outgrows the pants quickly. There are shooting pains, aching, and even cramping. The child seems dissatisfied with everything and is chilly.

- ***Phosphoric acid:** Pain in legs feels like someone is scraping them. Weakness with tearing pains. There may be a feeling like ants crawling under the skin of the legs.

If the cramping is paramount, alternate **Magnesium phos 6X** cell salt with the chosen remedy.

Dosing: Use the BLUE method. Observe and evaluate.

Note: *Osgood-Schlatter Disease—pain typically on the knees from overuse and strain during and after a growth spurt—is covered in **Chapter 22—Young Adults (ages 12-24) page 269.***

BLOWS TO THE MUSCLES

The most common remedies for blows to muscles are:

- **Arnica:** This is the first remedy to give for blows followed by bruising. The muscle feels very sore and beat up. Give the remedy every three to four hours or more frequently if the pain is severe.

- **Rhus tox:** This is the most common remedy for inflammation, stiffness, and tearing pains after an injury to the muscle, which usually leads to inflammation of the muscle tissue. The keynotes for choosing this remedy are: the area feels better from massage, hot applications, and sustained movement and is worse on the first movement or after resting. Give the remedy every three to four hours, and soak in a hot bath. Repeat as necessary.

BONE INJURIES AND FRACTURES

There are many different types of bone injuries and fractures. For example, a bone can be completely fractured or partially fractured in a variety of ways. Fractures can be crosswise, lengthwise, or broken in multiple pieces. Fractures can range from a small hairline fracture, to a compound fracture where a broken bone pierces the skin, to a massive break in the pelvis, which can be life-threatening. Homeopathy can reduce pain and swelling. It can also speed up the process of healing.

IT'S AN EMERGENCY WHEN

- The person develops breathing difficulties or has an obvious injury requiring medical attention.
- You suspect the person has a skull, neck, spine or hip fracture. Do not move them. You can then give a remedy while waiting for emergency assistance to arrive. If they become cold, cover them with a blanket.
- You suspect the person has broken their collarbone. This kind of fracture can puncture the adjacent lung so immobilize the arm and keep them as still as possible while awaiting emergency care. Only give **Arnica** until the emergency room physician has assessed whether or not there is a fracture. Then review other remedy possibilities in this section.
- You suspect the person has a broken rib. Immediately give **Bryonia**. To avoid puncturing the adjacent lung, keep them as still as possible while awaiting emergency care. Continue giving **Bryonia**, as needed.

WHEN TO CONTACT YOUR HEALTHCARE PROFESSIONAL

- You suspect a fracture. Look for the following symptoms: severe pain or swelling, deformity, weakness, inability to bear weight, shortening of a limb, or extreme tenderness.
- A crushed finger or toe does not respond to the remedies given. These areas are nerve rich, can be quite tender, and can take a while to resolve.

Important note: Because of their rapid-healing properties, the remedies *Symphytum or *Calcarea phos should NOT be used until a doctor confirms that the bones have been set in the right place.

Remedies to consider during the initial stage of healing for relieving pain from bone injuries include:

- **Arnica:** Start with this remedy, whether or not you suspect a break. It will help with shock, pain, swelling, and bruising and can speed the healing time. Give the remedy every 15 minutes for the first hour then every two to four hours for the first 24 hours.

- ***Eupatorium perf:** This remedy will help with pain. The person will complain of bone-breaking pain or intense aching deep in the bone. They moan a lot and are restless. They can be nauseous from the pain. The skin can feel quite sore around the bruised bone. Dose hourly until relieved then on an as needed basis.

- **Ruta:** This remedy will help with pain from bruised bones, breaks near a joint, and severe jawbone fractures. The pains are intense with a feeling of deep bruising, soreness, and aching. The person is restless, despairing, weak, and fretful. They can be weepy.

Special Notes: If bone pains do not respond to these remedies, after giving them hourly for six doses, have the limb checked in case there is a fracture to a bone or to a child's growth plate. Simple or hairline fractures will cause persistent, nagging pain, and can sometimes go unnoticed. If the pain does not subside, there is severe pain on using the limb, or there is pain from rotating the limb, keep the limb immobile and call a healthcare practitioner, or go to an urgent care facility. Know that hairline fractures may not show up on x-rays for up to six weeks, so if the pain continues, get the x-ray retaken. A bone fracture may also affect the periosteum, a fibrous, dense covering on the bone where tendons and muscles attach.

Remedies to consider for specific fractures of bones are:

- **Bryonia:** This remedy will help broken ribs and jawbones. The person does not want to move the injured part. Any motion brings much pain. They are irritable, grumpy, and want to be left alone. The person is worse from touch and slightest motion and better from rest, heat and pressure.

- **Hypericum:** This remedy will help heal a fracture of the face, jaw, fingers, toes, spine, or tailbone. The pains are violent, darting, and shooting upwards. They are very sensitive to touch. The person can be quite nervous, irritable, and fearful. The person is worse from cold, touch, motion and jarring and better from rubbing the area gently.

- ***Symphytum:** the remedy should NOT be used until the bones are set in the right place because of its rapid healing properties. This is a remedy for fractures of the face, skull, and shins. This remedy will also help if there is an injury to the lining of the bone (periosteum). The pains are intense, pricking, penetrating, and intensely sore. Reduces swelling. The person is worse from touch, stooping, and movement and better from rest.

Special Notes: To help the bone to repair quickly, you can use ***Symphytum** ONLY if the fracture is simple (a fracture of the bone only, without damage to the surrounding tissues or breaking of the skin), or if it is well set and no further surgery is needed. ***Symphytum** should NOT be used until the bones are set in the right place, because of its rapid healing properties. Give ***Symphytum** once a day for up to two weeks. In addition to helping the bones mend completely and quickly, this remedy alleviates soreness, tenderness, pain, and bruising. For extra support, consider the cell salt combination of ***Calc Flour 6X**, ***Calc Phos 6X** and ***Silicea 6X** three times a day for up to five days. If a break is slow to heal, you can give the homeopathic remedy ***Calcarea phos** once a week to assist with healing.

DISLOCATIONS

A dislocation is an injury to a joint, a place where two or more bones come together, in which the ends of your bones are forced from their normal positions. This painful injury temporarily deforms and immobilizes the joint. Dislocation can occur in the ankles, knees, shoulders, hips, elbows, jaw, and finger and toe joints. These joints are often swollen, possibly immobile, very painful, and visibly out of place.

Depending on its severity, a dislocation can cause damage to the surrounding muscles, ligaments, tendons, and nerves. A simple dislocation may resolve itself after some rest and taking a few doses of **Arnica**. If a doctor has to return the bones to their original positions, **Arnica** can be given hourly until the pain is relieved and the dislocation is resolved. Repeat only if there is a return of pain. Once the dislocation has been corrected and the pain has calmed down, give one dose of **Arnica** in the morning and one dose of **Rhus tox** in the afternoon, for three days. Only repeat beyond three days if there is a return of symptoms.

ITS AN EMERGENCY WHEN

- The person has a dislocated joint. Go to the emergency room to have the bones returned to their original position.

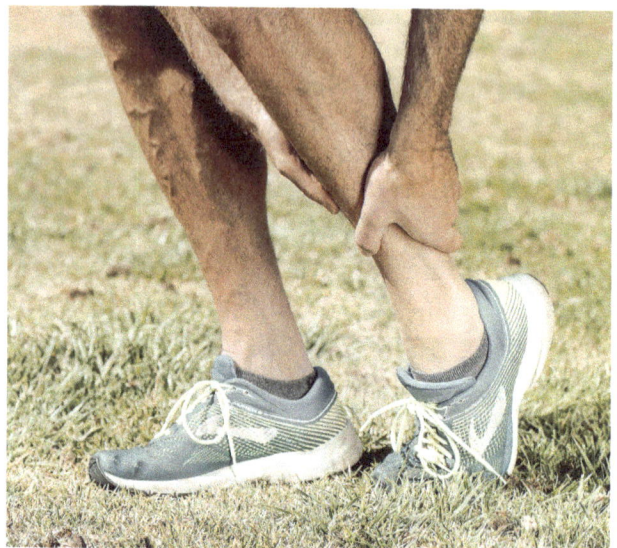

ADDITIONAL SUPPORT FOR DISLOCATIONS

- Treat the dislocated joint as a fracture and immobilize the joint.
- If a dislocated shoulder, place the arm in a sling and strap it with a triangular bandage snugly to the body.
- Administer **Arnica** 30c or 200c to control shock and hemorrhage, repeat every half hour up to four times, if needed, or until the dislocation can be reset. Stop giving if the person is recovering well, and then give only as needed.
- After relocation of the joint, give a dose of **Ruta** dry under the tongue every two to three hours or put the pellets in a water bottle where one sip is a dose. Shake the bottle once before each sip.

Remedies to consider while waiting for care or on the way to the hospital:

- **Arnica:** Give to control shock and hemorrhage; bruising, soft tissue trauma; those who need this commonly say "I'm fine, leave me alone." Give as soon as possible and repeat hourly if pain continues, until the dislocation has been resolved and pain has ameliorated.

- **Ruta:** Administer after a health care practitioner relocates the joint.

- **Bryonia:** Should be given if the area surrounding the joint becomes swollen, filled with fluid, and feels worse on the least movement.

Dosing: Use ORANGE method as a starting point. Observe and evaluate remedy and frequency.

SMASHED OR CRUSHED FINGERS OR TOES

Smashed or crushed fingers or toes, or a finger or toe that was stepped on, hit with a hammer or other heavy object, or got slammed in a door can benefit from a homeopathic remedy. The fingers or toes might look compressed, have an imprint, be pale or red, and be very sore.

WHEN TO CONTACT YOUR HEALTHCARE PROFESSIONAL

- If you suspect that a finger or toe might be broken.
- First, ice the finger or toe then elevate it and try to use it. This will help to get blood circulating again.
- The primary remedy for smashed or crushed fingers or toes is **Hypericum**, since it is indicated when there is injury to nerve-rich areas of the body. Give the remedy every 15 minutes for up to six doses. Re-evaluate if there is no response. Repeat only if symptoms return.

? WHAT'S THE FIRST REMEDY YOU THINK OF WHEN...

1. The person is in shock after an accident but denies there is anything wrong with them.
2. The person complains of intense bone pain.
3. The person has been vigorously exercising and gets a stitch on the left side.
4. Stiffness and pain around a joint is relieved by gentle motion.
5. A child complains of chest pains during a growth spurt.
6. The injury feels worse for even the slightest movement.
7. The person has fallen on their coccyx.
8. The fractured bones have begun to knit.
9. A gymnast complains of pain on the shin bone which gets worse from walking.
10. A muscle strain or injury is felt deep in the body.
11. A sprain which doesn't heal becomes chronic.
12. Sciatica feels better from warmth and pressure.
13. There is pain following abdominal surgery.
14. Bone pain is worse at night.

Answer key on page 324.

CHAPTER 18
Skin

Your skin is the body's largest organ. It plays a remarkable and multifaceted role, often serving as the first line of defense against external threats while also functioning as a remarkable barometer of our inner health. As we interact in the physical world, we frequently come upon issues that cause an immediate change in skin health such as splinters, puncture wounds, bites and stings, poison ivy, etc. Additionally, we are frequently exposed to allergens that cause a change in how the skin feels, its appearance, texture, or condition. Here we will look at some of the more common skin conditions and some simple homeopathic options to help in the healing process.

ACNE

Acne vulgaris is a common inflammatory skin issue affecting most adolescents. One common cause is increased hormone levels stimulating an oily secretion from the sebaceous gland that surrounds the hair follicle resulting in pimples. These often appear on the face, upper chest and/or back. Another cause is from a dysregulated microbiome.

Cases of acne can range from mild, moderate, to severe. Typical conventional treatments include topical creams and cleaners, oral antibiotics and sometimes steroids. Although not debilitating, the social and psychological impact it plays on adolescents can range from low self-esteem, social isolation, to anxiety or depression.

ADDITIONAL SUPPORT FOR ACNE

Supportive measures at home can include dietary changes such as:
- Drink an adequate amount of water.
- Ingest essential fatty acids through foods or supplements.
- Try a minimum two week to one month time of eliminating each of these things, one at a time, to see if there is any shift in acne or digestion. Choose the one you consume the most as that can be a possible antagonist.
  1. fatty, refined, fried, and processed foods
  2. gluten and dairy
  3. foods with chemicals and artificial dyes. This includes most food from fast food restaurants.
  4. foods with sugar and white flour
- Use witch hazel on a cotton ball to cleanse the face or use natural, non-fragrant soaps.
- Some remedies helpful in the treatment of acne are shared in the following chart. When treating a skin condition, use low potencies. Higher potencies should be used in complicated acne under the supervision of a professional homeopath.

COMMON REMEDIES FOR ACNE

	*Calcarea sulph	Hepar sulph	Nux vomica	Sepia	Silicea	Sulphur
Symptoms	Acne with pus filled pimples.	Sensitive to touch and can't stand a cold draft.	Eruptions with prickling, burning, and itching.	Yellow discoloration of face, yellow saddle across nose and down sides of face, large freckles. Itching.	Acne itches and burns only during daytime.	Skin is rough and unhealthy. Facial eruptions can be burning, itching, stinging, and aggravated by warmth.
Mood	Irritable. Argumentative. Jealous. Doesn't feel appreciated.	Irritable. Dissatisfied. Contradictory.	Irritable. Impatient. Mean. Easily offended. Never feels finished (work, stool, urinating).	Sadness and weeping often without knowing why. Indifference to loved ones.	Shy, timid, lack of self-confidence. Fear of pins and pointed objects. Failure and anticipation.	Critical. Selfish. Anxious.
Indications	Pimples and pustules on face. Pus is thick, yellow and bloody. Slow to heal with continuous discharges.	Skin is unhealthy, draining, moist and intensely sensitive to touch. Pus smells like old cheese. Heals slowly.	Acne from eating cheese. Pimples from overuse of alcohol.	Acne, worse before menses.	Pus is offensive. Perspiration is copious and offensive. The perspiration can eat through socks. Profuse perspiration on the head.	Pimply eruptions and pustules. Itching, burning. Red face. Itching is worse from bathing, heat, hot bed, night, and wool.
Worse	Cracked skin worse in winter or when washing. Drafts.	Hypersensitive to pain, touch, cold air, uncovering. Drafts.	Very chilly, worse cold, dry winds. Early morning. Unrefreshed, irritable, depressed, pains.	Evening. Fever.	Cold, damp and drafts. Feels extremely cold. Touch.	Warmth. Becoming warm in bed. Scratching and washing.
Better	Cold bathing and washing face. Walking in open air.	Wrapping up the head. Warmth.	Hot food, warm drinks. Warm applications.	Hot applications. Warm bed.	Heat. Warm room. Warm wraps covering head.	Dry weather. Cold air and applications.

Dosing: Use the BLUE method. Observe and evaluate.

CUTS AND ABRASIONS

A cut or laceration is typically caused by a sharp object such as a knife or shard of glass, and typically none of the skin is missing, just separated with clean edges. A surgical excision, like the wound left after surgical removal of a mole or skin cancer, is also considered a laceration. An abrasion is an open wound caused by friction or scraping and skin is missing or dislodged, like a flap of skin.

Treatment for a laceration typically depends on how deep it is. A deep laceration may reveal underlying tissues such as fat, tendon, muscle, or bone.

Treating a Laceration

The main concern with lacerations is blood loss, so it is important to control the bleeding as much as possible. Putting pressure directly on the laceration while holding it above the level of the heart for 15 minutes should be enough to stop bleeding. If not, try using pressure points. Tourniquets should be avoided unless immediate medical care is delayed and it's advised by the 911/Emergency operator. Tourniquets are typically viewed as a last resort.

IT'S AN EMERGENCY WHEN

- You have tried to control blood loss and the bleeding still will not stop, call 911. Remember, if you are not the victim, assume that all bodily fluids are dangerous. Practice universal precautions found at https://www.osha.gov/bloodborne-pathogens/worker-protections.

- **Calendula:** used as an ointment or taken internally in pellet form for open, torn, cut, lacerated, ragged, or suppurating wounds, especially when the pain is excessive and out of proportion to the extent of the injury.

Important note: make sure the wound is clean before topically applying **Calendula** ointment.

- **Staphysagria:** taken orally for post-surgical pain and healing of post-surgical incisions.

- **Hypericum:** especially for nerve damage or intense pain.

Dosing: Use the ORANGE method.
Observe and evaluate.

Additionally, you can crush two tablets of **Ferrum phos 6X** cell salt in a spoonful of water and apply to the wound.
*More about **cell salts** in **Chapter 3** starting on **page 39**.*

INFECTED WOUNDS

If, despite your best precautions, a wound turns red, hot, swollen, and painful, it has probably become infected.

IT'S AN EMERGENCY WHEN

- The wound site is very red, swollen, and/or hot, AND there are red streaks going up from the affected area. The person may or may not have a fever. DO NOT DELAY getting help.

Consider the following remedies:

- **Hepar sulph:** The first remedy to be thought of for early treatment of bacterial or fungal infections with pus formation. People needing **Hepar sulph** are always chilly, intensely dislike cold drafts, and are extremely "touchy."

- **Belladonna:** This is another remedy for the early stage of infection with sudden and rapid swelling and intense throbbing pains in a bright red wound.

- ***Calcarea sulph:** Much like **Hepar sulph**, only warmer individuals. Suppuration, the formation of pus, goes on and on instead of resolving, producing thick, yellow and even bloody pus.

- **Calendula:** Useful when the wound exudes clear fluid that starts to turn yellow or green or becomes brownish — these are signs that an infection is worsening rapidly.

- **Apis:** For a puncture wound that turns rosy red, swells with fluid (edema), and is very sensitive to the touch, think of **Apis**. Pains are burning or continuous, and the redness spreads out from the wound.

- **Silicea:** The person is very chilly, the suppuration unrelenting, and the wound will not heal. Like ***Calcarea sulph**, the pus refuses to resolve, but unlike that remedy **Silicea's** pus is a watery yellow.

- ***Pyrogenium:** Like **Hepar sulph** and **Silicea**, small cuts tend to become swollen and inflamed, with great pain and strong burning. The pulse is abnormally quick, even with little or no fever, or abnormally slow with a high fever. Discharges smell foul, suggesting sepsis is on the way, and there are red streaks extending from the wound. Give this remedy on the way to the hospital.

Dosing: Use the ORANGE method.
Observe and evaluate.

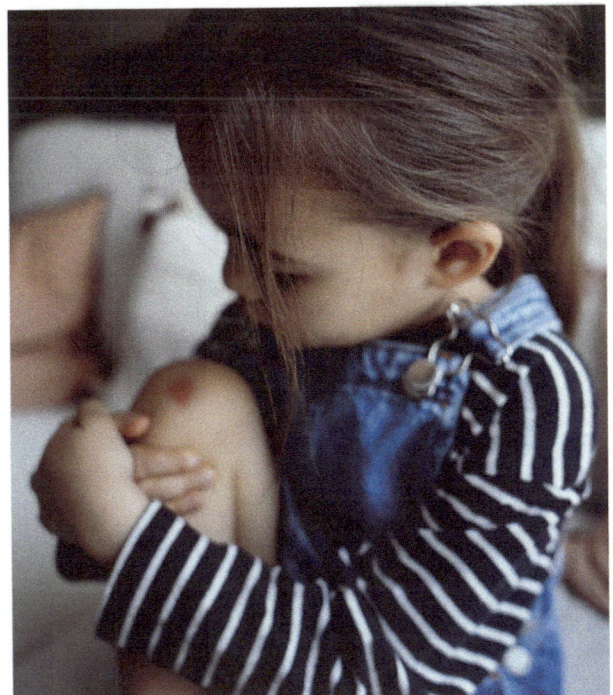

SPLINTERS

Splinters cause puncture wounds and bleed very little or not at all. The body can cause foreign objects to be expelled naturally; it surrounds the object with white blood cells, forming a pocket of pus. The area around the splinter swells, and eventually the body rejects both the splinter and the pus. This may take days, or even weeks.

For more review **Puncture Wounds** *in this chapter on* **page 207**.

For more review **Puncture Wounds** in this chapter on **page 207**.

🏥 IT'S AN EMERGENCY WHEN

- A large fishbone or chicken bone is caught in the throat and/or the person is choking. Call 911.
- The puncture site is very red, swollen, and/or hot, and there are red streaks going up from the affected area. The person may or may not have a fever.

💚 ADDITIONAL SUPPORT FOR SPLINTERS

- If a person has a glass splinter, it can be hard to see and remove because it can so easily break off. If the splinter or thorn is not too deep, use a sterilized needle and tweezers to remove it. Always allow a shallow wound to bleed for a short time. This is very cleansing for the wound and activates lymphocytes, the immune cells that produce antibodies.
- Cleanse the area with a **Hypercal solution** (see box below). This is a combination of **Hypericum tincture**, which heals damaged nerves, and **Calendula tincture**, which repairs damaged skin. This combination is invaluable when applied topically, as it brings about rapid healing.

> ### How to make a Calendula/Hypericum Solution
> Start by purchasing a "mother tincture" of each remedy. A mother tincture is made from a mixture of the original herb and alcohol or glycerin. Unlike the homeopathic form, which is drastically diluted, a mother tincture is a concentrated form of the active element of the herb.
> To prepare the solution, use a clean jar or bottle and distilled or spring water. Using very clean utensils, measure out one-part **Calendula tincture**, one-part **Hypericum tincture**, and eight-parts distilled water. Close the container and shake gently to blend. Place five drops of each tincture in a quarter-cup of spring water or boiled water that has been cooled and apply directly to the site. It will sting for a few seconds and then give relief. You can obtain these tinctures at any health food store, homeopathic pharmacies, or online. The wound must be clean before applying this solution.

- Be sure to watch for infections afterward.

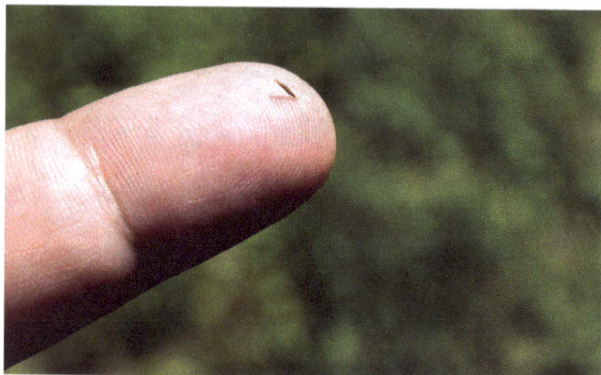

Remedies for different types of splinters:

- splinters of wood or glass: **Silicea**

- fishbone splinter in the throat: **Silicea**

- splinters or thorns under fingernails: **Ledum**

- splinter or thorn sites that are very sensitive and painful: **Hypericum**

Remedies to consider:

- **Silicea:** This is the most useful remedy to help expel foreign objects from the body, especially splinters. It promotes the painless expulsion of any foreign object, including fishbones caught in the throat. For minor punctures, it will expel the object without producing pus at the puncture site. For a deeper splinter, pus will form a creamy color.

- **Hypericum:** For tearing pain that shoots upward along the nerve pathways. Nerve pains are sharp and intense. This remedy is especially effective for splinters in nerve-rich areas, such as fingers or toes. The splinter area is very painful, tender, and inflamed, with burning heat of the skin. There is usually swelling. The person may experience numbness and tingling. This remedy can be alternated with any of the splinter remedies.

- **Ledum:** This is a good remedy if there are a lot of puncture lacerations. The site is puffy, tender, and very dark red or purple. The skin feels cold to the touch but feels better with cold applications. Pain may be throbbing, shooting, pricking, and or biting. Repeat up to four times a day, only if the pain returns or the person is complaining that the site feels cold.

Dosing: Use the **BROWN** method. Observe and evaluate. If giving **Hypericum**, this can be used every three hours if the site is extremely painful; then use on an as-needed basis.

BLISTERS from Friction

Blisters are a pocket of fluid between the upper layers of skin. They can be filled with pus, blood, or the clear, watery part of the blood called serum. They can appear as a single bubble or a cluster. Friction is a common cause—think of when you begin shoveling dirt or snow, or playing tennis or golf and your hand gets a blister, or you have a shoe that doesn't fit well and it rubs causing a blister. They are commonly found on your feet, toes, thumbs, or palms.

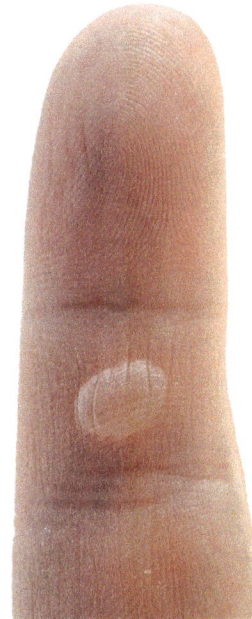

For more information about other types of blisters:

Blisters from Burns (*See Burns in Chapter 4—First Aid starting on page 54*).

Blisters from Poison Ivy (*See Poison Ivy later in this chapter starting on page 206*).

Blisters from Insect Bites (*See Bites and Stings later in this chapter starting on page 208*).

Blisters from Chicken Pox and Shingles (*See Chickenpox in Chapter 21—Childhood Ailments on page 254*).

Blisters of the Mouth and Lips (*See Mouth Sores in Chapter 9—Mouth and Teeth on page 106*).

Blisters of Hand, Foot and Mouth Disease (*See Hand Foot and Mouth Disease in Chapter 21—Childhood on page 256*).

♡ ADDITIONAL SUPPORT FOR SPORT-RELATED BLISTERS

- If you tend to blister easily, e.g., after running a long way or using an instrument repeatedly, consider applying a chafing cream or ointment like one of the **Badger® balms**.
- If you get blisters between your toes because your feet sweat, try **Silicea 6X** cell salt for daily use or the homeopathic remedy **Silicea** for occasional use, or use for prevention just before a race or competition.

TO POP OR NOT TO POP

- Resist the urge to pop the blister because it opens up the possibility for bacteria to enter the skin. Many blisters DO get better on their own-your skin absorbs the fluid and the blister flattens and peels off. Until that happens, you can use a donut-shaped piece of moleskin padding or band-aid or tape to help keep it from breaking. Keep the area clean and dry.
- IF, however, the blister is very large (bigger than a nickel) or so painful that you can't get around with it, you may need to puncture it to let the fluid drain. You can either go to a qualified practitioner, such as a foot doctor, and have them do it or you can use a sterile lancet or sterile needle to gently and carefully puncture it. Make sure to clean the area with alcohol before and after you puncture it. Once the fluid is released, gently wash the area with soap and water, dry it gently and completely and apply a topical **Calendula ointment** and band-aid. This keeps the bacteria out and helps the skin heal. Again, keep the area clean and dry and reapply the ointment and band-aid until the blister heals.

COMMON REMEDIES FOR SPORTS RELATED BLISTERS

	Arnica	Calendula	*Causticum	Silicea	Rhus tox	Sulphur
Symptoms	Symmetrical eruptions. Eruptions occur from trauma or contusion.	Blisters caused by friction, typically on hands or feet.	Blisters from a sunburn or on the heels of the feet.	Frictional blisters develop from shoes or a bat, golf club, or racquet causing friction against skin.	Skin feels tight. Burning especially after scratching.	Affinity for the skin. Skin may be rough, dry, and peeling.
Indications	Blister appears from friction or injury.	Excessive fluid under skin, surrounding area may be red. To aid in general healing.	Blisters that burn, itch, and/or bleed.	Stinging on touch. Blisters on feet from perspiration.	Blisters are red, swollen and intensely itchy.	Eruptions usually moist, and extremely itchy and burning.
Worse	Continuing to move with the affected part.		Heat of bed. Warm bathing.	Cold, bathing.	Cold air, uncovering, overuse, at night.	Heat, heat of bed, night, bathing.
Better	Relieving the part of any pressure.		Wet. Bathing affected part in cool water.	Warmth.	Hot water.	Cold applications.

Dosing: Use the BLUE method. Observe and evaluate. Blisters take a while to heal. If the pain, burning, itching or other sensations subside and the blister is healing, stop the remedy and take only if sensation returns and healing is hindered.

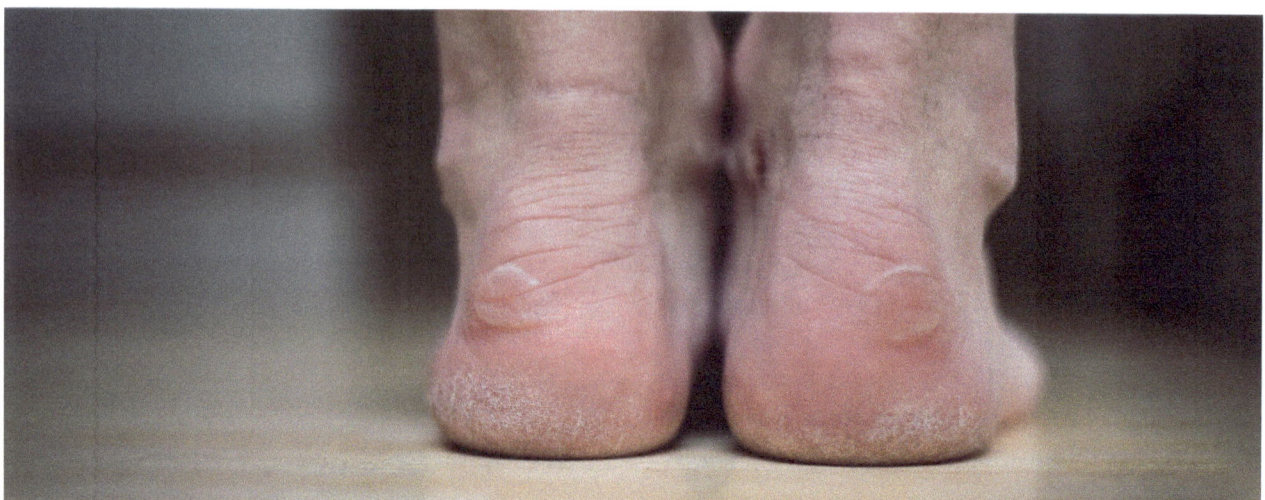

HIVES

Hives are also called urticaria. They are a histamine reaction consisting of itchy, stinging welts on the skin. They can be triggered by irritants such as poisonous plants, food intolerances, and animal dander. Hives can also be produced by an emotional upset.

IT'S AN EMERGENCY WHEN

- The person is experiencing anaphylactic shock, a serious life-threatening condition. DO NOT DELAY, as time is of the essence, especially if hives have come on very quickly and/or the throat is swelling. Give **Apis** on the way to the hospital (see below).

  Anaphylactic shock symptoms include: *The person may feel too warm, have the sensation of a lump in their throat or difficulty swallowing, breaking out in hives or localized redness, experiencing tingling or itching, or feeling the tongue and lips swelling. Blood pressure can drop dramatically, resulting in faintness; the pulse may become weak and rapid, with heart palpitations that can set off panic and agitation.*

- Call the hospital or local poison control center if you suspect that someone has eaten a poisonous plant. There are some plants for which you want to induce vomiting, and others for which you do not want the person to vomit.

Remedies to consider while you wait for care, or on the way to the hospital using the RED dosing method:

- **Apis:** This remedy can save a life in an extreme allergic reaction. Swelling is rapid, and there is no thirst. There may be panting and a feeling of not being able to get enough air or take another breath. Someone who needs **Apis** may be whiny, weepy, restless, anxious, irritable, and fidgety. On the other hand, they may be tired and want to lie down.

- ***Carbolic acid:** This remedy is for anaphylactic shock following a bee or wasp sting, with respiratory problems, fainting, swelling, and hives. The part affected will be weak, with intense itching and severe burning and pricking pains that come and go. There may be cold hands and feet, trembling, and profuse cold, clammy sweats. The person rapidly loses vitality and strength, even to the point of collapse. People needing ***Carbolic acid** are likely to have strong chemical and environmental sensitivities, and a very acute sense of smell can be a strong indicator for this remedy. If you or someone close to you has a known allergy that can cause anaphylactic shock, you might want to purchase this remedy to have on hand in an emergency.

ADDITIONAL SUPPORT FOR HIVES

- Baking soda or oatmeal baths and poultices (a healing paste) can be soothing for the swelling and itching. For a bath, use one cup of baking soda in a bathtub full of warm (not hot) water. For a poultice, mix one teaspoon of bottled spring water, or fresh water that has been boiled and cooled, with one teaspoon of baking soda or oatmeal, and put the paste on the affected area. Lightly cover the area with sterile gauze. Remove gauze and rinse with cool water when the itching has subsided, and the swelling has gone down. You can use cold compresses if it makes the person feel better.
- Have the person drink lots of water to flush out the histamine.
- Give high doses of vitamin C (to toleration), or foods rich in vitamin C, to continue the flushing out.
- If the allergic reaction is from pollen and you know what pollen they may be allergic to, find out when the pollen count is at its highest. The person should stay indoors as much as possible during that time.

WHEN TO CONTACT YOUR HEALTHCARE PROFESSIONAL

- If hives do not go away after giving well-chosen remedies and/or the person keeps having acute allergic reactions.

COMMON REMEDIES FOR HIVES

	Apis	Arsenicum	*Carbolic acid	Rhus tox	*Urtica
Onset	Rapid onset from contact with an allergen.	Eating shellfish. Dust, smoke, pesticides, poisonous plants, or animal dander.	Rapid weakness. Hives may spread over the entire body.	Rapid onset from contact with poisonous plants, poison ivy, or oak. Reaction to cold air or water.	Rapid onset from stinging nettles or eating shellfish.
Symptoms	Skin is itchy, swollen, puffy, sensitive, sore, hot, shiny rosy-red color. Large masses of hives, with burning, stinging, itching that is very intense at night. Sensitive to touch.	Many burning symptoms, however, the person is very chilly. Does not want to lie down for fear of suffocation. Feels weak and exhausted, but restless. Can have heart palpitations.	Hives severely sting, burn, and itch. Pricking pains come and go. Sense of smell becomes very acute. Face, ears, tongue, and throat may swell.	Intensely itchy, water-filled blisters or hives. Sensitivity to cold air. Skin can become red, infected, may become scaly. Glands, joints, or muscles around the affected area can become stiff and achy.	Itching with raised, pale welts on a background of red skin. Areas appear in blotches. Itching can be quite severe.
Mood	Whining, weepy, restless, anxious, irritable, fidgety, tired, and wants to lie down.	Anxious, irritable, oversensitive, needy, demanding. Can fear they are dying or will not get better.	Explosive temperament. Discontented, rude, and gloomy.	Extreme mental and physical restlessness, irritability. Cannot get comfortable. Anxious, may become confused and/or weepy.	Very restless.
Indications	Sensations of constriction, stiffness, swelling, redness, puffiness, especially of eyelids, lips, nose, mouth, and throat. No thirst. Can be drowsy. Contraindication: Do not give in combination with **Rhus tox**.	Burning sensations, but the person feels better with heat. Has frequent thirst for small amounts of water.	May break out into a cold, clammy sweat, or tremble. Rapidly lose vitality and strength, which may bring about collapse. Scratching temporarily relieves itching.	Even though the person feels worse with cold, they do crave cold drinks. Contraindication: Do not give in combination with **Apis**.	Feel hot in bed at night, with sweating. Can experience burning in throat. Very restless. Wants to rub affected area.
Worse	Heat in any form, touch, late afternoon, nighttime, pressure, after sleep, when lying down, especially on right side.	Physical exertion, after midnight, anything cold, and lying down.	Warm rooms, cold drafts, jarring.	Cold, damp, cold applications on skin, scratching, beginning to move after resting or sitting and nighttime.	Cold water, cool moist air, touch, nighttime, and strenuous exercise.
Better	Cold applications, cool air, cool baths, sitting up, cool drinks, and being uncovered.	Warmth, hot compresses, warm drinks, fresh air, sitting at a 45-degree angle, company.	Tepid temperatures, rest, strong green or black tea. Scratching.	Movement, limbering up, warm applications, and heat.	Lying down (but not on the affected parts) and rubbing the affected area.

Special Dosing: If the hives are severe, use the RED dosing method. If the condition is significant, use the ORANGE dosing method. If there has been no improvement after two hours, choose a new remedy. Observe and evaluate. **Other remedy to consider: *Histaminum.**

POISON IVY AND POISON OAK

Poison ivy and poison oak are known for causing severe inflammation of the skin if there is contact. Both plants contain saps that have a sticky, long-lasting, oily resin called urushiol. This resin is easily wiped from the plants to other objects. It causes an itchy, blistering rash on the skin after a person has come into contact with the oil of either of these plants. The allergic reaction typically begins 12 to 48 hours after exposure to the sap and lasts at least two or three weeks. Poison ivy is found in almost all of the United States. Poison oak is most common in the western United States. It is also found in some eastern states but is rarely found in midwestern states.

IT'S AN EMERGENCY WHEN

- A person has inhaled the smoke from burning poison ivy and is having difficulty breathing.
- The person has trouble breathing or swallowing.
- The eyelids have swollen shut.
- The person has swelling of the lips and itching in the throat. The reaction is severe or widespread.

ADDITIONAL SUPPORT FOR POISON IVY AND POISON OAK

- Even though the skin is itchy, it is best to try not to touch it and to leave it alone.
- Aloe Vera gel soothes the itch and is less astringent than calamine, but it can prolong the itching.
- Sometimes cool compresses feel better, but to others a hot shower can alleviate the itchiness.
- If there are blisters, avoid the sun. If blisters are open and oozing, cover lightly with gauze; when they crust over or start drying out, exposing the area to the air will speed healing. Do not pop the blisters open.

WHEN TO CONTACT YOUR HEALTHCARE PROFESSIONAL

- The skin continues to swell.
- The rash affects the eyes, mouth, or genitals.
- Blisters are oozing pus.
- The person develops a fever greater than 100 °F (37.7 °C).
- The rash has not gone away within a few weeks.
- There is severe itching that interferes with sleep.

Remedies to consider:

- **Rhus tox**: Hot, inflamed, dry, burning skin with a red rash; water-filled blisters that itch intensely and burn. Sensitivity to cold air. Skin may become scaly. Swelling, intense itching that is worse on hairy parts. Cannot rest in any position. Itching is better by taking a hot shower.

- ***Anacardium:** Intense itching, which is made worse by scratching. Burning; stinging; swelling. Redness of skin. Blisters with a discharge of yellow liquid that form crusts. Irritability is so intense from itching that it brings on cursing and swearing. Better from eating. If a scalding hot shower feels better, consider this remedy.

- ***Croton tiglium:** Itching of skin, but the scratching is painful because the area is so tender they are unable to scratch. Itching is better by gentle rubbing. Burning red skin. Blisters that ooze pus-colored or a clear discharge and then form crusts. Intense itching of genitals may occur. Sensation "as if the skin were hide-bound," meaning the skin has a tightness because of the swelling and feels as though it is going to explode. May also develop watery diarrhea.

Special Dosing: If the outbreak is severe, meaning if the person is having unusual swelling, having trouble breathing or swallowing, use the RED dosing method and go for emergency help. If the condition is significant, meaning visible over a large portion of the body and seems to be spreading, use the ORANGE dosing method. As the condition improves, move to the BLUE dosing method. Observe and evaluate.

PUNCTURE WOUNDS

A puncture wound is a wound that is deeper than it is wide; it is usually a small hole caused by a pointed object (nail, fishhook, etc.). It is important to gently press around the wound to encourage bleeding, which can be cleansing and greatly reduce the risk of the wound sealing in any sort of contamination. However, if the wound is bleeding excessively, take the appropriate measures to slow the bleeding. Soak the wound in clean water with a few drops of **Ledum tincture** or apply a **Ledum tincture** compress to reduce infection and promote healing.

*For more review **Splinters** in this chapter starting on **page 202**.* page 202

Remedies to consider:

- **Ledum:** In addition to using **Ledum tincture** directly on the wound, taking homeopathic **Ledum** internally is the most common protocol for puncture wounds. The leading indications that would require **Ledum** are redness, swelling, throbbing pain, and wound feels cold to the touch and is relieved by cool applications.

- **Apis:** Indicated if the puncture wound feels warm or hot with inflammation and stinging pains that are relieved by cool applications.

- **Hypericum:** Indicated if there is sharp shooting pain, especially for wounds that are in an area rich with nerves such as fingers and toes.

For puncture areas that have become infected, use **Hepar sulph** twice a day until resolved; it will keep the infection from spreading. The area becomes swollen, red, hot, sometimes hard, and extremely sensitive. The skin around the area is dry. The pains are sore, splinter-like, and sharp. The wound may be bloody, look abscessed, or ooze pus that is yellow or green and tends to smell like old, rotten cheese.

If you suspect a foreign object is in the wound, such as a splinter, see the section on **Splinters** in this chapter starting on **page 202**.

Dosing: Use the ORANGE dosing method to start. Observe and evaluate.

BITES AND STINGS FROM INSECTS AND SEA CREATURES

Bites and stings are common encounters in our natural world. Things like bug bites, bee stings, spider bites, cat or dog bites, jellyfish stings, sea urchin stings, snake bites and more will force us to stop and take action sooner rather than later. Since some people react more strongly than others to these influences, there are homeopathic remedies as well as other supportive suggestions here to help in most situations.

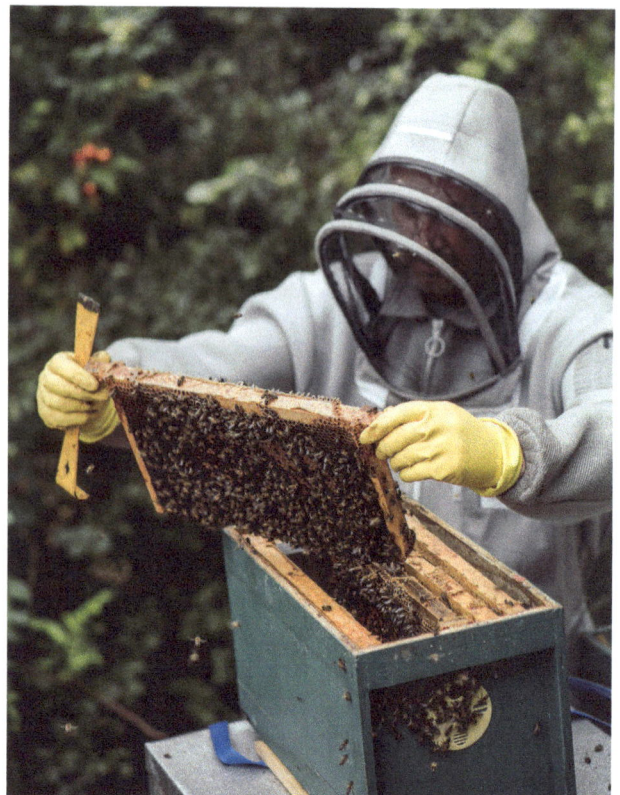

IT'S AN EMERGENCY WHEN

- The victim has been stung in the mouth or throat; airways can swell and obstruct breathing. Give **Apis** every 10 minutes, ice to suck on (if age appropriate), and take them to a hospital.
- You suspect that a bite is from a highly poisonous spider such as a black widow or brown recluse. Apply an ice pack to keep the poison from spreading and give the appropriate remedy on the way to the hospital. Some homeopaths recommend **Lachesis** as the first-aid remedy to take immediately after a black widow or brown recluse spider bite.
- The person has been bitten by a venomous snake.
- There are red streaks running up or outwards from the wound.
- The person has a high fever, is delirious or confused, feels faint, or loses consciousness after a bite.

GENERAL SUPPORT FOR MOST BITES AND STINGS

- Clean all wounds by washing the area with mild soap and running water. If running water is not available, use a sterile cloth with soap and water. Wipe away from the wound, not into it. Keep all wounds clean and dry. If the wound does not have any redness, you can apply sterile gauze soaked in five drops of **Calendula tincture** to a quarter-cup of bottled spring water or fresh water that has been boiled and cooled.
- Externally apply **Calendula cream** or apply a few drops of **Hypercal** to bites and stings from mosquitoes, bees, wasps, hornets, and fleas. **Hypercal** is a combination of **Hypericum tincture**, which heals damaged nerves, and **Calendula tincture**, which repairs damaged skin. This combination is invaluable when applied topically, as it not only brings about rapid healing but also helps to prevent scarring. Apply it to the skin with a sterile cloth or cotton ball on an as-needed basis until healed. This solution stings at first but then takes the pain and stinging away. The skin must be clean and disinfected before applying this solution. *See **How to Make Hypercal Solution** on **page 202** in this chapter.*

ADDITIONAL SUPPORT FOR BITES AND STINGS FROM INSECTS AND SEA CREATURES

- **Bee stings:** If a bee stinger remains in the skin, remove it as soon as possible by carefully scraping a sterilized needle across the skin. Do not pull the stinger out with fingers or tweezers, as this can squeeze more venom into the puncture. Clean the wound. A paste of baking soda and water feels best on the sting. Use an ice pack to reduce swelling and prevent the venom from spreading to surrounding tissues. You can crush a few pellets of **Apis** in half an ounce of spring water and apply directly onto the sting. If a person is extremely reactive to bee stings, ask your homeopath for a higher potency of **Apis** and always carry it with you.

- **Spider bites:** Spider bites can cause both swelling and pain. All spiders are poisonous to varying degrees. The bite can be anything from a tiny red welt to a very toxic reaction including redness, heat and swelling. Apply an ice pack to keep the poison from spreading. There are usually two puncture wounds if the bite is from a spider. Seek immediate medical attention if you suspect the spider was a dangerous variety such as a brown recluse or black widow. Baking soda or oatmeal baths can soothe the swelling and itching. Use one cup of either and add to warm bath water (not hot). Consider **Ledum, Arsenicum,** or **Lachesis.**

- **Jellyfish stings:** Rinse the sting with seawater. (Fresh water will increase the pain.) Do not apply ice packs or rub the area. Apply white vinegar or isopropyl alcohol (except in the eye area). Flush eye-area stings with one gallon of fresh water. Use one-part vinegar to four parts of water for mouth-area stings. However, do not use vinegar if there is any swelling in the mouth or throat or if there is difficulty swallowing. Carefully remove any tentacles with tweezers, while wearing gloves. Apply a paste of baking soda, mud, or shaving cream to the injury and then shave any hair from the area with a knife or razor and reapply the vinegar or alcohol. The paste will absorb any additional toxin discharge during the shaving.

- **Sea Urchin stings:** Remove any spines carefully with tweezers while wearing gloves. You probably cannot get the entire spine out so get out what you can. Do not dig too deeply. Do this as soon as possible to reduce pain and start the healing process. Cover the area immediately with a clean cloth soaked in white vinegar, hot water or saline solution and leave it on for as long as possible. Have the person soak the affected area in the hottest water they can tolerate for 20 to 40 minutes. This eases the pain and will help to alleviate soreness on the following day. Soak the area with the vinegar cloth again, all night if possible. Watch for infection. There may be a dark discoloration immediately after the sting. Any stingers that are not removed will dissolve on their own; giving a small extra dose of vitamin D can speed this process. All sea urchins are poisonous to varying degrees, but there are a few deadly varieties. If you suspect the person has been stung by a deadly one, seek immediate medical attention.

A FEW ADDITIONAL TIPS

- Use all-natural insect repellents (avoid using chemical-based insect repellents).
- Do not use bug sprays to kill insects because it is toxic and can be harmful if inhaled (especially for children).
- For mild itching from insect bites or stings, **Sting-Stop homeopathic gel** is an excellent topical, as is calamine lotion. A dab of tea tree oil will also alleviate itching as well as prevent infection.

There are two main remedies appropriate for most insect bites and stings:

- **Apis:** This remedy is not just for bee stings but for any insect bite or sea creature sting with swelling; the bites feel better from cold applications.

- **Ledum:** For insect bites or stings of any kind without significant swelling, including mosquito, flea, or tick bites.

Additionally, **Lachesis** can be considered for infected wounds and ulcers that heal slowly. The wound may appear dark red, bluish, or purplish. The swollen bite site may seep dark, bloody pus. Pain may have a burning, throbbing, or shooting quality. The person may feel worse at night and from heat, pressure, or touch.

If the person is not responding to **Apis** or **Ledum**, consider one of the other remedies in the following chart as the remedy of choice depends on the creature creating the injury.

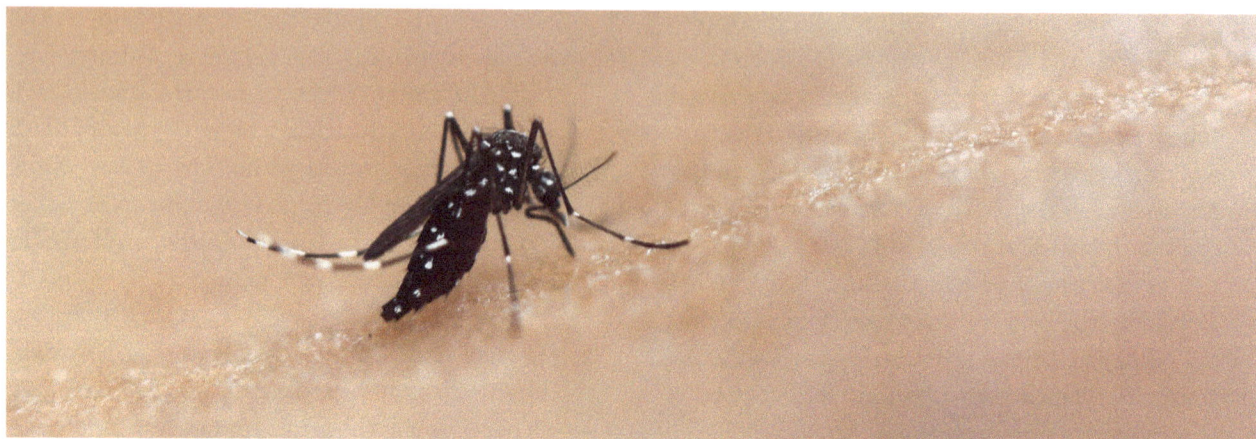

COMMON REMEDIES FOR BITES AND STINGS

	Apis	Arsenicum	Hypericum	Ledum	Silicea	*Urtica
Cause	Bee Sting Wasp Sting Hornet Sting Jellyfish Sting Spider Bite	Black Fly Bites Spider Bite	Bee Sting Wasp Sting Hornet Sting	Bee Sting Wasp Sting Hornet Sting Spider Bite	Sea Urchin Sting	Bee Sting Jellyfish Sting Spider Bite
Symptoms	Skin is rose-colored, puffy, very sensitive to touch with burning, hot, piercing, stinging pains. May not be thirsty.	If itching is maddening. Discomfort, swelling and pain. Swollen lymph nodes, fever, nausea, and headaches.	Severe, tearing pains that shoot upward along the nerve pathways. Nerve pains are sharp and intense. Usually swelling and a heightened sense of pain, smell, and hearing.	Site is puffy, tender, dark red or purple. May be twitching around the site. Throbbing, shooting, pricking pains, numbness. Foul smelling pus if infected.	Redness and swelling around puncture wound. If the spine is embedded in the wound, **Silicea** will help to expel it from the body.	Intense itching with raised, pale welts on a background of red skin.
Mood	Weepy, restless, fidgety, anxious. Wants to lie down. Doesn't want to be left alone.	Restlessness.	Nervous and depressed. May seem confused, forgetful, and have a wild, staring look on the face. Constantly drowsy.	Angry, anxious, and want to be left alone.	Anxiety and sensitivity to pain.	Restlessness.
Indications	Stings with rapid swelling.	Tiny puncture wounds or a huge swelling on the skin.	Stings to nerve rich areas such as fingers, toes, eyes or lips.	Skin feels cold to the touch; however, feels better with cold applications.	Specifically, if stung by a sea urchin or if any part of any sting is embedded in the body.	Raised welts which may or may not be fluid filled.
Worse	Any form of heat or pressure and after sleep.	Cold.	Pressure, touch, cold, and damp.	Touch, being exposed.	Washing and uncovering.	Cold water, touch, nighttime.
Better	Cold applications, cool bathing, cold drinks, being uncovered.	Warmth.	Rubbing.	Cold applications and rest.	Warmth and wrapping.	Lying down, rubbing the affected parts.

Dosing: If the condition is severe, give the remedy using the ORANGE method. Otherwise, give the remedy hourly until there is improvement. You may need to repeat the remedy two to three times per day for a few days. Observe and evaluate.

BITES FROM ANIMALS

Besides pain from an animal bite, the major concern is a bite becoming infected. Bacteria from the animal's mouth can enter the wound and begin growing. An infection, if left unchecked, can cause tissue damage or even life-threatening problems. The seriousness of a bite depends on the location and what type of animal has bitten the person. Infections occur more frequently from cat bites because cats have sharp, pointed teeth that cause deep wounds. The skin can close over quickly and trap bacteria under the skin.

Rabies is a rare but potentially fatal infection that may result from wild animals such as bats, skunks, raccoons, and foxes. Bites from these animals need immediate emergency treatment and should be reported to your public health department.

Snakebites aren't very common, and most snakes in North America are not venomous. Snakes will not bite humans unless they feel threatened, so leaving them alone is the best strategy for preventing a bite. Symptoms of snakebites can include bleeding, pain, swelling, redness, and itching near the bite area.

IT'S AN EMERGENCY WHEN

- There is any snakebite, whether you think the snake is venomous or not. Give **Ledum** every 10 minutes on the way to the hospital or while you wait for care. Also consider giving **Bach Rescue Remedy®** to reduce anxiety.
- The person has a high fever, is delirious or confused, feels faint, or loses consciousness after a bite.
- There is bleeding that is difficult to control.
- After a bite to the finger(s), there is loss of finger motion or if the finger(s) is unusually pale, severely red, or numb.
- There are red streaks leading away from the wound, up the limb and toward the heart.
- There are swollen glands around the elbow or in the armpit.
- The person has a fever, is unusually tired, has night sweats, and/or shakes.

GENERAL SUPPORT FOR BITES FROM ANIMALS

- Clean all wounds by washing the area with mild soap and running water. If running water is not available, use a sterile cloth with soap and water. Wipe away from the wound, not into it. Keep all wounds clean and dry. If the wound does not have any redness, you can apply sterile gauze soaked in one teaspoon of **Calendula tincture** (found in health food stores or natural pharmacies) to one pint (two cups) of spring water or water that has been boiled and cooled. Apply a new dressing once a day. If the area is inflamed and not healing, it is important to note that some bite wounds may take time to heal.
- A snake bite causes swelling, intense pain, and redness or blueness of the skin that looks like a bad bruise. There may be a fever, with muscle or abdominal cramping. Sometimes there are burning pains or sensations throughout the body or in certain parts. Apply an ice pack to keep the venom from spreading, keep the area immobilized, and give the appropriate remedies on the way to the hospital. It is important to follow up with your healthcare practitioner because chronic symptoms can appear long after the bite has occurred.
- Trauma after being bitten by an animal is common, especially if the bite is from a family pet. If the person is extremely afraid of the animal, give **Aconite** every two hours, for three doses. If they feel abused by the animal and/or can no longer trust it, **Staphysagria** will help resolve the trauma.

ADDITIONAL SUPPORT FOR BITES FROM ANIMALS

- **Cat bites:** Cat bites are painful wounds that often get infected. Speed is essential in treating them. Prepare a solution of pure water and three pellets each of **Ledum, Hypericum, Calendula** and **Lachesis** all in 30c potency. Succuss (shake vigorously) ten times; take a big sip internally (that's a dose) every 10-15 minutes for an hour as well as applying the solution to the wound. If the bite is shallow and addressed immediately, a few doses may be enough. Otherwise, take as needed for 3-7 days until there is no more pain or sign of infection. If the injured area becomes hot and red or there are red streaks spreading out from the bite, immediately go to the hospital. This can become a life threatening situation.

- **Dog bites:** Dog bites carry less risk of infection than cat bites but may be very painful. If the wound is red, hot, and swollen, use **Apis**; if it is cold to the touch, with pains that shoot upward, use **Ledum**. For gaping, exquisitely painful wounds, especially if on the hands or soles, use **Hypericum**.

- **Wild animals or non-venomous snake bites:** Treat them as you would a cat bite, because the risk of infection is high. Check with your healthcare provider right away if bitten by a possum, raccoon, fox, etc.

- **Tick bites:** For tick bites, start with **Ledum**. At the site of the bite there will be redness, possibly surrounded by a light-colored border, maybe even the famous bulls-eye rash, and perhaps some swelling and itching. For chronic Lyme treatment, see a healthcare professional and/or professional homeopath.

WHEN TO CONTACT YOUR HEALTHCARE PROFESSIONAL

- There is severe swelling.
- There is deep red or purple skin.
- There is heat around the wound.
- There is continued pain beyond 24 hours.
- There is drainage from the wound.
- There is a bulls-eye rash after a tick bite.

Here is a brief overview of remedies useful for specific types of animal bites:

- Cats and Rodents: **Arsenicum, Hypericum, Lachesis,** or **Ledum.**

- Dogs and Horses: **Arnica** or ***Bellis per** if it is a deeply bruised wound. If the bite has drawn blood, you may also need **Apis, Arsenicum, Hypericum, Lachesis,** or **Ledum.**

- Snakes: Snake bites are puncture wounds and may be poisonous. Emergency care is needed.

COMMON REMEDIES FOR ANIMAL BITES—part 1

	Apis	Arnica	Arsenicum	*Carbolic acid
Onset	Snake, dog, or horse bites.	Deeply bruised wound from a dog or horse.	Cat, rodent, dog, horse, or snake bite.	Snake bite.
Symptoms	Skin is puffy, rosy-colored, and very sensitive to touch, with burning, hot, piercing, stinging pains. Not thirsty.	Pains are sore, aching with bruised feeling. Skin is black and blue. May be tingling.	Swelling and burning pain. If wound becomes infected, it oozes foul, yellow pus.	Inflammation, burning, tingling and numbness. Bites may form very itchy burning blisters with smelly, clear fluid.
Mood	Weepy, restless, fidgety, anxious, irritable, scared to be alone, wants to lie down.	Does not want to be touched, fussed over, approached by anyone. Says they are okay, so they will be left alone.	Anxious irritable, over-sensitive, needy, may fear they are dying.	Least amount of mental exertion leaves them exhausted.
Indications	For puncture wounds with rapid swelling.	For bruising and swelling from a bite that has not broken the skin.	Puncture wounds with burning symptoms.	Rapidly lose vitality and strength to the point of collapse. Can break out into a cold sweat. Cold hands and feet.
Worse	Heat in any form, touch, pressure, after sleeping.	Touch, jarring and motion.	Physical exertion, after midnight, anything cold, and lying down.	Warm rooms, cold drafts, jarring.
Better	Cold applications, cool air, drinks, and bathing. Being uncovered, sitting up.	Lying stretched out or with head low, and not talking.	Warmth, hot compresses, warm drinks, sitting at a 45-degree angle, fresh air, and company.	Tepid temperatures, rest, strong green or black tea, and scratching gives temporary relief.

COMMON REMEDIES FOR ANIMAL BITES—part 2

	Hypericum	Ledum	Lachesis
Onset	Cat, rodent, dog, horse, or snake bite.	Cat, rodent, dog, horse or snake bite.	Snake, cat, rodent, dog, or horse bite.
Symptoms	Severe, tearing pains that shoot upward along nerve pathways. Pain is sharp and intense. Heightened sense of pain, smell, and hearing. Usually swelling.	Site is puffy, tender, dark red or purple. Pains are throbbing, shooting, pricking. Numbness. If infected, pus smells foul. May twitch around the site.	Wound is dark red, bluish, or purplish. Burning, throbbing, tightness, fullness. May bleed dark thin blood.
Mood	Nervous, drowsy, depressed. Can seem confused, forgetful. May have a wild, staring look on their face.	Angry, anxious, and wants to be left alone.	Tense, nervous, excitable, talkative, jumping from one topic to another.
Indications	Bites in nerve rich areas such a fingers, toes, eyes, or lips.	Skin feels cold to the touch, but site feels better with cold applications.	Affected area feels like it is going to burst open.
Worse	Pressure, touch, cold, and damp.	Night, heat of bed, warmth of covers, warm air.	Touch, heat, night, constriction, pressure, tight clothing.
Better	Rubbing.	Cold applications, cold air, cool bathing and rest.	Allowing wound to discharge, open air, and cold drinks.

Note: Bites that become infected may need **Hepar sulph** or ***Pyrogen**.

Dosing: If the pain is severe, use the RED dosing method to start. If the condition is improving but still painful, use the ORANGE dosing method. As the condition improves, move to the BLUE dosing method. Observe and evaluate.

FUNGAL INFECTIONS

Fungal infections can be itchy and annoying. Common fungal infections include Athlete's Foot, Ringworm, and Jock Itch. Healthy people who drink adequate amounts of water and eat a healthy organic diet are more resistant. Wearing sweaty, wet clothing in the summertime or wearing several layers of clothing in the wintertime causes an increased incidence of jock itch, such as in hot yoga and exercisers who wear sweat suits. Being barefoot in public showers, wearing sweaty socks for a long period of time, and a diet high in sugar are some other common causes of fungal infections.

Fungal skin and nail infections may look bad, but they rarely lead to more than itching and irritation. Still, you can take plenty of precautionary measures to prevent them.

RINGWORM

Ringworm of the body (tinea corporis) is another form of athlete's foot as is jock itch (tinea cruris) and ringworm of the scalp (tinea capitis). It is a fungal infection that develops on the top layer of your skin. It's characterized by a red circular rash with clearer skin in the middle that may or may not itch. Ringworm gets its name because of its appearance. No actual worm is involved. Ringworm often spreads by direct skin-to-skin contact with an infected person or animal. The symptoms of athlete's foot and ringworm are very similar. There's intense burning, stinging, redness, and itching. It also may cause flaking and/or peeling of the skin in some people.

ATHLETE'S FOOT

Athlete's foot, also known as tinea pedis, is a contagious fungal infection affecting the skin between the toes. It can also spread to the toenails and the hands. It is called "athlete's foot" because it's commonly seen in athletes. Athlete's foot is not serious, but sometimes it's hard to alleviate.

This fungal infection involves itchy, burning, cracking, and peeling feet. Athlete's foot is a form of ringworm that usually develops between the toes. It can spread via wet locker room floors and contaminated towels and shoes. Prevent it by wearing shower shoes at the gym, washing your feet daily, drying them well especially between the toes, and wearing clean, dry socks.

JOCK ITCH

Jock Itch (tinea cruris) can affect both men and women. It causes a raised, itchy, red, often ring-shaped skin rash in warm, moist areas, such as the genitals, inner thighs, and buttocks. Jock itch gets its name because it is common in people who sweat a lot, as do athletes. It also is more likely to occur in people who are overweight.

Jock itch is another type of ringworm, and it can be caused by sweating and the humid environment often created by athletic gear. You can prevent it by keeping your groin clean and dry, changing into dry, clean clothes and underwear after exercise or practice, and avoiding tight clothing. The fungus that most commonly causes jock itch is called trichophyton rubrum. It also causes fungal infections of the toes and body. Jock itch involving the scrotum or penis is most likely candida albicans, the same type of yeast that causes vaginal yeast infections.

Symptoms:

- itchy or burning sensations on the affected area

- red skin

- ring-shaped skin rash

- may consist of a line of small, raised blisters

- flaky or scaly look to the skin in the affected area

Jock itch is contagious and may be spread through contact with towels, clothes, etc., contaminated with fungal microorganisms. As with athletes foot, using public showers raises the chances of getting jock itch.

ADDITIONAL SUPPORT FOR FUNGAL INFECTIONS

- Keep skin clean and dry. Shower after practice or competition, and change clothes including underwear and socks.
- Let your sneakers air out and wash them regularly; consider having two pairs of shoes to rotate, if you need them daily.
- Take your shoes off at home to expose your feet to the air.
- Make sure showers and towels are clean as well.
- Keeping the skin, clothes, sheet, and covers clean will help to heal the skin.
- Use clean clothes and towels with every practice/competition. Re-wearing sweaty sweatshirts or gym clothes or sharing towels puts you at risk of developing this infection.
- Wear shower shoes, such as flip flops, in any communal locker room.
- Avoid sitting on wet benches at a gym.
- Take along an extra towel and fold it over to sit on.
- Don't share workout mats or towels.
- Wash your hands before and after a workout, and don't forget to wipe down gym equipment with some tea tree oil in the water before and after using it.
- Keep your groin area clean and dry to prevent jock itch from developing.
- Dry yourself thoroughly after showering; consider, as well, using a cornstarch-based powder in the groin area.
- Choose looser clothes in breathable fabrics like cotton and wash all clothes after exercise or a workout.

WHEN TO CONTACT YOUR HEALTHCARE PROFESSIONAL

- The skin condition fails to improve, or becomes chronic.

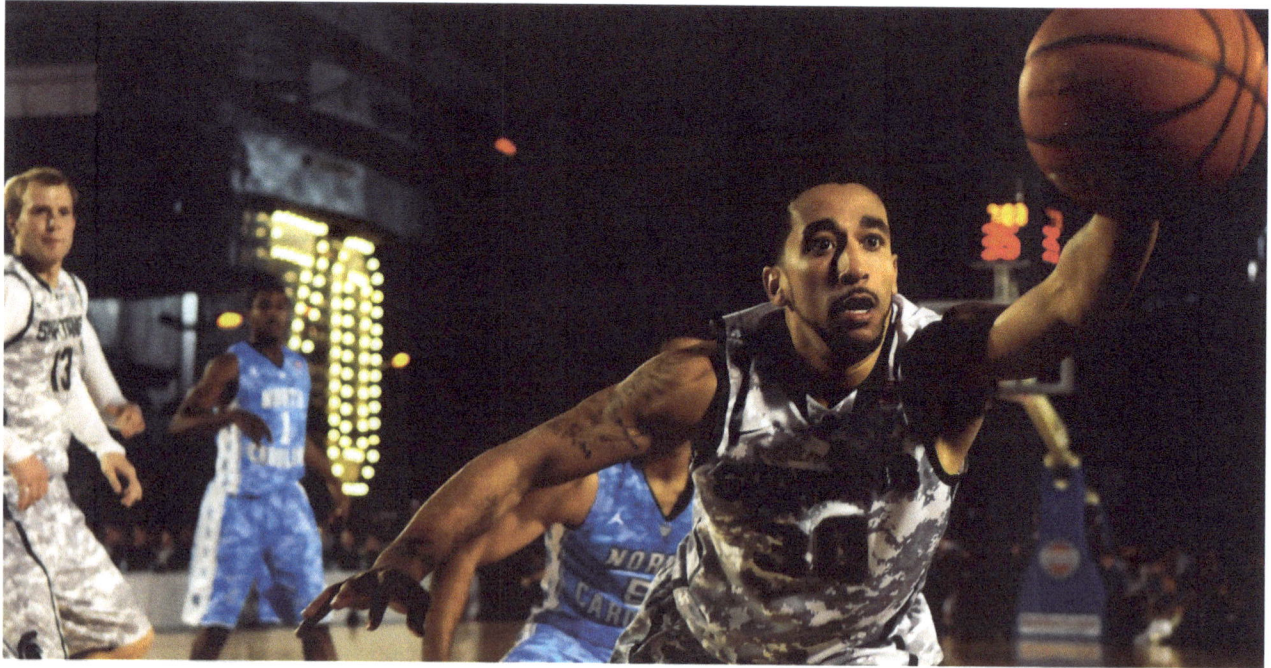

COMMON REMEDIES FOR FUNGAL INFECTIONS—part 1

	*Baryta carb	Graphites	*Petroleum	Sepia
Symptoms	Intolerable itching. Burning sensation and needle-like pricking with violent itching. Oozing athlete's foot.	Itching with moist eruptions. Odorous discharge. Thick water honey-like sticky fluid. Athlete's foot with cracks. Dry rough skin, cracks between toes. #1 remedy for athlete's foot.	Rough and cracked skin. Deep cracks in folds of skin (especially around toes.) Skin is hard, raw, cracks easily and bleeds. Greenish crusts with burning, itching and bleeding.	Top remedy for ringworm on any part of the body, but particularly in the bends of knees and elbows. Isolated ring-shaped spots on the skin. Itching, but scratching brings no relief. Can turn into burning sensations. Affected skin is raw, rough, and hard. With athlete's foot can cause thickening of the soles of the feet.
Mood	Poor self confidence. Anxiety about the future. Oversensitive. Critical.	Sensitive, irritable.	Anxiety in a crowd. Worried without a cause. Long lasting fear. Inconsolable. Low-spirited. Irritable, easily offended. Quarelsome in the morning.	Testy, excitable, sensitive. Hard and indifferent to loved ones. Worse in company, yet dreads being alone. Spiteful and blunt around people. Tearful, careworn, and pathetic.
Indications	Pricking sensation like needles that itch as well. Moisture and soreness between scrotum and thighs. Skin injuries taking a long time to heal.	Itching with moist eruptions. Odorous discharge. Thick water honey-like sticky fluid.	Severe itching, will scratch until skin bleeds. Deep cracks between toes. Burning and itching of skin. Stinging and red. Offensive foot sweat. Thickened skin that is hard and splitting.	Ringworm in isolated spots. Tends to be worse in the flexures (bends of the elbows and knees). Itching vesicles (fluid-filled bumps). Not relieved by scratching.
Worse	Thinking of symptoms. Company. Sitting. Cold and damp. Suppressed foot sweat.	Warmth of bed, hot drinks, scratching.	Dampness, cold weather, winter, changing weather, and during thunderstorms. Vexation and touch.	Cold wind, snowy air, snowfall, before thunderstorms. At seaside. Coition or sexual excess. After first sleep. After eating. 3-5 PM.
Better	Walking in open air. Cold food. Warm wraps. Alone.	Cold. Open air.	Warm air, dry weather.	Strong movement, exercise, dance, especially once warmed up. Pressure, warmth of bed, warm room, hot applications, sitting with legs crossed.

COMMON REMEDIES FOR FUNGAL INFECTIONS—part 2

	Silicea	Sulphur	*Thuja
Symptoms	Ringworm presents as crops of boils with foul pus on feet and toes. Intensely itchy, especially in the daytime and evening. Skin fungus that comes on from excess sweating that smells foul as is the case with jock itch.	Intense burning and itching. Sensitivity to washing and air. Painful cracking of the skin. Scratching the itch causes a burning sensation. Soreness in folds of skin.	Profuse perspiration on the scrotum and inside of the thighs. Erosion and rawness between legs and on sides of the scrotum, with a constant oozing of moisture. This emits a sweetish smell and stains clothes yellow. Pungent odor-sweet or burnt. Eruptions cause violent itching or burning.
Mood	Rose-colored blotches. Eruptions itch and burn. Sensitive foul spongy skin on feet, toes and nails. Skin can be dry and cracked.	Mechanical thinking, inquiring minds, philosophical, reclusive, extroverted, practical idealist.	Low self-esteem. Feels worthless. Tries to fit in by imitating behavior of popular or successful people around them.
Indications	Sensitivity to cold.	Dry, scaly, unhealthy skin. Every little injury suppurates. Itching and burning. Must scratch until it bleeds. Scratched skin ulcerates and exudes an offensive discharge. Often a history of skin affections being suppressed with topical medications.	Intense itching that burns violently after scratching or bathing. Sometimes oozes moisture. Bleeding readily. Luxuriant growth of hair on parts usually not covered by hair. Skin looks oily or greasy. Sensation of needle-pricking.
Worse	Cold, but worse from heated stuffy rooms. Cold, damp, and changes of weather. Excess stress. Thinking about problems. Suppression of sweat. Lying down.	Night. Heating up in bed. Bathing. Overexertion. Milk. 11 PM.	Cold, damp air or weather. After vaccinations. Left side. 3 AM or 3 PM. Scratching and cold bathing.
Better	Warmth, warm wraps. Summer. Profuse urination.	Open air, dry weather. Motion. Drawing up of affected limbs. Cold applications.	Warmth, warm wrappings, warm moisture. Motion. Rubbing . Rest.

Other remedy to consider: *Tellurium.
Dosing: Use the BLUE method. Observe and evaluate.

BOILS

A boil is a painful infection of a hair follicle or oil glands and the surrounding skin. A boil stands out as a small and hard red bump. As white blood cells rush to the site of the infection, the boil fills with pus and becomes more tender. Soon thereafter, a boil usually forms a head that bursts open and discharges.

ADDITIONAL SUPPORT FOR BOILS

- Keep the area clean and apply **Calendula lotion** throughout the treatment.
- Warm saltwater soaks, if possible, or application with a clean cloth can soothe a painful boil.
- When the boil comes to a head, it will burst, and it is best to let it drain naturally. Never pinch or squeeze it.

WHEN TO CONTACT YOUR HEALTHCARE PROFESSIONAL

- There are recurrent boils. It can be a symptom of underlying disorders that carry the bacteria.

Remedies to consider:

- **Belladonna:** This is the first remedy used when the boil is hot, red, and coming on fast. There may be fever, flushing of the face, and swollen glands.

- **Hepar Sulph:** This boil is hard and very painful. The area is very tender to the touch. This remedy helps the boil mature and release its pus and heal. As it is discharging, it may smell like rotten cheese. The glands may be swollen. The person may be chilly and irritable.

- **Silicea:** This boil tends to be hard and continues to ooze. This remedy helps the slow forming boil come to a head and discharge. The person is sensitive and quiet.

Dosing: Use the **BLUE** method. Observe and evaluate.

? WHAT'S THE FIRST REMEDY YOU THINK OF WHEN...

1. The skin has acne as a result of eating cheese with eruptions that burn or itch.
2. An open wound is suppurating and especially painful with torn or lacerated skin.
3. Splinters that are from wood or glass cannot be removed because there is not enough above the surface to grab with tweezers.
4. There is acne with offensive pus and the person perspires copiously and offensively.
5. A puncture wound is puffy, possibly purple with shooting, biting or pricking pains.
6. Blisters caused by friction typically occur on the hands or feet with excessive fluid under the skin.
7. The site of a splinter is extremely sensitive and painful.
8. The skin has itchy pimply eruptions that burn. The face can also be red and is aggravated by warmth.
9. Hives from contact with an allergen causes swelling that is itchy, puffy, sensitive and sore.
10. Poison ivy or oak that causes hive-like eruptions on the skin. They are intensely itchy and come on as water-filled blisters.
11. Blisters that come on from poison ivy or poison oak that discharge yellow liquid that form crusts and are intensely itchy.
12. There is a sweet smell coming from the groin area with a rawness and itching that is worse from bathing or scratching.
13. A boil that comes on from an ingrown hair that is painful and contains pus.
14. There is a fungal infection that is burning and itching, and the person tends to scratch it until it bleeds.

Answer key on page 324.

CHAPTER 19
Mind and Emotions

Being human, we experience a wide range of emotional issues that can significantly impact our well-being and daily lives. These often manifest as disruptions in one's emotional state, mood, or overall mental health. Common emotional issues include shock, fear, anxiety, rage/anger, irritability, grief, humiliation, insomnia and stress. The severity of these issues depends on multiple factors including genetics, one's life experiences and sensitivities, environmental stressors, and the individual's coping mechanisms. In this chapter, we will explore the many ways humans experience emotions and provide homeopathic options that may provide some relief.

EMOTIONAL SHOCK AND FRIGHT

If a person has experienced an intense emotion such as fright, they may be experiencing an emotional shock. It is important to know what remedy to give if a person is in a state of shock.

*Please review **Shock** in **Chapter 4—First Aid for Injuries** on **page 47**.*

WHEN TO CONTACT YOUR HEALTHCARE PROFESSIONAL

- If the person continues to experience fright after giving well-chosen remedies.

There are two generally recommended remedies for shock:

- **Aconite:** The person is very fearful, anxious, extremely reactive to pain, and inconsolable. They feel death is imminent, and they are quite restless with anxiety. Their eyes may have a glassy appearance and/or pupils can be dilated. They are likely to be screaming, crying out, and trembling with terror and pain.

- **Arnica:** The person is stunned, irritable when offered help, exhausted, and uncooperative. They say they are fine and don't want to be touched. They may complain of pain but will maintain that not much is wrong with them. They feel like they have been beaten up and want to be left alone.

Dosing: Use the ORANGE method. If after four doses there is no improvement, reevaluate.

Note: After giving **Aconite** or **Arnica**, the person may need one of the remedies found in the charts that follow. If a person keeps reliving a trauma, consider ***Stramonium**. A person needing ***Stramonium** keeps re-experiencing the initial fright and may exhibit hysteria, talkativeness, rage, loud laughter, or a fear that they are going to die. The person needing this remedy may be afraid of the dark and not want to sleep alone. They can also wake screaming from nightmares.

ANXIETY AND FEARS

There are many reasons why a person may feel anxious and many ways they show their anxieties. In this chapter, we look at two specific types of anxiety – school anxiety and performance anxiety. Then below that section, you will find information about other fears and frights.

HOMESICKNESS

See **Chapter 22—Young Adults** starting on **page 264**.

SCHOOL ANXIETY

Children can exhibit various behaviors and feelings as they adjust to separating from their parents and their home to a group situation with their peers. Listen to your child to understand their fears. Talking to them and reassuring them will go a long way in giving them the confidence they need to feel comfortable in this entirely new setting.

Though most people think of school anxiety for children, adults can also feel anxious when they return to school, especially if they haven't been in a classroom in a long time. You can adapt these remedy pictures for an adult in a similar situation, be it in a classroom or other new environment.

ADDITIONAL SUPPORT FOR SCHOOL ANXIETY

- Be as reassuring and loving as possible. Expect the child may be upset and that it's ok, especially on the first few days. Let them 'feel to heal', hear all of their concerns, no matter how trivial they seem.
- Help your child understand that school is their work, like adults have theirs.
- If possible, arrange for a walk through the school and the classroom beforehand, so it's familiar to the child on day one.
- Allow the child to participate in the decisions about what they wear, what they bring for lunch, what supplies they buy, etc.
- If very anxious, allow the child to bring a favorite stuffed animal to school to provide comfort and company and make sure it is okay with the school that the child will have the stuffed animal, so it doesn't create another stressful situation.
- Connect with a school counselor if the child continues to have a hard time adjusting.

WHEN TO CONTACT YOUR HEALTHCARE PROFESSIONAL

- If the situation doesn't resolve in a week or two, then consult with a professional homeopath and/or a mental health professional.

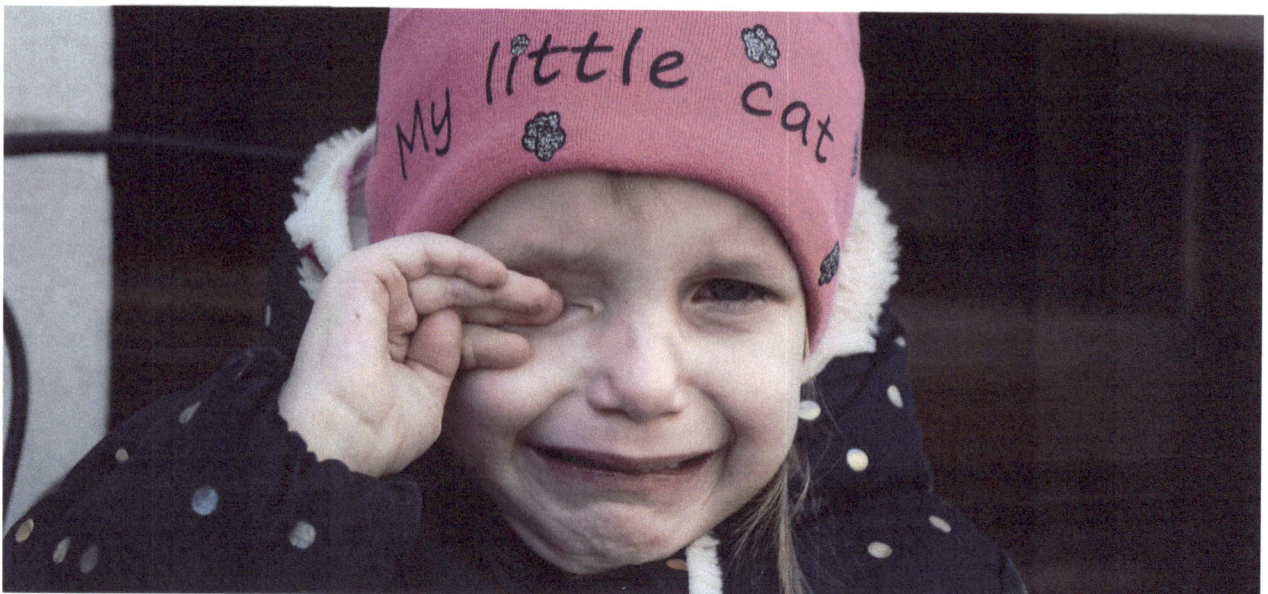

COMMON REMEDIES FOR SCHOOL ANXIETY

	Arsenicum	*Baryta carb	Calcarea carb	*Calcarea phos	Ignatia	Natrum mur	Pulsatilla
Onset	Anticipatory anxiety.	Homesickness, developmental delay.	Any change in routine.	Dissatisfaction with new circumstances.	Grief, separation, being reprimanded.	Depressions, grief sadness and/or feelings of loss.	Separation anxiety.
Symptoms	Anxious, irritable, nervous, restless with exhaustion.	Sits alone, dreads new situations.	Dreads new situations, head sweats, cold clammy feet, inner trembling.	Wants to be here then there, can't wake up. Desire to travel.	Sighing, trembling, rigid, over-sensitive to pain, sore throat.	Headaches. Craves salt. Sad, but cannot cry.	Clingy, tearful, whiny. Symptoms change frequently.
Mood	Impatient, demanding, doesn't like to be left alone.	Timid, shy of strangers, fear of being laughed at. Lack of self-confidence, anxiety about the future.	Whimpering, fear of being looked at. Nightmares. Fear of monsters.	Easily frustrated, fatigue, mentally irritable. Homesickness.	Hysterical. Nervous, moody, weepy, grieving, sad, laughing, sobbing.	Irritable, easily offended. Serious, introverted, abrupt, absent-minded, hurt feelings. Fear of rejection.	Timid, mild, weeps easily. Changeable moods. Feels alone in the world. Craves sympathy. Fear of abandonment.
Indications	Burning pains. Diarrhea and/or vomiting. Respiratory symptoms. Thirsty for frequent small sips.	Hides behind furniture or a parent. Mental fatigue, weak, enlarged glands, mental and physical immaturity.	Anxiety with sour stomach, sour perspiration, craves eggs.	Stomach aches, headaches, growing pains. Possible loss of body fluids. Anxious expression on face.	Unpredictable.	Oversensitivity. Awkward. Wants to be alone.	Emotional roller-coaster. Thirstless.
Worse	Cold, after midnight, being alone, exhaustion.	Thinking about school, washing, cold, mental exertion.	Cold, wet, bathing. Mornings. Exertion.	Mornings. Damp, cold, drafts, melting snow. Weather change. Exertion.	Mornings. Grief. Odors. Open air. After meals.	Sun, consolation. After eating.	Heat. After eating rich foods. Evening. Lying on one side.
Better	Warmth, head elevated, motion, lying down.	Walking in open air, warmth, holding mom's hand, reassurance.	Warmth and dry climate. Lying on painful side. Reassurance, knowing what is going to happen at school.	Warmth. Dry. Motion.	While eating, change of position, warmth and walking. Being alone.	Open air. Cold bathing. Tight clothing.	Open air. Motion. Cold food and drinks. Consolation.

Dosing: Use the **BROWN** method. Observe and evaluate.

PERFORMANCE ANXIETY

If you dread the thought of getting up in front of a group of people and performing, you are not alone. Millions of people, especially athletes, presenters, musicians, actors, and public speakers suffer from performance anxiety, commonly called "stage fright."

Performance anxiety can prevent a person from doing what they enjoy and can affect one's success. It may also cause a concurrent physical symptom such as sweating, diarrhea, a speech impediment, or possibly fainting.

Homeopathic remedies are very useful for this situation and can be used for any performance anxiety such as before interviews, taking college entrance exams, driver's tests, sports tryouts, etc.

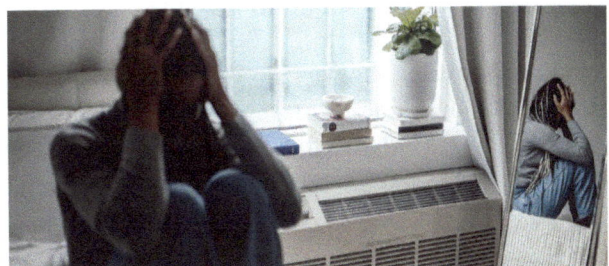

❤ ADDITIONAL SUPPORT FOR PERFORMANCE ANXIETY

- Getting control of one's breath is helpful in calming the nervous system. Take slow and deep breaths into the belly and exhale just as slowly, repeatedly.
- Try a cool compress to the forehead.
- Before the event, have the person sit in a quiet place and visualize over and over again the event going just the way they would like.
- Add two drops of **Bach Flower Rescue Remedy®** liquid (can be found online or in a health food store) added to some spring water for the person to sip. This can be repeated as often as necessary starting two hours before the event.

The most common remedies for performance anxiety are:

- **Argentum nit:** The person asks questions such as "What if I forget my lines/the answers/my speech?" "What if I faint?" "What if I make a mistake?" "What if I flunk?" There is lots of worry, such as about getting to the event on time. The heart starts beating hard and fast. They are in a hurry, talk fast, and desire sweets. Their imaginations might be overly active, or they might want to carry a "good luck charm" or exhibit other superstitious behaviors.

- **Gelsemium:** The person says things such as: I am really scared or I feel dizzy/weak/chilly/shaky. They become indifferent to their surroundings and look dull and droopy. They are emotionally delicate, exhausted, and want to be left alone. They usually have sticky and clammy sweat. There is no thirst, so encourage them to drink. They may have been worrying about the ordeal for weeks prior to the actual event. This remedy can also be used for school anxiety if the remedy picture fits.

- **Lycopodium:** The person says things such as "I know I am going to make a fool of myself", or "everyone will be laughing at me," or "I know I am going to fail", or "I can't do this". They get so anxious about the upcoming situation that they lose their self-esteem and may fear that they are

going to break down. They can have indigestion, gas, and/or diarrhea. They are irritable but don't want to be left alone. Even though they get so anxious, they love applause and thrive on appreciation.

Consider **Phosphorus** as they too can have great anxiety and many fears as seen in those needing this remedy.

Other remedies to consider if there is speech stammering or stuttering:

- ***Agaricus:** Mainly a neurologic remedy for twitching, spasms, convulsions, and stammering/stuttering in speech with grimacing of the mouth likely when beginning to speak. They have a great aversion to speaking.

- ***Causticum:** Stammering/stuttering on account of excitement or anger over injustices toward themselves or others.

- ***Stramonium:** Usually some fears, violence, or convulsions are evident; the person lives under the impression of an immediate danger. There may be incomprehensible speech or stammering/stuttering.

APPREHENSION ABOUT THE DENTIST/DOCTOR

If the person feels anxious before going to the dentist or doctor, consider taking a well-selected remedy before the appointment. This can really help to keep the person calm and less fearful. These remedy suggestions can also be considered for other medical visits if the person is apprehensive.

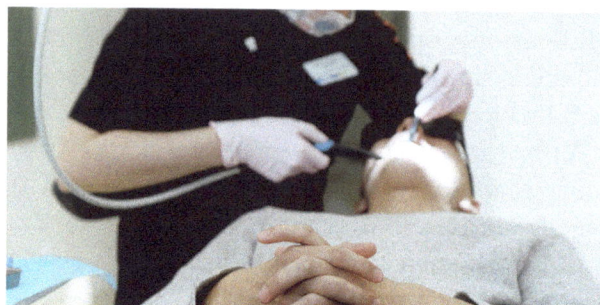

COMMON REMEDIES FOR APPREHENSION ABOUT THE DENTIST (DOCTOR)

	Aconite	Argentum nit	Chamomilla	*Coffea	Gelsemium	Pulsatilla
Symptoms	Intense anxiety, fear something bad will happen.	Fidgety and restless with many fears.	Fear of pain.	Hyperactive with anxiety.	Weak and wobbly with anxiety.	State of anxiety.
Mood	Intensely afraid.	Very anxious.	Inconsolable. Irritable. Restless.	Agitated.	Afraid of pain.	Clingy. Crying.
Indications	Panicky feeling. Restlessness. Bites nails or hand.	Anxious concerning many activities. Superstitious dread.	Temper tantrum.	Can't sleep from worry. Child may run about.	Panic attack. Worry or fear. Has a hard time concentrating.	Thirstless.
Worse	Being touched.	Anything warm.	Nothing soothes.	Stimulation.	Anticipation.	Warm closed room. Evening.
Better	Sitting still.	Open air. Cold water.	Being held.	Being quiet.	Continued motion. Open air.	Open air, fresh cool air. Company for support and sympathy.

Special Dosing Instructions: Give the chosen remedy the night before the appointment and then again 30 minutes before the appointment.

OTHER FEARS AND FRIGHTS

Acute fears will be addressed here. Phobias, which are deep-seated, chronically ingrained fears, should be dealt with by a professional homeopath. Any of the following fears can develop into a phobia:

- fear of seeing the doctor or dentist, or going to the hospital: **Aconite, Argentum nit, Gelsemium**

- fear of flying in airplanes: **Aconite, Argentum nit, Gelsemium, Rhus tox**

- fear and anxiety before performances, tests, etc.: **Argentum nit, Gelsemium**

- fear which produces a sudden histamine reaction (hives/anaphylaxis): **Apis**

- fear of being in a crowd or crowded room: **Aconite, Gelsemium**

- claustrophobia: **Aconite, Argentum nit**

- fear of death: **Aconite**

Another source of fear may originate from a fright—a sudden emotion that arises from being threatened or attacked. It can bring about feelings of terror, fear, anxiety, panic, or dread. It can even cause a histamine reaction that produces welts on the skin or hives. It is important to keep your children from viewing movies or TV programs with scary, grotesque, or violent images. This can cause frightful imagery in your child's mind and can cause nightmares in younger children. If they see a scary movie or TV show and are now acting afraid and/or fearful, look to the following remedies.

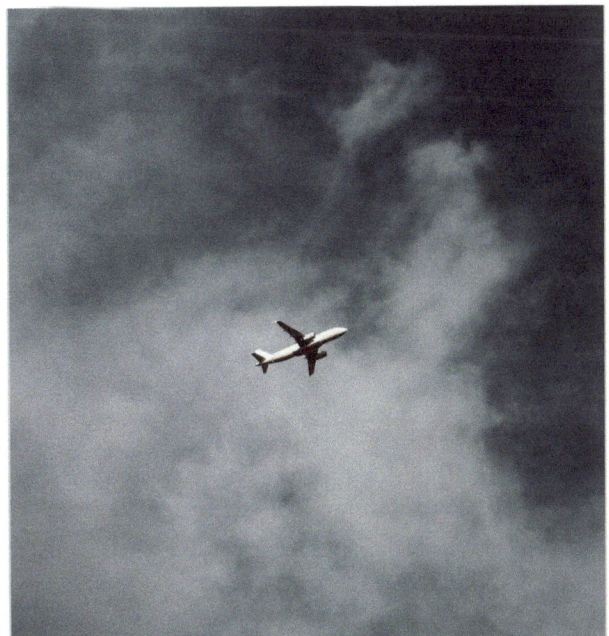

COMMON REMEDIES FOR FEARS AND FRIGHT

	Aconite	Apis	Argentum nit	Gelsemium	Pulsatilla	Rhus tox
Onset	Fear of flying on airplanes, nightmares from scary movies or stories, which can lead to fear of the dark and/or ghosts. For after effects from any sudden fright.	ONLY if any strong fright or rage has caused a sudden histamine reaction which produces hives.	Fear of flying, heights, claustro-phobia, failure, fear of being alone, doctors, losing control.	Fear of doctors and dentists because they don't want to be left alone or examined. Fears flying because of fear of mechanical or pilot failure. Fears public per-formance, tests, crowds, getting over-excited.	Fright from movies or TV, especially if an animal has been hurt, killed or abandoned. Any disturbing impressions such as witnessing a bad car accident. Fear of crowds, narrow places, and being alone in the dark.	Fear of flying, because there's a lack of fresh air. Cannot sit still for long periods of time. Cannot get negative pictures from a trauma out of their head, such as after a bad car accident. Fear of being poisoned.
Symptoms	Rapid pulse, profuse perspi-ration, extreme reaction to pain. Dilated pupils. Easily startled.	Skin becomes puffy, red, swollen, hot and itchy. Rosy red, sensitive, sore skin. Can also have hives, breathing prob-lems, swelling of face and tongue, nausea, blurred vision, diarrhea with cramps or headache.	Once the door is locked on the plane, fear there is no escape. Think they can't do anything right. Fear of losing control. Don't want to go to the doctor because they fear disease. Usually a great desire for sweets.	Reactions become slow, sluggish, and heavy with great weakness. Dullness, confusion, exhaus-tion, trembling, and sometimes dizziness. Eyelids are droopy and become drowsy.	Deeply disturbed and very sensitive to impressions. Cries easily. Emotions rise to a certain pitch, then suddenly cease. Must have sympathy. Needs attention and gentleness.	Mentally and emotionally, becomes stiff, cloudy, confused, and forgetful. Extreme restless-ness and continue change of position. Great apprehension at night. Answers slowly or hastily or reluctantly. Fears are worse at night
Mood	Fearful, anxious, panicked, restless, inconsolable.	Moody, dramatic and oversensitive to pain. May become hysterical.	Anxious, nervous, easily excitable, trembling, timid, and impulsive. Has sense that time is going too slowly and want everybody to hurry up.	Weak, tired, delicate, timid, excitable, angers easily. Wants to be quiet and left alone.	Weepy, whiny, whimpering, fretful, but affectionate. Mild, timid, easily offended, irritable. Wants attention. May feel sorry for self.	Anxious, sad, restless, fearful. Inclination to cry. Confused.
Indications	Likely to be screaming and crying out in terror or pain. Afraid of crowds and death, because they are sure they are going to die.	Awkward, can be listless or become irritable if disturbed, but do not want to be left alone.	May pace up and down in a panic. May become so anxious they get diarrhea that is frequent, watery, and smelly. May talk fast, in a childish way.	May stutter or get diarrhea. Head may ache at the forehead and/or the back of the head. May completely freeze up mentally and physically in a public perfor-mance situation.	Very changeable moods. Emotions are all over the place, especially after an emotional trauma.	Helplessness and despondency. May burst into tears but not be able to tell you why they are crying.
Worse	Fright, shock, getting chilled, pressure, touch, noise, light, excitement, music, smoke, evening and night.	Heat in any form, touch, late afternoon, lying down, pressure, after sleeping and on the right side.	Mental strain, worry, apprehen-sion, night, sugar, sweets, crowds, warmth in any form, suspense.	Emotions, excitement, shocks, bad news, surprise. Thinking about ailments. Hot room. Physical exertion.	Warm stuffy rooms, during menses, twilight and evening. Sunlight. Lying down. Dehydration. Excessive joy. Rich food.	Initial motion. After rest. Night. Exposure to wet, cold, and getting chilled. Lying on back or right side. Over-exertion.
Better	Open air, rest, warmth.	Cold applications, cool air, cool bathing, cool drinks. Sitting up. Being uncovered.	Fresh cool, open air. Motion. Pressure.	Bending forward while sitting, lying down with head slightly elevated, fresh air. Urination. Sweating.	Intake of liquids. Walking or any motion in cool, fresh, open air. Cool applications. Gentle massage. Erect posture. Gentle encourage-ment. Consolation.	Continue motion. Heat, hot bath, warm applications. Rubbing, stretching limbs, changing position, and walking.

Dosing: If symptoms are intense, use the ORANGE method. If the symptoms are present but not seemingly as urgent, use the BLUE dosing method. Observe and evaluate.

RAGE, ANGER, AND IRRITABILITY

Rage is a powerful, intense emotion expressed in sudden and extreme anger. The person is usually in a state of fury, frenzy, and wrath, brought on by frustration, pain, feeling overwhelmed, grief, loss, low blood sugar, poor diet, hormone fluctuations and more. It can even cause a histamine reaction that produces welts on the skin or hives. It is normal for most two-year-old's and some teenagers to throw temper tantrums; however, it is not as common or acceptable for adults. A fit of rage can be quite distressing. Rudeness, verbal abuse, or violence should always be addressed and when appropriate, not tolerated. If an adult is in a chronic state of rage, a consultation with a professional homeopath is advised. In addition to homeopathy, the person may need help from a mental health provider or may need to take some training in learning how to manage their anger.

♡ ADDITIONAL SUPPORT FOR RAGE, ANGER AND IRRITABILITY

- The quickest way to get someone to calm down is to establish calm eye contact and have them take slow, deep, rhythmic breaths into their belly. Keep the focus on the breath.
- Listen to the person and talk it out with them. Understanding is needed without judgment or criticism. The person's fears or feelings should not be minimized. The person should not be forced to talk if they are not ready. It can be helpful for an older child to write or draw pictures about what they are experiencing.
- In many cases, tranquilizers or antidepressants deaden the feelings and have the potential to cause detrimental side effects. It is important for a person to learn how to deal with and express emotions appropriately.
- For intense emotions, try some spring water with two drops of **Bach Flower Rescue Remedy®**, which can be found in a health food store. This can be repeated as often as necessary to reduce one's stress level.
- Consider meeting with a professional homeopath or mental health counselor for personalized support.

🩺 WHEN TO CONTACT A HEALTHCARE PROFESSIONAL

- If temper tantrums persist or become destructive or violent.
- Depression or anger should not be allowed to become chronic. Psychological counseling should be sought.
- The person has not responded to well indicated remedies—there may be a deeper seated problem that needs to be addressed. Or a higher dose remedy may be needed. If either of these is the case, consider contacting a professional homeopath.

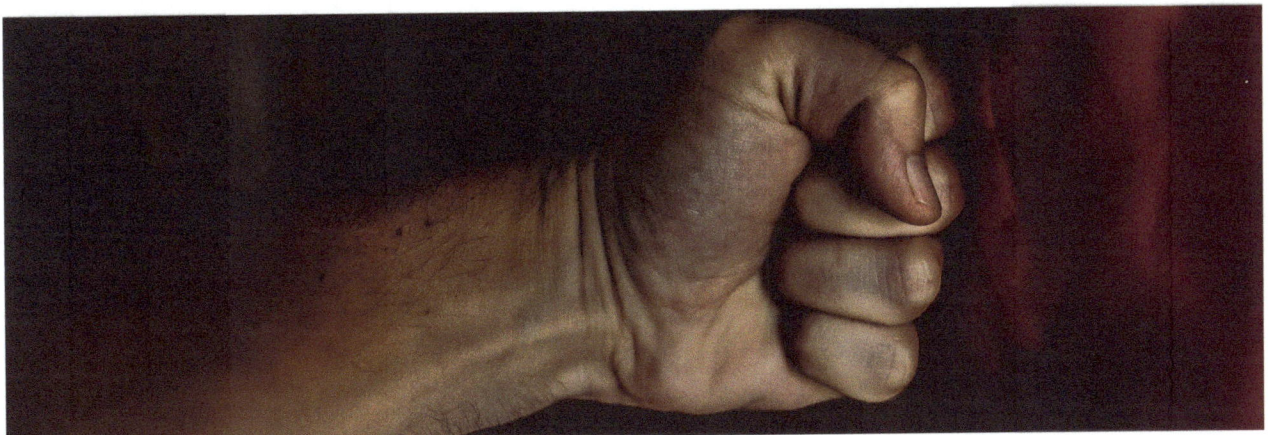

COMMON REMEDIES FOR RAGE, ANGER, AND IRRITABILITY

	Apis	Arsenicum	Belladonna	Ignatia	Nux vomica	Staphysagria
Onset	After a bout of rage.	After a bout of rage.	From excitement, fright, fear or anger.	After a bout of rage, grief, reprimand, homesickness or humiliation.	After a bout of rage. Chronic stress. Wounded honor. Overindulgence in food or drinks.	After a bout of humiliation, criticism, shame, or rage.
Symptoms	Skin eruptions that itch, are red and swollen.	Anxiety with moaning, restlessness, and exhaustion after the slightest exertion. Burning pains.	Symptoms appear and disappear suddenly. Easily angered with desire to hit or bite. Sudden rageful behavior with possible violence. Crying. Howling.	Very sensitive, especially to pain. Sigh a lot and yawn. Loss of appetite. Can have strange sensations anywhere in the body. Throat can be sore, chest tight, cramping of muscles, numbness or tingling of the nerves, spasms, or a stomachache.	Irritable. Chilly, constipated. Hypersensitive to noise and light.	Feels disempowered, downtrodden, inadequate, indignant. Sadness with crying or tries to keep up cheerful, pleasant appearance. Constant seething, trembling, irritability. Sensitive. Suppressed anger. History of emotional or physical abuse. Urinary tract infections.
Mood	Irritability and violent anger. Feels everything is going wrong.	Anxious, irritable, oversensitive, needy demanding. They worry a lot. Want company.	Angry, irritable. May seem delirious and utter silly talk. May be exhausted.	Grieve quietly, unless hysterical. Do not want sympathy, and may become antisocial. Nervous, excitable, anxious, introspective, easily frustrated, moody, and weepy.	Irritable, very angry, impatient, stubborn, easily offended, mischievous, and very competitive.	Sensitive to rude treatment and criticism. Irritable, indignant, sad, gloomy, nervous, easily excitable.
Indications	Ailments from jealousy, fright, anger, hearing bad news. Skin eruptions.	Fastidious. Gets upset about dirt, germs, disorder, and wants surroundings orderly and neat. Fault finding, selfish, suspicious. Anguish and restlessness. Can have suicidal impulses.	Anger accompanied by a flushed face, glaring eyes, pupils dilated, throbbing carotid arteries. Excited mental state.	Can be hysterically crying. Do not want sympathy, and may become antisocial. Nervous, excitable, anxious, introspective, easily frustrated, moody, and weepy.	Oversensitive to noises, odors, light. Hangover. Time passes too slowly. Pessimistic. Fault finding. Over-sensitive to pain. Type A personality.	Throws things in anger. Headaches "like a block of wood" in the forehead or occiput. After a bout of rage. Can have menstrual cramps, cessation of periods, or bladder infections.
Worse	Suppressed emotions. Warm applications on skin.	Physical exertion, disorder, after midnight, cold air, cold drinks.	Being spoken to, even kindly. In a quiet place. In bed.	Strong emotions, worry, open cold air, strong odors, morning after breakfast, coffee, extreme heat, being overworked. Being consoled.	Early morning, cold, cold weather, drafts, noise, touch, odors, rich food, coffee, stimulants, alcohol.	Suppressed anger and abuse, sleep. Sexual excess, touch, tobacco.
Better	Cool applications on skin.	Warmth, warm drinks, lying down, fresh air, company, order. Reassurance they are going to get better.	Sitting upright. Drawing head back. In a warm room.	Eating, pressure, deep breathing, being alone, calmness, temperate weather.	Open air, sleep, strong pressure, warmth, hot drinks.	After breakfast. Night. Warmth.

Dosing: If the episode is intense, use the ORANGE method. If onset is less intense but present, consider the BLUE method. Observe and evaluate. Consider making an appointment with a professional homeopath as rage, anger and irritability may need more than what a remedy kit can offer.

GRIEF

Grief is an emotional state frequently caused by some form of loss. It could be from losing family members, friends, partners, a pet, a home, a job, etc. Some people are so sensitive that a movie or TV program can evoke this emotion. A teenager may need one of these remedies if they have broken up with their girlfriend or boyfriend. Grief can be manifested by uncontrollable crying, hysterical sobbing, long bouts of weeping or wailing, fear of being alone, much sighing, becoming quieter than usual, withdrawing, and/or depression. The most common remedies for grief are **Ignatia** and **Natrum mur**.

See more specific information about these remedies on the charts that follow.

HUMILIATION

Humiliation from severe criticism, name calling or being bullied can damage a person's dignity, pride, and self-esteem. It brings up feelings of shame, disgrace, embarrassment, and dishonor. It is very important not to ignore the person, thinking that they have to find their own way or toughen up.

A child or adolescent will feel further victimized if the parents do not step in and support them. It may be necessary to take further steps with the school or other parents to remedy the situation. Remember that your child or adolescent may be the victim of humiliation not only from other children or adolescents but also siblings, coaches, babysitters, teachers, or other family members. Along with giving a remedy, it is important to teach the child or adolescent coping skills. Professional help may be needed. This kind of situation should not be allowed to continue because the child may develop unhealthy emotional coping patterns and be affected by long-term stress.

These remedies will be helpful for adults as well. However, if an adult is in a chronic state of humiliation, a constitutional consultation with a professional homeopath will be needed. The most common remedies for humiliation are **Ignatia** and **Staphysagria**.

See more specific information about these remedies that can be found on the charts that follow.

STRESS

Stress is a fact of life, and we all deal differently with the stresses we experience. For a healthy person, some stress should be tolerable, but when it becomes overwhelming, it can present problems. Reactions to stress vary from mental or emotional symptoms to physical ailments. Anger, crying, irritability, headaches, frequent infections and exhaustion could all be manifestations of a person's response to life's stresses.

If the person can identify their stressors, sometimes there are simple things that can be addressed to lower one's stress level such as correcting a poor diet, getting more sleep, meditating regularly or adding exercise to their life. Other times, the support of a homeopathic remedy can lend assistance. Chronic stress may need the attention of a professional homeopath.

It's interesting to note that the body will speak what is on the mind, so when a person is under high stress, their body may begin producing symptoms of illness. It is important to inquire what was going on in the person's life when the symptoms began.

If a child is unhappy at school, they may develop headaches, stomach aches, anxiety, or sleep difficulties. It is important to recognize these symptoms when they appear and not let them become chronic. A child should be encouraged to safely talk about how they are feeling. If necessary, intervention may be needed with help from teachers, coaches, school counselors, etc. Children can be victims of bullying, which may leave a child terrified to go to school. Speaking with other parents can be helpful in addressing the situation.

Children (and adults) with little to no downtime are more stressed than those with some downtime. It is ideal to spend some of our time engaging in activities we enjoy or find interesting. Stress accumulates when we spend too much of our time doing things we do not enjoy or things that overburden us. If a child is forced to participate in too many sports, dance, or academic activities, they will exhibit symptoms of stress. It is important to work towards a healthy balance of activities and downtime.

Teenagers inherently deal with many temptations. In this frantic-paced digital world, it is easy for a teen to feel a lot of pressure to perform or conform. They can easily become scared, overwhelmed, and intimidated.

Parents need to help their teenagers develop healthy eating habits, encourage outdoor activities, avoid playing too many video games, limit computer time, restrain from watching too much TV, discourage staying up too late, and provide sound advice about drugs and alcohol.

Any teenager who has suffered an emotional shock, e.g., divorce or death of a friend or loved one, will more than likely need psychological help as well as a professional homeopath for support. Emotional stress can be quite intense at this time of development, and homeopathic remedies can keep your teenager more balanced. It is important; however, not to give a remedy for every little emotional upset. If a teen has been brooding for weeks, is intensely overreacting to situations, or is dealing with big distress in their lives, a homeopathic remedy may be in order.

Adults may feel the pressures of work and family and become a workaholic or develop illnesses, anxiety, insomnia and/or seek other inappropriate alternatives to de-stress their mind, such as pornography, drugs, and/or alcohol. A parent may be trying to "keep up with it all" and have no time for self-care. Stress can also become an issue due to lack of sleep, an unhealthy diet, lack of exercise, or not drinking enough water. These things should be addressed along with taking an appropriate remedy. If a person's stress is overwhelming, and the remedies here aren't helping, consider consulting with a professional homeopath. Once again, it's useful to find a healthy balance of work, family, downtime, and doing the activities that are most enjoyable to reduce one's stress.

ADDITIONAL SUPPORT FOR STRESS

- There are many self-care strategies that can be used regularly to reduce or keep stress at bay. They all help to calm the nervous system. Simple and easily accessible activities like taking a walk outside or doing some gentle exercise, listening to favorite music, meditating, doing yoga or Tai Chi, learning pranayama (deep breathing techniques), getting together with a good friend, getting enough sleep, eating a healthy diet and more. The options are there if the person is willing.
- Remind the person to tap into a support system of others including parents, trusted family members, friends, a spiritual or school counselor, or a psychologist to help reduce one's feelings of stress.
- In many cases, tranquilizers or antidepressants deaden the feelings and have the potential to cause detrimental side effects. It is important for a person to learn how to deal with and express emotions appropriately.
- For intense emotions, try some spring water with two drops of **Bach Flower Rescue Remedy®**, which can be found in a health food store. This can be repeated as often as necessary to reduce one's stress level.
- Consider meeting with a professional homeopath or mental health counselor for personalized support.

WHEN TO CONTACT YOUR HEALTHCARE PROFESSIONAL

- The person becomes withdrawn, irritable, rude, arrogant, dictatorial, bullying, or violent. They may have an unexpressed emotional conflict that they do not know how to deal with.
- The person talks about or threatens suicide or homicide.
- The person isn't sleeping well and is having trouble functioning.
- The person has not responded to well indicated remedies—there may be a deeper seated problem that needs to be addressed. Or a higher dose of a remedy may be needed. If either of these is the case, consider contacting a professional homeopath.

COMMON REMEDIES FOR STRESS

	Arnica	Arsenicum	Ignatia	Natrum mur	Nux vomica	Pulsatilla	Staphysagria
Onset	After trauma. Shock.	Hearing bad news, feeling stressed.	Grief, insults, heartbreak, reprimands.	Grief, disappointed love, anger. Embarrassment, hurt feelings.	Overworking, overeating, overdrinking or any overindulgence.	Grief or any emotional trauma.	Humiliation, criticism, shame or rage.
Symptoms	Sunken, pale, or red face. Stunned, exhausted, feels beat up and sore. Irritable when offered help. Wants to be left alone and doesn't want to be touched.	Depressed. Anxiety with moaning, restlessness. Exhaustion after the slightest exertion. Anxiety with cough. Burning pains.	Very sensitive, especially to pain. Sighs and yawns a lot. Loss of appetite. Can have strange sensations anywhere in the body. Throat can be sore or feel there is a lump in the throat. Chest tight, cramping of muscles, numbness or tingling of the nerves, spasms, or stomach ache.	Chilly, sleepless. Dwells on past unpleasant memories. Emotionally sensitive to all sorts of influences. Finds it hard to cry. Wants to be alone to cry. Sensitivity to being teased.	Irritable. Chilly. Constipated. Hypersensitive to noise and light.	Grief with lots of weeping. Cries readily. Changeable moods. Craves sympathy.	Feels disempowered, downtrodden, inadequate, indignant. Sadness with crying, constant seething, trembling, anger. Sensitive, irritable. Suppressed anger. History of emotional or physical abuse. Urinary tract infections.
Mood	Fear of being touched. Wants to be left alone. Denial of illness or suffering. Shock.	Anxious, irritable, over-sensitive, needy, demanding. Worry a lot. May feel they are dying and won't get better. Want company to be nearby.	Grieves quietly, or alone. Does not want sympathy and may become antisocial. Nervous, excitable, anxious, introspective, easily frustrated, moody, and weepy.	Irritable, angry, serious, anxious, abrupt, absent-minded, and confused. Depression and introversion from hurt emotions.	Irritable, angry, impatient, spiteful, stubborn, easily offended, mischievous, and very competitive.	Weepy, whiny, whimpering, fretful, suspicious, affectionate. Wants attention. Fears to be alone. May feel sorry for self.	Extremely touchy and sensitive, especially to rude treatment and criticism. Irritable, indignant, sad, gloomy, nervous, and easily excitable.
Indications	Acts like a wounded animal wanting to go to a corner and lick their wounds. Sensitive to pain. Nervous shock.	Fastidious about dirt and germs. Has fixed ideas about things. Fault-finding, cowardly, malicious, selfish, suspicious. Anguish with restlessness. Can have suicidal impulses.	Can be hysterically crying one moment, laughing the next, furious the next, distant the next, anxious the next, and restless the next. May sob when trying not to cry.	May get a sore throat from trying to hold back crying. Averse to consolation. Can have a tendency to get canker sores and fever blisters when stressed. Tends to be constipated and have greasy skin. Can be quite awkward, hasty, and drop things.	Oversensitive to noises, odors, light. Hangovers. Time passes too slowly. Pessimistic. Fault-finding. Oversensitive to pain. Digestive issues. Can be a driven Type A personality.	Likes to stretch feet. Moody. Desires sympathy. Needs attention and gentleness. Needs to be gently encouraged out of their self-pity. Wants head high, one pillow is not enough. Thirstless.	Throws things in anger. Headaches "like a block of wood" in the forehead or occiput. With stress, may have menstrual cramps, cessation of periods, or bladder infections.
Worse	Touch, jarring, too many questions.	Physical exertion, after midnight, cold air, cold drinks.	Strong emotions, worry, open cold air, strong odors, morning after breakfast, coffee, extreme heat, being overworked, being consoled.	Eating too much salt. 9-11 AM. Heat of the sun, summer, violent emotions, fat, acid foods, sex, noise, pressure, and a full moon.	Early morning, cold weather, drafts, touch, odors, rich food, coffee, stimulants, and alcohol.	Warm, stuffy rooms, morning, twilight, getting overheated. Fatty or rich foods, dairy products, tea. Sun and thunderstorms.	Suppressed anger and abuse, sleep. Sexual excess, touch, and tobacco.
Better	Lying with head low, lying outstretched. Being left alone.	Warmth. Warm drinks. Lying down, fresh air, company, order. Reassurance they are going to get better.	Eating, pressure, deep breathing, being alone, patience with their hypersensitivity. Temperate weather.	Open air, cool bathing, sweating, rest, deep breathing, rubbing, and long talks.	Open air, sleep, strong pressure, warmth, and hot drinks.	Cool fresh open air, rest, rubbing, sympathy, gentleness, being held or hugged, erect posture, after a good cry.	After breakfast. Night. Warmth. Stretching.

Dosing: If feelings are very intense, use the ORANGE dosing method. If feelings are not unusually intense but present, use the BLUE dosing method. Observe and evaluate.

INSOMNIA

Insomnia is a common sleep disorder that can make it difficult to fall asleep, difficult to stay asleep, or cause the person to wake up too early and not be able to get back to sleep. It can also cause an inability to sleep at all. The person with insomnia may still feel tired when they wake up. Insomnia can sap not only one's energy level and mood but also one's health, work performance, and quality of life.

At some point, many adults experience short-term (acute) insomnia, which may last for days or weeks. It's usually the result of stress or a traumatic event, but some people have long-term (chronic) insomnia that lasts for a month or more. Insomnia may be the primary problem or it may be associated with other medical conditions or medications. Chronic insomnia is usually a result of stress, life events, environmental influences or habits that disrupt sleep. Treating the underlying cause can help resolve insomnia.

Symptoms of insomnia include:

- difficulty falling asleep at night

- waking up frequently during the night and not being able to go back to sleep

- waking up too early in the morning and not being able to go back to sleep

- not feeling well-rested after a night's sleep

- frequent daytime tiredness or sleepiness

- irritability, depression, and/or anxiety

- difficulty paying attention, focusing on tasks, or remembering

- increased errors or accidents

- increased need to nap during the day, which may negatively affect nighttime sleep

- ongoing worries about sleep

Possible causes of insomnia:

- Stress: concerns about work, school, health, finances, or family can keep your mind active at night. Stressful life events or trauma may lead to insomnia.

- Travel or work schedule: your circadian rhythms act as an internal clock, guiding such things as your sleep-wake cycle, metabolism, and body temperature. Disrupting your body's circadian rhythms can result in insomnia. Causes include jet lag from traveling, working a late or early shift, or frequently changing shifts.

- Poor sleep habits: poor sleep habits include an irregular bedtime schedule, naps, stimulating activities before bed, an uncomfortable sleep environment, and using your bed for work, eating, or watching TV. Use of computers, televisions, video games, smartphones, or other screens just before bed can interfere with your sleep cycle.

- Aging: as we age, changes in our hormones, such as the levels of melatonin and cortisol, can play a role in disrupting ones sleep. Older adults are more likely to take longer to fall asleep, wake up more frequently throughout the night and spend more time napping during the day compared with younger adults. Seemingly, most people need a little less sleep as they age. *For more info on **Insomnia and Aging**, see the box on the next page.*

Additional causes of insomnia include:

- Anxiety disorders, such as post-traumatic stress disorder, may disrupt sleep. Insomnia often accompanies other mental health disorders.

- Many prescription drugs can interfere with sleep, such as certain antidepressants and medications for asthma or blood pressure. Some over-the-counter medications contain caffeine and other stimulants that can disrupt sleep.

- Medical conditions linked with insomnia include chronic pain, cancer, diabetes, heart disease, asthma, gastro-esophageal reflux disease (GERD), overactive thyroid, sleep apnea, restless leg syndrome, Parkinson's disease, and Alzheimer's disease.

• Caffeine, chocolate, nicotine and alcohol can interfere with sleep. Coffee, tea, cola, and other caffeinated drinks are stimulants. Drinking them in the late afternoon or evening can keep you from falling asleep at night. Some find their sleep adversely affected by chocolate, as the theobromine in cacao is closely related to caffeine. Nicotine in tobacco products is another stimulant that can interfere with sleep. Alcohol may help you fall asleep, but it prevents deeper stages of sleep and often causes awakening in the middle of the night.

ADDITIONAL SUPPORT FOR INSOMNIA

• Create and religiously follow a realistic wake/sleep schedule providing sufficient hours of sleep. The body likes a regular bedtime and wake time.
• Avoid using electronics at least one hour before bed including watching television, using a cell phone or computer. The content you watch before bed can stimulate the brain making it hard to fall asleep. Also, the light from the device affects your melatonin levels, fooling your mind into thinking it's still daytime.
• Reduce your overall stress through regular exercise, meditation, yoga, and/or deep breathing exercises.
• Check medications for their potential effects on sleep.
• Sleep in a cool, completely dark room.
• Limit or restrict products with caffeine after 12pm.
• Limit or restrict drinking anything two hours before your bedtime to avoid having to wake to urinate in the night.
• Consider these useful supplements: **Avena sativa tincture** or **Passiflora tincture**, B vitamins, chelated magnesium or magnesium orotate before bedtime, and melatonin is also a possible option before bedtime.

WHEN TO CONTACT YOUR HEALTHCARE PROFESSIONAL

• Despite remedies and lifestyle changes, insomnia makes it hard to function during the day.
• The person suspects they may have sleep apnea.

INSOMNIA AND AGING

Insomnia becomes more common as we age. As you get older, you may experience:
• Changes in sleep patterns. Sleep often becomes less deep as you age, so noise or other changes in your environment are more likely to wake you. With age, your internal clock often advances, so you get tired earlier in the evening and wake up earlier in the morning.
• Changes in activity. You may be less physically or socially active. A lack of activity can interfere with a good night's sleep.
• Changes in health. Depression or anxiety as well as chronic pain from conditions such as arthritis or back problems can interfere with sleep. Sleep apnea and restless leg syndrome become more common with age. With age, the body produces less of an antidiuretic hormone and the bladder loses holding capacity, creating a need to urinate during the night, which can disrupt sleep. Certain medical conditions may exacerbate this.
• Changes during perimenopause and in menopause due to hormonal changes that affect the sleep and wake cycle.
• More medications. Older people often are prescribed more medications, which increase the chances of insomnia as a side effect.

COMMON REMEDIES FOR INSOMNIA

	Arnica	*Cocculus	*Coffea	Gelsemium	*Kali phos	Nux vomica	Pulsatilla
Symptoms	Overtired, but can't sleep.	Sleepless from exhaustion.	Inability to sleep due to overactive mind.	Insomnia. Anticipation.	Inability to sleep due to overworking.	Difficulty maintaining sleep. Sleepless from business worries.	Difficulty maintaining sleep.
Mood	Often says they're fine (even though you see they aren't fine) and pushes through any situation.	Mildness, sensitive to rudeness, cares for others, serious, introverted, sentimental.	Anxious, energetic, and very tired at the same time—much like someone who drank too much coffee.	Feeling of weakness, not being able to cope with daily life, responsibilities, work. Anticipatory anxieties. Desire to be left alone. Avoids people and distresses of life. Fear of taking on new tasks, exams, and crowds.	Stress may be related to studies, business or health issues.	Very irritable, sensitive to all impressions. Competitive. Fanatical, nervous and excitable. Angry and impatient.	Fixed ideas, forsaken feeling, mild-mannered, but can be irritable. Easily moved to laughter or tears.
Indications	Jet lag.	Often comes on from loss of sleep associated with nursing an ill person. Sleep may be interrupted by waking and startling. Sleepless due to many cares and worries. Jet lag.	Can't sleep because of excitement and euphoria or feelings of being uptight and extremely sensitive. All senses are very acute and wake at the slightest sound. Mind is overactive and dreams are vivid. When the person lies down to attempt to sleep, the mind is awake with a flow of ideas.	Often dull and drowsy, maybe even trembling. Can't get fully to sleep. The body is still and may appear asleep from the outside, but they are on the edge of sleep internally. Sometimes starting on falling asleep. May have restless sleep. May feel nervous anticipating an upcoming event.	Sleeplessness from nervous fatigue, over-studying, or excess mental work. Insomnia induced by a depleted mind.	Falls asleep easily, but wakes around 3 AM and unable to fall back asleep. Insomnia from abuse of stimulants like caffeine, tobacco, and/or from business tensions. Sleep disturbed because of nightmares and anxious, amorous, or hurried dreams. Dreams of misfortune like accidents.	Cannot fall asleep for long hours after retiring to bed. When it's time to get up in the morning, the person goes into a sound sleep.
Worse	Overexertion, touch, motion, alcohol, damp, cold, and evening. Night, noises.	Motion of boat, cars, swimming, loss of sleep, touch, noise, emotions, anxiety, talking, laughing, crying, and coffee.	Noise, touch, air, cold, wind, mental exertion, emotions, overeating, alcohol, narcotics, night, and excessive emotions.	Emotions, dread, shock, ordeals, surprise, when thinking of the ailments, bad news.	Slightest causes, excitement, worry, mental or physical exertion, touch, pain, cold air, puberty, sex.	Early morning, cold, open air, coffee, alcohol, drugs, and overeating. Noise, odors, touch.	Sun, warm room, warm air. Clothes, bed, rest, ice cream, eggs, and pastry.
Better	Lying down or lying with head low or outstretched. Cold, stimulating weather. Motion.	Sitting in a warm room. Lying quietly. Open air.	Lying down, sleep, warmth.	Profuse urination, sweating, shaking, alcoholic drinks, mental efforts, bending forward, continued motion.	Sleep, eating, gentle motion, leaning against something.	When allowed to finish task at hand. Naps, resting, strong pressure and after dinner.	Consolation, cold, open air, uncovering, erect posture, after a good cry. Cold applications.

Special dosing: Give chosen remedy once before bed for three days. If there is no change in sleep, choose a new remedy. Continue with the remedy that's working until symptoms have subsided then stop taking the remedy and only repeat if the symptoms return.

Other remedies to consider for insomnia include **Staphysagria** for those who are sleepless after a fit of anger or after a dispute in which their honor was wounded and they suppressed their anger or ***Capsicum** for sleeplessness due to homesickness. Additionally, **Kali Phos 6X** cell salt can help with stress that interferes with sleep. *For more options, see **Chapter 3—Cell Salts** on **page 39.***

FATIGUE

Symptoms of fatigue are extreme tiredness, typically resulting from mental or physical exertion or illness. Most of the time fatigue can be traced to one or more of your habits or routines, particularly lack of exercise, one's diet or poor sleep. It's also commonly related to depression. On occasion, fatigue is a symptom of other underlying conditions that require medical treatment. Taking an honest inventory of things that might be responsible for your fatigue is often the first step toward relief. If well-chosen remedies are not helping, consider contacting a professional homeopath for a more in-depth view of your situation.

Fatigue may be related to any of the following:

- abuse of alcohol or drugs
- exhaustion—mentally or physically
- excess physical activity
- jet lag
- lack of physical activity
- lack of sleep
- medications
- unhealthy eating habits
- recovery from a recent illness
- too much caffeine
- dehydration
- heart issues
- sleep apnea
- Vitamin B12 deficiency
- overwork
- excess worry
- anemia
- thyroid issues
- depression
- dealing with pain
- menopause

♡ ADDITIONAL SUPPORT FOR FATIGUE

- Eat a healthy diet with a variety of fresh organic fruits and vegetables. Avoid all processed foods, sugar and sugary drinks.
- Exercise some daily to get your circulation going and improve your metabolism.
- Drink plenty of water.
- Limit caffeine.
- Take time for the things you enjoy.
- Prioritize and maintain a consistent sleep schedule.
- Manage stress through mindfulness practices such as meditation, yoga, breath work, etc.
- Consider taking cell salts **Calc Phos 6X** and **Calc Flour 6X** twice daily for up to two months to strengthen a weak back.

WHEN TO CONTACT YOUR HEALTHCARE PROFESSIONAL

- The symptoms are not relieved within a few days of rest, well-chosen remedies and diet of healthy food and water.

COMMON REMEDIES FOR FATIGUE

	Arsenicum	Gelsemium	*Kali phos	*Phosphoricum acidum	Phosphorus	*Picricum acidum	Sepia
Symptoms	Anxious and fretful about survival issues like health, money, and having a roof over head, even about things being out of place. Extreme exhaustion that seems out of proportion, like why would someone stay in bed for a week with a cold.	Weakness, seen on all levels -mental, emotional, and physical- an all-pervading weakness.	Mental and physical exhaustion, especially after a period of stress and overexertion. Needed for students who have made some type of enormous exertion and have a type of mental breakdown. Being up late hours. Caring for a loved one.	Fatigue that lingers from an acute or long-term health issue. From grief or from profuse urination. Weight loss, accompanied by weakness. Dark circles around the eyes.	Sudden weakness or collapse, aggravated by motion or mental fatigue. Weakness from hunger.	Ailments from mental work, collapse, mainly in the area of intellectual functioning. Cause is often mental exertion. Collapse usually caused by physical exertion. Great dullness and tiredness that comes on after exerting the mind in any way. Mind becomes dull, unable to concentrate for a few minutes. May become confused.	Females who are exhausted and feel overworked, plus are having hormonal symptoms, including weepiness and irritability with loved ones, and feels at the end of her rope. Burned out.

Dosing: Use the BLUE method for up to three days. Observe and evaluate.

? WHAT'S THE FIRST REMEDY YOU THINK OF WHEN...

1. A person has lost a loved one recently.
2. Someone says they're fine and that nothing's wrong when it's clear that they have been injured.
3. Bullying from criticism results in humiliation and shame.
4. A traumatic experience induces a state of shock.
5. A student has anxiety from being in school.
6. A performer has anxiety prior to an engagement.
7. Insomnia occurs from stress.
8. Long hours have been spent caring for another.
9. A workaholic person who craves coffee and alcohol and is irritable and stressed.
10. Unresolved anger results in sleeplessness.

Answer key on page 324.

CHAPTER 20
The First Three Years Ages 0-3

Homeopathy is an invaluable gift to families with young children. Because the remedies are gentle, non-toxic and non-invasive, they can be safely used to alleviate many regular and acute childhood ailments. With homeopathic remedies in your toolbox, you can soothe many common newborn and baby discomforts naturally. The remedies also boost immune response, decreasing the need for chemical medicines.

*For more information about providing remedies to infants, see **Special Dosing Instructions for Infants, Young Children or Pets** under **How to Administer a Remedy** in **Chapter 2** on **page 35**.*

In addition to the material provided in this chapter, www.healthychildren.org can provide more medical information about each childhood issue.

AFTER BIRTH AND CIRCUMCISION SUPPORT

Bringing a child into the world is an amazing feat of humankind. The process is expected to go smoothly, but sometimes there are unexpected complications that can make the birthing process more stressful. As a new little human, your baby may react to these things just like adults do, but they can't say how they feel, rather they demonstrate their feelings through behaviors. If after tending to all your baby's apparent needs—feeding, burping, diaper changing, cuddling, etc.—and your baby still seems constantly uncomfortable, difficult to please, or appears to be wrestling with continued pain for no apparent reason, she/he might need some additional support.

If you want to find a remedy to support the baby, it's important to ask the mother, father or other loved one in the room if there were any issues or unusual incidents that occurred during the pregnancy or delivery. This information can provide a possible cause for the infant's persistent discomfort.

If the child has been circumcised, there may be a need for some additional support. **Arnica** can be used for any inflammation or pain for a few days after the procedure and **Calendula** can be used for overall healing.

ADDITIONAL SUPPORT FOR CIRCUMCISION

- Keep the affected area clean.
- Placing ice wrapped in a cloth to the affected area can reduce swelling
- Applying **Calendula ointment** topically, after the incision is closed, will help speed the healing of the skin.

WHEN TO CONTACT YOUR HEALTHCARE PROFESSIONAL

- If the circumcision wound is not healing properly.

COMMON REMEDIES FOR AFTER BIRTH AND CIRCUMCISION SUPPORT

After	Aconite	*Borax	*Nux mochata	Staphysagria	*Stramonium
Symptoms	Sensitive to noise.	Sensitive to downward motion. Easily startled when put down.	Chilly. Colic with much gas. Excessive sleepiness.	Incredibly sensitive to pain, noise, touch or odors.	Inconsolable crying all night. Does not want to be alone. Terrified of the dark. Screams bloody murder upon waking.
Mood	Fearful, anxious, restless.	Anxious look in the eyes.	Nurses for a few minutes, then falls back asleep because they are so exhausted.	Sleepy all day and awake all night.	Terror in the eyes which are wide open with dilated pupils.
Indications	Look of terror in eyes. Can be brought on especially after a fast labor or circumcision. Even a fast labor that scares the mother.	Look of fright. Wants to be carried day and night. Might turn blue. Any downward motion is unwelcome.	Trauma causing baby to be so sleepy that they cannot latch on to the breast.	Especially helpful after circumcision or any surgical intervention.	For baby boys after circumcision.

Special Dosing: For infants, dilute the remedy in four ounces of water, stir it up and give 1/4 teaspoon every 15 minutes for one hour (or place liquid on lips), then once per hour as needed. Another option is to place one pellet in between the infant's lower lip and gum. If the baby falls asleep in between doses, just resume once they wake. If there is no change in comfort after four doses, choose another remedy.

TEETHING

Teething (dentition) babies can experience gum discomfort in the mouth. If your baby is particularly uncomfortable, below are commonly used remedies to aid in difficult dentition.

ADDITIONAL SUPPORT FOR TEETHING

- Provide a frozen teething ring, a frozen bagel or a fat, long cold peeled carrot for your child to chew on. It can be soothing to their gums. However, you MUST NOT leave a child unattended as they can be choking hazards.

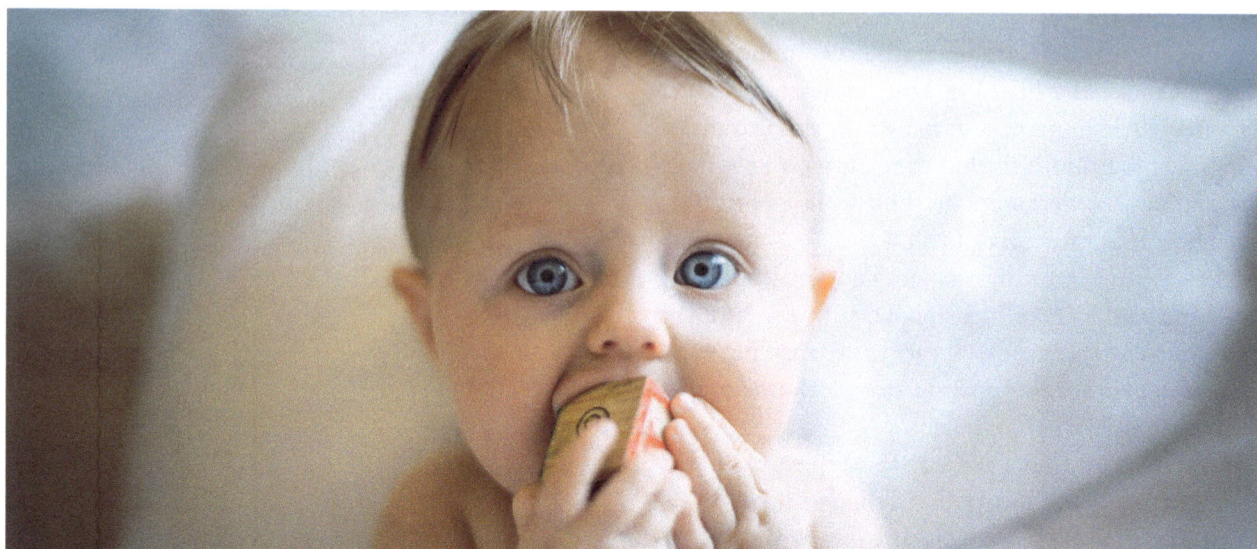

COMMON REMEDIES FOR TEETHING

	Belladonna	Calcarea carb	*Calcarea phos	Chamomilla	Silicea
Onset	Great and sudden pain.	Late dentition and teething.	Delayed or late dentition.	First remedy to consider for teething difficulties. If this remedy fails, try Belladonna next.	Painful and delayed teething.
Symptoms	Screaming, kicking, twitching. Desires lemonade.	Head perspiration. Grinding of gums or teeth at night.	Diarrhea with teething, accompanied by lots of gassiness.	Rocking and being carried relieves temporarily. Does not want to be put down. Slight relief from cold applications. Can have greenish diarrhea, like chopped grass.	Diarrhea. Sweating of head/neck area. Aggravation from milk.
Mood	Restlessness.	Uncomfortable, whining.	Restlessness, never satisfied.	Extreme impatience and irritability. Demands something and then refuses it when it is offered.	Irritable. Sensitive. Anxious, but wants to do things by themselves.
Indications	Flushed red face, gums and lips. Dry heat.	Fingers in mouth to relieve sensation. Sour smelling stool and perspiration.	In emaciated, weak infants late in learning to walk.	Great pain, aggravation from touch. One cheek hot and red, the other pale.	Foul smelling diarrhea with much gassiness.
Worse	Drafts. Being touched, noise, sudden jarring motion.	Cold, drafts, damp weather	Constant change of position.	Cold open air, wind, touch and 9 PM.	Damp, cold weather. Baths. Mornings.
Better	Partially sitting up. Bending backwards. Pressure. Eating lemons or drinking lemonade.	Dry weather. Warmth. Lying on painful side.	Dry, warm weather. Riding in a car.	Being carried or rocked. Cold applications. Wind.	Dry weather. Wrapping up.

Dosing: Start with the BLUE dosing method. However, if symptoms are intense, give remedy once an hour for four doses. Observe and evaluate.

COLIC IN NEWBORNS

Colic is a period of intense fussiness usually in the late afternoon or early evening at a time when parents are tired and need a break! Your baby spends the day absorbing the stimulation of the world and some need to release it by fussing and crying. It helps them release tension while shutting out sights, sounds, and other sensations that may be too intense. In infants who experience colic, it typically lasts from a few weeks to a few months. It often resolves on its own as the infant matures over those initial few months after birth.

If your child is intensely fussy all day as well, digestive discomfort may be more the issue. This can be a result of a combination of any of these three factors: 1) immature digestive organs, 2) quick eating combined with quick let down of the mother's milk (fast consumption) and/or 3) an intolerance to a food or other ingredient in the mother's milk or formula.

ADDITIONAL SUPPORT FOR COLIC

- Make sure the baby has been fed, burped, has had a wet diaper recently and had an appropriate stool.
- If you're breastfeeding and you notice your baby's fussiness is worse after eating a certain food, avoid that food. Some common offenders include dairy, wheat, sugar, soy, eggs, corn, beef and nuts.
- If you're feeding formula, again notice if your baby is seemingly not digesting it well or reacting to it. Consult with your healthcare provider on making appropriate changes to the formula provided.
- "Bicycle" the baby's legs and gently squeeze/push the legs bent into the abdomen. These motions help release the pent up emotions from the day.
- If your baby enjoys touch, consider gently and slowly massaging your baby to calm their nervous system down.

WHEN TO CONTACT YOUR HEALTHCARE PROFESSIONAL

- The baby is lethargic and/or is passing bloody stool.
- If the baby is constantly screaming and not responding to remedies.
- If the baby is vomiting or has constant diarrhea and/or is not urinating or gaining weight.

COMMON REMEDIES FOR COLIC IN NEWBORNS

	Chamomilla	*Colocynthis	Lycopodium	Magnesium phos	Nux vomica	Pulsatilla
Onset	Cold wind. Anger. Nursing mom drinks coffee and/or alcohol.	Overexcitement. Nursing mom eats cheese, unripe or rotten fruit, or too much fruit.	Wet weather. Nursing mom eats oysters, milk, peas, beans, or raw cabbage.	Cold baths. Cold drinks.	Overfeeding. Nursing mom ingests spicy, rich food, stimulants, or alcohol.	Nursing mom ingests fatty, rich food, or ice cream.
Symptoms	Screams, shrieks. May arch back in pain. One cheek red and hot, the other pale. Gassy, but passing gas does not relieve the pain. Greenish diarrhea that smells like rotten eggs.	Twists and doubles up. Sudden, violent, severe, cutting pain, usually moves from left to right. Watery, sour, yellowish diarrhea with gas and pain.	Much loud gas and belching, even after slightest amount of breast milk or formula. Very hungry, but doesn't nurse long.	Crampy pain with lots of trapped gas. Burps and passes gas without relief. Draws all limbs into body due to pain or lies curled in fetal position on their side.	Trapped gas with constipation. Strains and grunts with no bowel movement, even though stool may be soft. May retch without vomiting.	Gas. Possible vomiting long after eating. Hiccups soon after eating. Rumbling and gurgling noises in abdomen. Diarrhea alternates with constipation. No two stools look alike.
Mood	Wants to be held, but only for a while. Nothing pleases them. Angry, irritable. Sensitive to odors and noise. Starts to nurse, then turns away. May bite nipple.	Extremely restless. Oversensitive, easily irritated. Infant sometimes moans.	Wakes irritable and angry. Look of anxiety or worry with a wrinkled brow.	Irritable. Wants to be nurtured.	Angry, irritable, tense. Fitful with intermittent crying. Has an angry sounding cry.	Cries a lot until picked up, weepy and clingy. Eats constantly, not because of hunger, but from craving comfort. Moods change often. Has a piteous sounding cry.
Indications	Hot. Thirsty. Over-tired, but cannot sleep due to pain. Cries out in sleep.	Wants to lie on abdomen and screams if moved.	Long and lean infants. Bloated abdomen.	Abdomen is very bloated.	Disrupted sleep. Stuffed up nose. Face pinched. Arches back. Chilly.	Face may have visible small veins. Usually thirstless. May be plump infant.
Worse	Cold open air, wind. Touch. Anger. Night, especially around 9 PM.	Night.	4 AM or 4-8 PM. Warm room. Strangers. Too tight diapers or clothing.	Cold drafts. Being uncovered. Open air.	After eating. Morning, 3 AM. Noise, odors, light, touch. Too tight diapers or clothing.	Warm, stuffy room. Evening time.
Better	Being rocked or carried. In mild weather. Warm (not hot) applications on abdomen.	Warmth. Drawing knees to belly. Firm pressure on abdomen by putting infant over the top of your shoulder.	Warm (not hot) applications on abdomen.	Knees to chest. Warm baths. Gentle pressure and rubbing. Warm covers.	Passing gas or stool. Warmth of bed.	In parent's arms. Outdoors, fresh air. Gentle motion. A soothing voice.

Dosing: Use the **BLUE** method. Observe and evaluate.

CONSTIPATION IN NEWBORNS AND BABIES

Constipation is a condition of the bowels in which the stool is dry and hardened. Evacuation is sluggish, difficult, infrequent or inactive. It is a result of slowness or inaction of peristalsis, the wave-like contraction of the colon that moves waste material through to the rectum and out of the body. This can be due to a not fully developed digestive tract, or weak smooth muscle in the intestines. Cramping intestines can produce an urging to eliminate, with an inability to push waste out.

Painful cramping, bloating and trapped gas are all symptoms of constipation. If you observe your baby crying and bending double, or lying on his/her stomach for relief, combined with an inability to produce stool at least once a day, they are experiencing constipation.

SUPPORTIVE MEASURES FOR CONSTIPATION IN NEWBORNS AND BABIES

- Keep the baby and nursing mother hydrated. Also for the nursing mother include fiber, fruits and vegetables in the diet.
- Refrain from using aluminum pans; even in trace amounts as aluminum can cause constipation.
- Gently massage the baby's belly in an upward motion when they are laying on their back, starting on the left over the upper abdomen (as the adult is looking at the child) and down the right side, following the digestion route.
- "Bicycle" the baby's legs when they are laying on their back and gently squeeze/push the legs bent into the abdomen. These motions help stimulate the digestive contractions to "get things moving."

WHEN TO CONTACT YOUR HEALTHCARE PROFESSIONAL

- The constipation becomes a chronic situation that remains unaffected by remedies.
- If the child is in pain and has not had a bowel movement in 24+ hours.
- If the difficult stool, once passed, is white, gray, hard, black or accompanied by blood.
- If the constipation is accompanied by fever and pain or if the child's eyes or skin have a yellow hue.

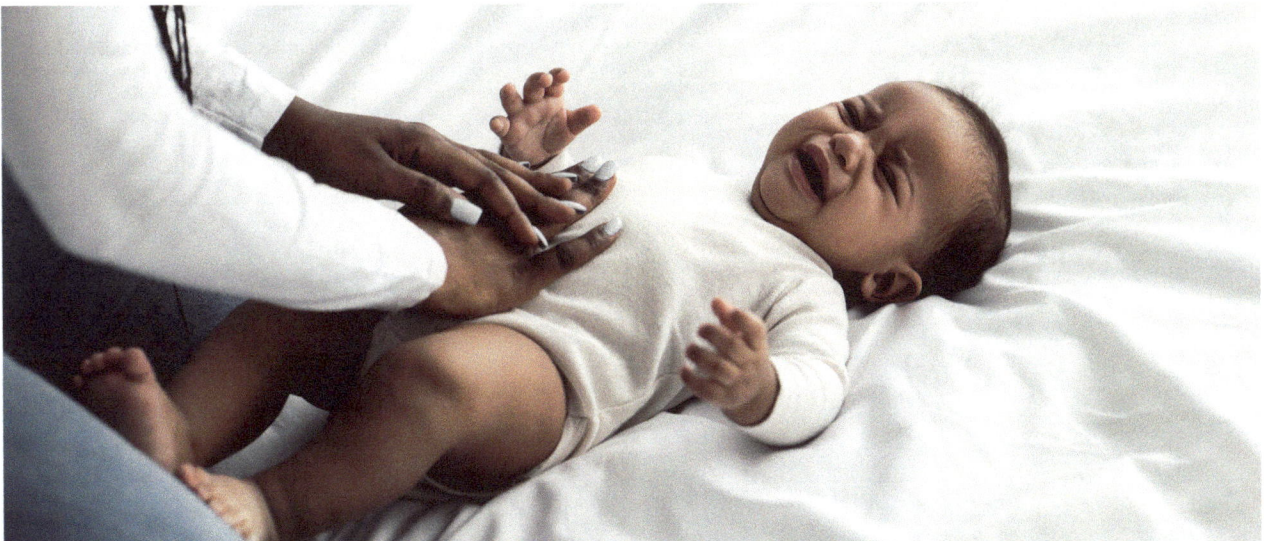

COMMON REMEDIES FOR CONSTIPATION IN NEWBORNS AND BABIES

	*Alumina	Bryonia	Calcarea carb	Lycopodium	Natrum mur	Nux vomica	Silicea
Onset	Generally formula fed infants. Newborns with delicate digestion.	Dehydration.	Stubborn constipation with no urge. Even though constipated, seems to feel okay.	Very little urge for a bowel movement.	Constipation may alternate with days of watery diarrhea.	Constant desire to pass a stool with much painful straining, but little or no result. Constipation alternates with diarrhea.	Because rectum does not have enough strength for contracting, stool starts to come out, but then recedes. Can also be due to spasms of the sphincter muscle.
Symptoms	Stool is small, dry, hard balls. Skin and mucous membranes are dry.	Stool large, dry, hard, may have burnt appearance. White coating on tongue. Extremely thirsty, craves cold drinks.	Stools look like clay. All discharges smell sour. Abdomen is bloated, large and hard. Stool may be hard in the beginning followed by diarrhea full of undigested food.	Small, hard stools. Abdomen is very bloated. Rumbling with lots of gas.	Hard, dry, and crumbly stools. Little balls passed with much straining. Only passes small amounts at a time.	Stools are large, hard and dark.	Strains and strains to pass a hard stool, exhausted afterwards. Anus looks sore and oozes mucus.
Mood	Dull, sluggish, lack energy.	Does not want to be carried or moved. Wants complete stillness. Very grumpy and irritable. Seems uncomfortable.	Fearful, restless, crying out at night. Slow, easy-going, but usually obstinate.	Anxious or worried look with wrinkled brow. Wakes irritable and angry.	Tends to be weepy and sensitive. Doesn't like much physical contact. Wants to be left alone when upset.	Very irritable, impatient. Easily exhausted. Cries at slightest cause.	Delicate and very sensitive to cold. Needs lots of patient handling. Generally subdued, but can become surprisingly fussy.
Indications	Intense straining and trembling, even if stool is soft. Apparent pain during elimination. Bright red blood may be present.	Difficulty getting stool out. Dryness of mouth, tongue, rectum, and skin. Weakness from slightest exertion.	May have a large head. May be plump and large generally. Can expel a surprisingly large stool.	Urge for bowel movement, but can't get anything out.	Stool coated with glassy-looking mucus. Anus looks sore after passing a stool. May experience rectal bleeding.	Wakes in early morning with rumbling gas pains. May have upset stomach. Chilly.	Chilly with sour smelling sweat.
Worse	On left side when urge comes on. Starchy foods, especially potatoes. Aluminum cookware. Dry weather. Upon waking.	Any motion or exertion, touch. Excessive warmth or light. Early morning.	Cold, damp. Movement. Teething. Full moon.	4 AM or 4-8 PM. After eating. Warm rooms. Tight diapers or clothing. Strangers.	Between 9-11 AM. Lying down. Sympathy. Touch and pressure. Heat.	4 AM. Getting chilled, uncovering, and drafts. Loss of sleep.	Left side. Cold air, drafts, damp, uncovering. Morning. Loud noises. Teething. During full moon.

Dosing: Use the **BLUE** method. Observe and evaluate.

DIARRHEA AND VOMITING IN NEWBORNS AND BABIES

Diarrhea is characterized by increased frequency and fluidity of bowel evacuations, while vomiting is a regurgitation or throwing up of the stomach's contents. These conditions can easily cause dehydration, which is especially dangerous for newborns and infants. Both conditions are often due to bacteria or viruses in food — otherwise known as food-borne illnesses. Diarrhea and vomiting can also be associated with intolerance or allergy to something in the baby's diet such as formula, food or mother's milk.

A food-borne illness, motion sickness or intense, spasmodic coughing can cause vomiting.

Symptoms the body might present during dehydration are:

- infrequent wet diapers

- listlessness

- pale skin

- the eyes and fontanel (soft spot on top of the head) can look or feel sunken

- the urine will have a strong odor

- no urination at all

- the skin may have decreased rebound (doesn't spring back when pressed in or pulled upward)

SUPPORTIVE MEASURES FOR DIARRHEA AND VOMITING IN NEWBORNS AND BABIES

- Keep the child hydrated—continue to nurse an infant and encourage an older child to drink small sips of diluted apple or watermelon juice.
- Feed your toddler a B.R.A.T. diet as it helps the intestines bind: Bananas, Rice, Applesauce, and Toast. If the baby is nursing, continue nursing.
- Do not advance the diet too quickly or in too large of amounts; after a heavy loss of fluids, the digestive system improves gradually.

WHEN TO CONTACT YOUR HEALTHCARE PROFESSIONAL

- If the skin doesn't rebound (no spring back after being pressed with a finger on the shin-bone area) after attempting to rehydrate.
- If your baby will not nurse or drink.
- If there is any fever in an infant.
- If there is a fever in older children who are listless and not eating, drinking, playing or eliminating urine or stool.
- If there is blood in the stool or vomit.
- If vomiting doesn't cease or occurs after a head or abdominal injury.
- If there's been no response to remedies after 24 hours.

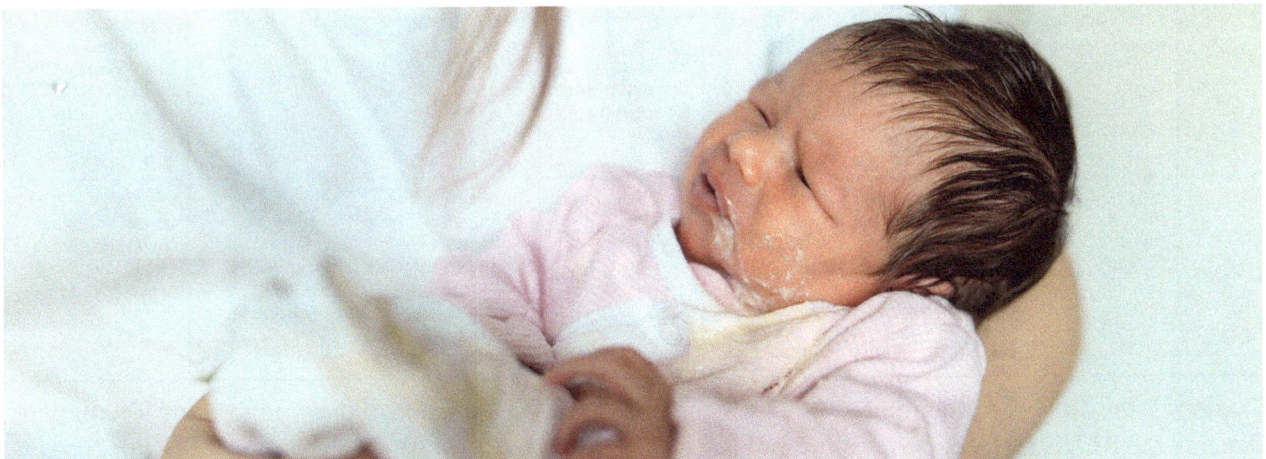

COMMON REMEDIES FOR VOMITING AND DIARRHEA IN NEWBORNS

	Argentum nit	Arsenicum	Carbo veg	Ipecac	Nux vomica	Phosphorus	*Veratrum
Onset	Vomiting preceded by loud belching. Diarrhea is common in babies who are being weaned from breast milk.	Nursing mother has food poisoning. Diarrhea after eating. A sense the baby has anxiety.	Nursing mother has food poisoning. Gas on passing foul-smelling stools.	Constant vomiting that does not appear to relieve.	Sudden diarrhea after anger. Also when nursing mother eats an offensive food or changes her diet.	Vomits by mouthfuls.	Nursing mother has food poisoning. Abdominal pain and cramping with extreme exhaustion. Unquenchable thirst which is soon vomited.
Symptoms	Vomit is full of thick mucus. Diarrhea is noisy, watery, and foul-smelling, with green stools that look like chopped spinach.	Foul smelling stools that seem to burn the anus. Simultaneous diarrhea and vomiting. Abdomen sensitive to touch. Chilly. Weakness from passing stool.	Curl up with pain. Cold to the touch with cold sweats. Not interested in eating.	Vomiting of food, bile, green mucus, and/or bright red blood. Overfilling of stomach causes much crying and vomiting. Yellow or green, very offensive smelling stools, can be streaked with blood.	Much gas and bloating. Stool seems to relieve but then has another stool.	May vomit bile or blood. Vomit may look like coffee grounds. Lots of belching.	Diarrhea and vomiting at the same time. Intense chills and cold sweat. Sweat on forehead while vomiting or passing stool. Odorless, watery stools that look like rice water, or watery yellow or green stools. Violent, projectile vomiting.
Mood	Anxious and fidgety.	Anxious and restless. Not very interested in eating. Weak energy, but demanding.	Appears anxious, irritable and sluggish.	Appears angry and complains with a lot of screaming and howling. Nothing pleases them.	Appears angry, acts irritable. Very sensitive. Hypersensitive to light, odors, touch and sound.	Affectionate and cheerful, later becoming upset and irritable. Wants attention and consolation.	Restless, moody, tearful.
Indications	Severe bloating and passing of loud gas. Diarrhea passed with much gas.	Retching after eating. Very watery, brown, yellow, or black slimy stools that may contain undigested food. Foul-smelling stools in small quantities. Cramping in abdomen.	Sour belching. Restricted breathing. Belly is very tender. Bad breath. Pale face that sometimes has a bluish tint.	Face pale, may have dark circles around eyes. Twitches. Hiccups. Increased salivation.	Much retching of sour-smelling vomit. Can be bilious.	Exhausting diarrhea that may be bloody. Watery and painless, with green mucus or grey/bluish, pasty color. Great weakness afterwards.	Apparent pain in abdomen before passing stool, weak afterwards. Frequent stools that blast out. Forehead, hands, feet, breath, and abdomen are cold. Vomit is slimy, and may be yellow, green or black.
Worse	Heat. Too much excitement. Lying on left side. Nursing mother is eating a lot of sugar.	Midnight to 2 AM. Cold food or drinks. Getting chilled. After nursing mother eats bad food (rotten meat, fish, or fruit).	Loss of fluids. Nursing mother has eaten rotten fish or meat (especially poultry), butter, fats, milk. Lying down.	Nursing mother eats bad food, unripe fruit, pork, ice cream, rich foods, pastries, sweets, berries. Overeating. Heat.	Nursing mother eats rich, spicy or junk food, fats, or impure water. Morning. After eating. Touch.	Evening. Touch. Odors. Light. Lying on the left side.	Nursing mother eats spoiled meats, fruits, potatoes, or green vegetables. Exertion. Cold, wet weather. Touch and pressure. Night.
Better	Fresh air, motion. Passing gas and burping.	Heat and warm applications to the abdomen.	Cool, fresh air, fanning. Elevating feet. Passing gas and burping.	Open air. Rest.	Temporarily, after a stool or vomiting. Heat. Nursing after vomiting subsides. Quiet, calm surroundings.	Sleep. Consolation. Low lights and darkness. Open air. Cool applications.	Warmth, covering. Lying down. Babies feel better if carried around, but not rocked.

Dosing: If the diarrhea or vomiting are persistent, use the ORANGE method. If the symptoms are intermittent, then use the BLUE method. Observe and evaluate.

EYE CONDITIONS IN NEWBORNS AND BABIES

Some newborns and babies have underdeveloped tear ducts and they can become blocked. Eye conditions can also be the result of a birth trauma or injury, or a symptom of infection. Sometimes it can be accompanied by a state of little to no energy, along with a fever. The eye is not red or swollen, just tearing. Warm compresses can help most eye conditions, unless the eye seems to feel worse from heat.

WHEN TO CONTACT YOUR HEALTHCARE PROVIDER

- If the tear duct remains blocked as evidence of the affected eye(s) tearing.

COMMON REMEDIES FOR EYE CONDITIONS IN NEWBORNS AND BABIES

	Apis	Argentum nit	Arsenicum	Calcarea carb	Pulsatilla	Silicea	Staphysagria
Onset	Blocked tear duct, conjunctivitis.	Conjunctivitis or blocked tear duct. Commonly presents shortly after birth.	Conjunctivitis.	Conjunctivitis or blocked tear duct. After exposure to cold.	Conjunctivitis, blocked tear duct. Sticky eyes in newborns.	Blocked tear duct. A foreign body lodged in the eye tissue.	Cuts or incisions to eye.
Symptoms	Puffiness and swelling around eyes. Redness.	Eyelid is red, swollen, sore, thick. Discharge is profuse and full of yellow pus. Thick crust on edges of eyelids upon waking; can become glued together.	Burning pain in eyes and eyelids. Eyes bright red and bloodshot, sometimes with dark rings or puffiness. Eyelids red, crusty and ulcerated.	Sore, watery eyes that ooze yellow or foul-smelling discharge. Eyes glued together after sleeping. Itchy and swollen. Discharge appears gritty.	Profuse, thick, yellow or yellow-green eye discharge which may be smelly. Discharge in corners of eyes, thick upon waking, then watery for rest of the day.	Noticeable inflammation of the eye. Swelling of tear duct. Stricture of tear duct. Seems averse to daylight.	Soreness and redness of eyelids. Sometimes there are no complaints.
Mood	Restless.	Irritable, seems anxious, weepy.	Seems anxious, restless.	May be happy go lucky despite eye issue, not a care in the world. Or could be trembling with terror and be clingy.	May be weepy, upset and clingy.	Mad and upset about eye, demanding attention to clear the issue.	Crying sounds angry.
Indications	Discharge clear or full of pus. Much itching, especially at night. Eyes bloodshot.	Swelling, inflammation, redness on inner corner of eye.	Extreme sensitivity to light. Eyelid may be spasming.	Chilly. Sensitivity to light, dilated pupils. May be squinting.	Itchy eyes cause a lot of rubbing.	Sensitivity to daylight. Eyes very tender to touch, especially when closed.	Eye appears itchy or seems that there is a sensation of something in the eye.
Worse	Late afternoon, sun, right eye, heat.	Warm rooms, heat. Upon waking.	Evening, cold damp. Upon waking. Light. On right side.	Open air. Early morning, cold, damp. When accompanied by common cold. Any eye movement.	Evening time. Warm, stuffy rooms, warm wind.	Cold, damp. Fresh air. Touch.	Angry crying.
Better	Cool applications, cool air.	Cool applications. Light pressure. Fresh air.	Warm applications. Lying down.	Rest. Warmth.	Temperate fresh air, cool applications.	Heat, warm rooms. Rest.	Cool and warm applications.

In addition to the remedies listed, **Mercurius** and **Natrum mur** are also worth considering for blocked tear ducts that are not moving in a healing direction.

Dosing: Use the BLUE method. Observe and evaluate.

COMMON COLDS IN NEWBORNS AND BABIES

Colds are difficult for newborns and babies since they haven't yet learned how to blow their nose, clear their nasal passages, or breathe through their mouths. A cold makes it difficult for babies to breathe easily and so they can be uncomfortable and sleep poorly. Eating is difficult if they can't draw air through their nasal passages.
For more on treating colds, see **Common Colds and Sinusitis** *in* **Chapter 8—Nose** *starting on* **page 91.**

♥ ADDITIONAL SUPPORT FOR COMMON COLDS IN NEWBORNS AND BABIES

- Use a bulb syringe, purchased at any pharmacy, to suck out mucus that the baby does not yet have the coordination to dispel. Do this frequently so the mucus does not drain down the back of the throat.
- A nursing mother should avoid dairy products, which are mucus producing, until the cold subsides.

⚕ WHEN TO CONTACT YOUR HEALTHCARE PROFESSIONAL

- If the newborn has any fever.

COMMON REMEDIES FOR COMMON COLDS IN NEWBORNS AND BABIES

	Aconite	Bryonia	Hepar sulph	Mercurius	Pulsatilla
Onset	Comes on suddenly, from a chill.	More gradual onset.	Oversensitive to pain, touch, cold.	Sensitive to temperature changes.	Nose gets stuffy when returning indoors after being outdoors.
Symptoms	Restlessness, tossing about. One cheek red, the other pale. Strong and frequent thirst or desire to nurse.	Does not want to be moved, wants to lay still. Very thirsty.	Sweaty, but chilly, wants to be kept warm and covered up at all times.	Hard, swollen glands under ears and down sides of the neck. Excess salivation/ drool. Offensive smelling breath.	Nose discharge is colored or yellow/green. Cold extends to the eyes with tearing and mild swelling.
Mood	Anxious look in their eyes.	Fussy.	Irritable.	Timid, restless, discontented.	Weepy, oscillating between fine and unhappy. Wants to be carried, cuddled and receive a lot of attention.
Indications	Comes on after being out in cold dry wind.	Dry lips and stuffed up nose. Tends to be constipated with dry, hard stools.	Touch with cold hands will make baby scream. Breath rattles and may be accompanied by a cough.	Sweaty. Smelly. Usually has diarrhea.	Happier and more comfortable in fresh air or with the windows open.
Worse	Night. From being chilled. From noise. During teething.	Motion. Exertion. Heat. From becoming chilled.	Cold dry air, drafts. Cold drinks and food.	Night. Sweating. Sensitive to drafts.	Warmth of any kind. Evening.
Better	Open air. Rest. Warmth. Perspiration.	Pressure. When quiet and resting. Cold air.	Heat. Warm applications to head. Warm, damp weather.	Moderate temperature. Rest. Morning. Scratching.	Cold, fresh open air. Uncovering. Cold drinks and food.

Dosing: Use the **BLUE** method. Observe and evaluate.

CRADLE CAP

Cradle cap, also called milk crust, is crusty, white or yellow scales on the baby's scalp. It can appear at birth or develop soon after. Cradle cap can last for more than two years if not addressed. It can be uncomfortable and itchy for the baby.

ADDITIONAL SUPPORT FOR CRADLE CAP

- To relieve and loosen the scales, gently rub organic olive or coconut oil on the baby's head.

WHEN TO CONTACT YOUR HEALTHCARE PROFESSIONAL

- You don't see improvement, consider seeking constitutional care for your baby from a professional homeopath.
- If the area is inflamed or swollen.

Remedies to consider:

- **Calcarea carb**: Children needing this remedy tend to scratch their heads on being disturbed or awakened out of sleep; have itchiness, especially at night. They have thick foul milk crusts on the scalp accompanied by swollen glands on the sides of the neck.

- **Silicea**: Children needing this remedy have moist, crusty eruptions on their scalp and a profusely sweaty head.

Dosing: Use the BLUE method. Observe and evaluate. This condition improves gradually so have patience with the process.

DIAPER RASH

A self-explanatory term, this is the rash that forms on the baby's genitals and/or rear end, or in the creases between the legs and hips, where the diaper touches the skin. It can be the body's reaction to something eaten, the wearing of a diaper soaked in urine or feces too long, and/or from diapers made with chlorine in the linings.

ADDITIONAL SUPPORT FOR DIAPER RASH

- Change diapers immediately when wet or containing stool.
- Replace wipes with water to which a few drops of **Calendula tincture** have been added.
- Dry area thoroughly.
- Allow child to go diaperless for as long as you can manage.
- If breastfeeding, avoid spicy foods and citrus.
- Using a mild soap, keep the area clean.
- You can use a hair dryer on the cool setting to completely dry the baby's bottom before putting on another diaper.
- Apply an organic egg white on the skin to serve as a barrier between the skin and diaper.
- **Calendula ointment** or cream applied externally is helpful—avoid the gel as it may sting. Organic coconut or olive oil can be soothing as well.

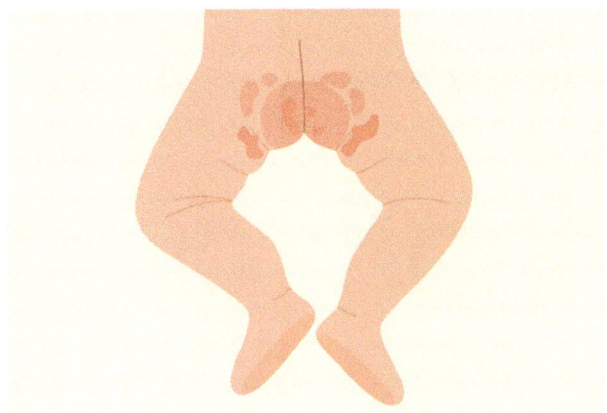

WHEN TO CONTACT YOUR HEALTHCARE PROFESSIONAL

- The rash is very uncomfortable and does not respond to remedies.
- If the child has had a rash, warts or skin infections since birth.
- If there is a cottage cheese-like discharge, it can be evidence of yeast as well.
- If there are blisters that ooze pus, or swollen lymph nodes in the groin.

COMMON REMEDIES FOR DIAPER RASH

	Calcarea carb	*Graphites	Hepar sulph	*Petroleum	Sulphur
Symptoms	Unhealthy looking skin; flaccid. Nettle (fine) rash.	Thick, sticky, honey-colored oozing that may form yellow crusts. May see streaks of blood.	Skin oozes pus that smells like old, rotten cheese.	Skin extremely sensitive, raw, burning, itchy. Slow to heal, especially in skin folds and around scrotum. Skin may crack and bleed.	Very itchy, burning, red diaper rash.
Mood	Chilly, fussy babies.	Startles easily.	Extremely sensitive, physically and emotionally.	Very irritable, physically and emotionally.	Irritated by heat.
Indications	Itching in cold air. Thick or fine rash, very pink or red.	In folds of skin. Will not want a warm bath. Skin is dry, inflamed, raw, itchy, and cracked.	Skin is very tender and extremely chilly. Averse to cold.	If rash improves without a diaper.	Bright red rash around anus. Raw skin can break open and bleed. Needs to be cool.
Worse	Cold air. Bathing.	Cold, drafts. Suppression of symptoms.	Cold air, drafts, water.	Motion, touch.	Heat, warm bathing.
Better	Heat. Dry weather.	Open air, touch, eating.	Warm bathing.	Warm air, dry weather.	Cool air.

Dosing: Use the **BLUE** method. Observe and evaluate.

FEVERS

See **Chapter 5—Head** starting on **page 69**.

HAND, FOOT AND MOUTH DISEASE (HFM)

See **Chapter 21—Childhood (Ages 3-12)** on **page 256**.

JAUNDICE

This is a common newborn condition due to an early delivery, inefficient filtering of bilirubin out of the blood before birth and/or inefficient filtering of the waste products from mom in the womb. Baby's skin will be yellowish in color. It occurs within the first day or two after birth.

Extent of jaundice

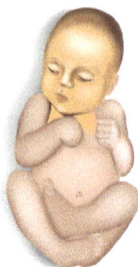

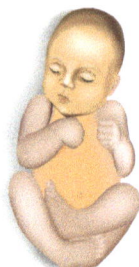

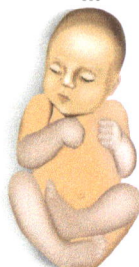

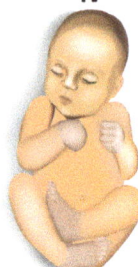

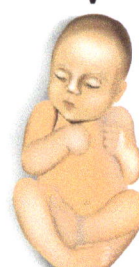

Grade I	II	III	IV	V
Face and neck only	Chest and back	Abdomen below umbilicus to knees	Arms and legs below knees	Hands and feet

ADDITIONAL SUPPORT FOR JAUNDICE

- Consider placing the baby undressed in front of a window drenched with natural sunlight.
- It has been shown to be helpful for the mom and baby to lie skin to skin.

WHEN TO CONTACT YOUR HEALTHCARE PROFESSIONAL

- Baby starts to have an odd or unusual appearance or behavior.
- Jaundice continues longer than 14 days.
- Jaundice worsens.
- The whites of the eyes become yellow.
- The skin of their tummy or legs look yellow.
- Taking inadequate nourishment or suckles weakly.
- You feel your child needs medical attention (for whatever reason).

The remedy ***Chelidonium** is the go-to remedy for this condition. If the newborn is not helped with this remedy and the jaundice persists more than a few days, consider consulting a professional homeopath.

MEASLES

See *Chapter 21—Childhood (Ages 3-12)* on *page 257*.

MUMPS

See *Chapter 21—Childhood (Ages 3-12)* on *page 258*.

RUBELLA (GERMAN MEASLES)

See *Chapter 21—Childhood (Ages 3-12)* on *page 260*.

SCARLET FEVER

See *Chapter 21—Childhood (Ages 3-12)* on *page 261*.

WHOOPING COUGH

See *Chapter 10—Throat and Chest* on *page 122*.

RESTLESSNESS, ANXIETY, OR OVER-STIMULATION

When timings of any regular schedule are off; for example, if she/he has been on a long car trip or journey, a baby can become overstimulated. Indications include arching the head back, looking at everything, making noise, and just not settling down/unable to sleep. If this is the case, you can try a dose of ***Coffea**, but if the state persists, it's best to consult a professional homeopath. **Special Dosing:** Give one dose. Observe and evaluate.

THRUSH

Thrush, which is a yeast infection in the mouth of a newborn, can be passed back and forth between mother and infant repeatedly if not treated. White patches appear in the child's mouth (tongue, cheeks or gums). The baby may have swallowed candida during the birth process. Antibiotic treatment of mother and/or child can also be contributing factors. The baby is uncomfortable nursing due to rawness or soreness in the mouth.

ADDITIONAL SUPPORT FOR THRUSH

- It would be helpful if the mother can add fermented foods, such as yogurt with live cultures into her own diet and eliminate regular dairy, gluten and sugar, because yeast feeds on sugar.
- The mother should be checked for a breast or yeast infection as well.

COMMON REMEDIES FOR THRUSH IN NEWBORNS

	*Borax	*Kali mur	Mercurius	Natrum mur
Symptoms	Canker sores, white spots/patches in the mouth.	White ulcers in mouth. Swollen glands in the neck.	Canker sores in mouth or on tongue. Moist, heavy, yellow-coated tongue. Very thirsty.	Mouth sore where nipple touches it. Gums red. Breath hot and foul.
Mood	Fear of any downward motion. Startles easily.	Irritable and discontented.	Restlessness. Weepy. Moaning in pain.	Dislikes being handled or carried.
Indications	Mouth feels hot to the mother's nipple. Can even refuse to nurse due to pain.	Gray, whitish coating of base of tongue. Gums shiny and red.	Much salivation with canker sores. Foul breath and sweat.	Lips and corners of mouth dry and cracked.

Dosing: Use the BLUE method. Observe and evaluate.

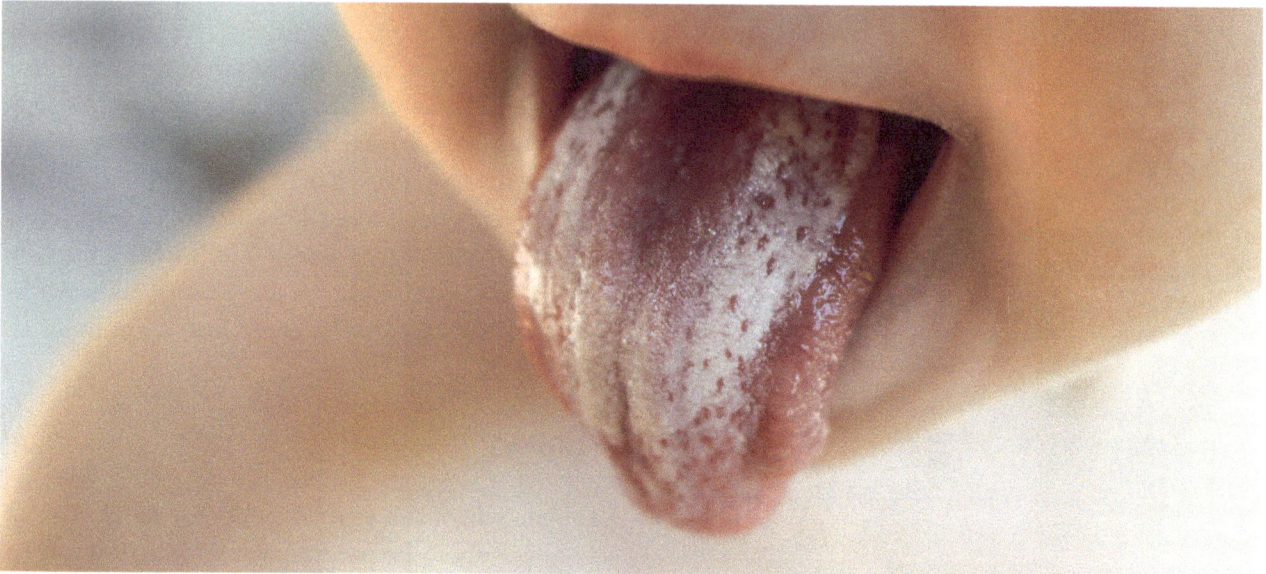

VACCINE REACTIONS

Anything beyond a slight fever and swelling/pain/redness at the vaccination site is considered a vaccine reaction. That can range from, for example, high fever to seizures, to high pitched shrieking or changes in behavior following an immunization. The objective of giving a remedy before an immunization helps to optimize the body's overall immune response.

♥ ADDITIONAL SUPPORT FOR EASING VACCINE REACTIONS

- It's advantageous to let a fever under 103 °F (39.4 °C) run its course without suppression. Fever is a body's natural reaction and immune response. However, make sure to keep the child hydrated.
- Consider giving some Vitamin C to help aid in clearing any toxins out of the body.
- The most common go-to remedy to give before and after receiving a vaccine is *Thuja. Arnica can help with soreness and Ledum can help with the possible lingering pain from the puncture.
- If there are lingering symptoms after a vaccine, consider seeing a professional homeopath or another healthcare provider.

Dosing: Use the BLUE method for several days. Observe and evaluate.

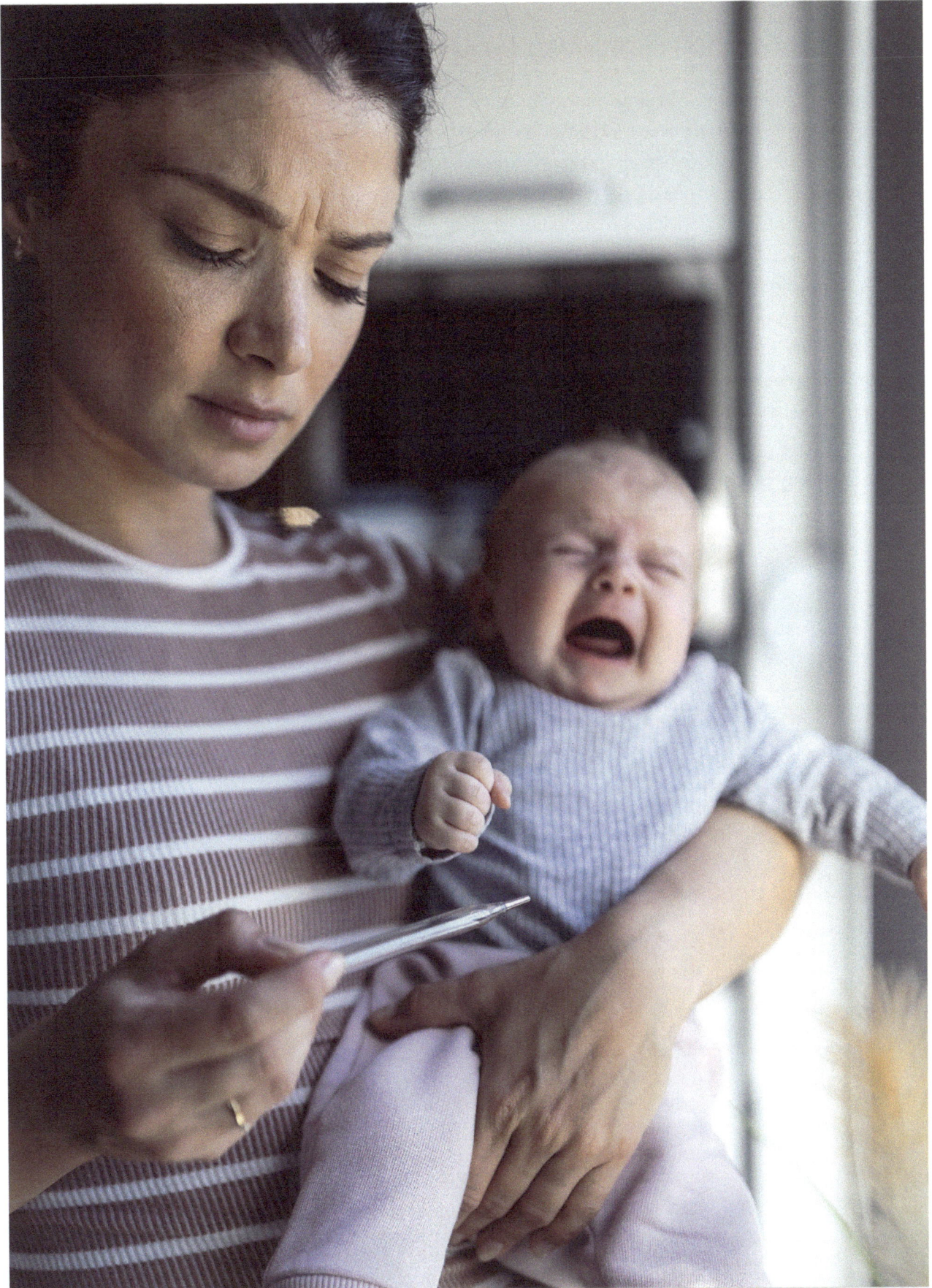

? WHAT'S THE FIRST REMEDY YOU THINK OF WHEN...

1. Your recently circumcised infant looks petrified.

2. Your teething child seems to be in pain and has extreme impatience and irritability.

3. Your newborn is colicky, especially around 9pm and nothing seems to please them.

4. Your colicky newborn has a lot of gas and burping and only nurses for a short time.

5. Your newborn is typically easy-going but when constipated has sour-smelling discharges with a bloated belly.

6. The baby has persistent diarrhea and repeated vomiting after the nursing mom got food poisoning.

7. Your angry and crying baby is hiccuping, vomiting yellow/green and doesn't seem relieved by it.

8. Your clingy and weepy baby seems to have a cold and is congested more when returning back inside.

9. Your baby has a red diaper rash that is itchy and bright red around the anus. Warm bathing makes it worse.

10. Your baby has thrush with excess salivation with the canker sores with bad breath and sweat.

Answer key on page 324.

CHAPTER 21
Childhood Ages 3-12

If you ask any homeopath how they got started using homeopathy, a vast majority will say it was when their child was little. It's the parents and caregivers who come to homeopathy because they want to help their child (and their family members) heal more naturally and in a most compassionate and supportive way. This chapter will help guide you to learn about some useful options for caring for your child.

In addition to the material provided in this chapter, www.healthychildren.org can provide more medical information about each childhood issue.

COMMON INFECTIOUS CHILDHOOD DISEASES

Childhood diseases can be scary for any parent; this is especially true for new parents or when the child is an infant. The symptoms can be a bit unnerving. Yet, they give the immune system an opportunity to strengthen, and after recovering from a childhood disease, many children often experience a growth spurt.

Note: A child who doesn't recover well from a childhood illness could benefit greatly from constitutional care of a professional homeopath.

CARING FOR A SICK CHILD

It is an art to care for a sick child in a way that reduces anxieties and fears and leaves pleasant memories of comforting healing rituals and extra love. In our modern-day, fast-paced life, you may feel overwhelmed when a child falls ill, especially if you work outside of the home. However, when your child becomes ill, it is a time to slow life down in order to prioritize the health and well-being of your child while attempting to maintain your sanity and that of the rest of the family.

While it is best for the caregiver to be a family member, ask alternative helpers to be on "standby" in case of emergency. Calling upon close friends or neighbors may help to ease the pressure and stress until a parent or other familiar caregiver can arrange to be at home with your child.

When your child is sick:
- Take the opportunity to make it a special time by giving extra comfort and cuddles.

- Use a reassuring and comforting voice to ensure that everything is going to be alright. Share with the child, if age appropriate, what is happening in their body, why you are doing certain things, and how soon they can look forward to feeling better.

- Keep them close by and not isolated by making up a bed on the sofa in a common area of the home.

- The atmosphere should be kept low stress, with few comings and only quiet activities such as soothing music and reading. Tell stories, play board games, or draw. A little TV or a movie may help with boredom, but too much is overstimulating and can keep them from sleeping and deeply resting.

- Allow time for extra rest—it is proven that healing takes place quicker and is more complete when the child gets extra sleep.

- Offer nutritious light snacks, soups, or pureed vegetables, and fruits. You do not need to insist that a sick child eat, especially if they don't want to. A brief fast can help in the healing process.

- Encourage them to drink plenty of water or diluted fruit juices. If they do not want to drink, they can suck on ice cubes (if age appropriate) or frozen juice bars. Small children with a fever, especially infants under six months old, must be watched carefully because they are vulnerable to becoming quickly dehydrated. If a baby is being breastfed it's important to allow him/her to nurse as often as they ask.

Sometimes when children are sick, they can become demanding and regress temporarily (e.g., sucking thumb, bedwetting). It's extremely important to be patient with them until they are well again and address those issues after they have had time to recover, if necessary. The behavior might shift back once the child is well again.

> **Important note:** Never give a child aspirin during or after a childhood illness as this can cause serious complications.

SCHOOL ANXIETY

See **Chapter 19—Mind and Emotions** on **page 220**.

BEDWETTING (ENURESIS)

Bedwetting is also known as nocturnal enuresis. It can be a significant source of embarrassment and make traveling or sleepovers very challenging for children.

The physical causes can be such things as:

- genetic factors (it tends to run in families)

- difficulties waking up from sleep

- slower than normal development of the central nervous system—this reduces the child's ability to stop the bladder from emptying at night

- hormonal factors (not enough antidiuretic hormone—this hormone reduces the amount of urine made by the kidneys)

- urinary tract infections

- abnormalities in the urethral valves in boys or in the ureter in girls or boys

- abnormalities in the spinal cord

Bedwetting can lead to additional problems because of the guilt and embarrassment a child feels. Parents should refrain from making the child feel guilty about something he or she can't control. Because bedwetting is a very emotionally stressful problem for older children, psychological counseling may be in order.

If bedwetting tends to run in a family, it is important that a parent share that they too wet the bed as a child. It also helps the child know that they can get "better" faster if the child, the family, the doctor, and/or the psychologist all work together. A few dry nights can work wonders to help the child feel better.

ADDITIONAL SUPPORT FOR BEDWETTING

If a medical professional has eliminated physiological symptoms as a cause, the following measures can help in addition to homeopathic remedies:

- Change the diet, eliminating caffeine, dairy products, anything with artificial sweeteners, citrus fruits, and/or any juices that cause an increase in passing of urine, also known as a diuretic effect.
- Begin bladder training exercises to help the child withstand longer periods of time between trips to the bathroom.
- Limit how much the child drinks, mostly two hours before bedtime.
- Provide emotional support and positive reinforcement to the child.

WHEN TO CONTACT YOUR HEALTHCARE PROFESSIONAL

- Parents suspect any of the mentioned physical conditions exists.
- Parents suspect this is having a detrimental effect on their child.
- There is any possibility of inappropriate sexual touching in the child's life.
- The well indicated homeopathic remedies are not eliminating the bedwetting.

COMMON REMEDIES FOR BEDWETTING

	Arsenicum	*Causticum	*Kreosotum	Lycopodium	Pulsatilla	Sepia
Symptoms	Bedwetting in nervous, anxious, restless and fastidious children. Often very chilly and irritable. Usually wets the bed between 1-2 AM.	Useful in children who wet the bed, especially in the first sleep. Often the urine passes so easily that the child is unaware of it. Can also leak urine on laughing or coughing.	Urine flows during first deep sleep, from which the child is roused with difficulty. Wakes with urging, but cannot hold the urine or dreams they are urinating and wets the bed.	Involuntary urination during sleep. Passes enormous quantities of clear urine. Can also have red sand in urine (in which case a urine sample should be lab tested for infection). Typically the child craves sweets, likes hot drinks. Tendency to feel worse from 4-8 PM and is irritable on waking.	For children who are gentle, sensitive, weepy and want affection. They might sleep on their back with arms above their head or on their abdomen. They want open windows or fan when sleeping.	Involuntary urination as soon as the child goes to sleep at night. Child is often indifferent, does not like sympathy and often wants to be alone. Possible history of sexual abuse. *If you suspect this, contact your healthcare provider to investigate.

Special dosing: Give the chosen remedy half an hour before bedtime for up to one week. If there is no change, re-evaluate and try another remedy. If no change then, consult a professional homeopath or your healthcare provider.

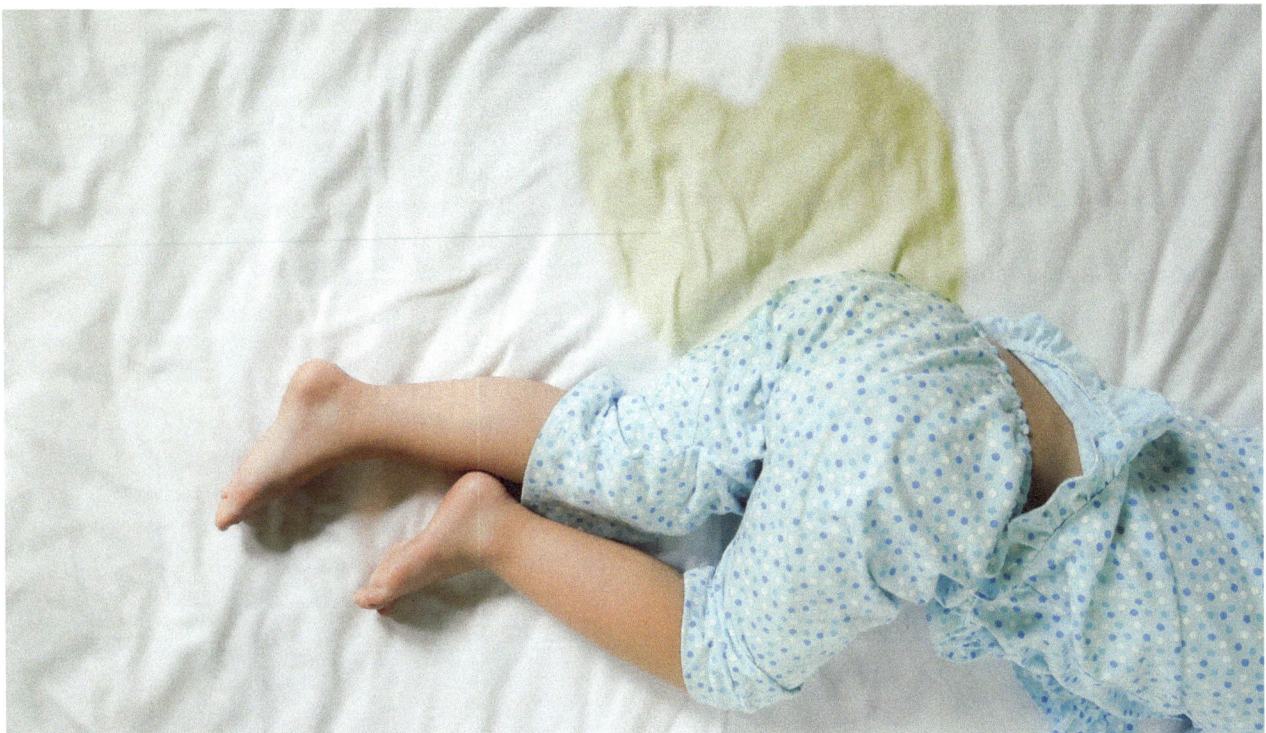

CONSTIPATION

See **Chapter 12—Stool Issues** on **page 137**.

COUGHS

See **Chapter 10—Throat and Chest** on **page 115**.

CHICKENPOX

Chickenpox is caused by a virus called varicella. It generally occurs in a mild form in babies and young children — the younger they are, the milder it is. Some babies have only a couple of spots while older children may experience the symptoms more intensely. Nowadays, chickenpox is less common because of the varicella vaccine that is now included on the childhood vaccine schedule.

Chickenpox starts with some small water blisters on the head or trunk, then progresses through these five phases:

1. small red bumps

2. thin-walled water blisters

3. cloudy blisters

4. open sores, and finally

5. dry brown crusts

Common symptoms include:

• fever

• flu-like aches

• headaches

• loss of appetite

• itchy skin

The incubation period (time between exposure to the chickenpox infection and the appearance of the first symptoms) is 7 to 21 days. Chickenpox is infectious a few days before the rash appears and until the last spot or blister has formed a scab.

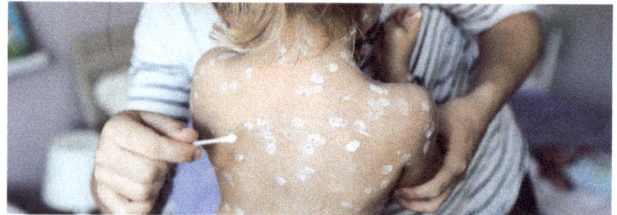

IT'S AN EMERGENCY WHEN

• The child has a fever of 104°F (40 °C) for more than four hours.
• A baby is under three months old and has any rise in temperature.
• There is a lack of reaction and/or the child is listless or limp.
• The child has trouble breathing.

ADDITIONAL SUPPORT FOR CHICKENPOX

• A chickenpox rash can be itchy, but scratching can leave scars. To help prevent children from scratching their rash, dress your child in loose cotton clothing, cut their fingernails, and/or have them wear mittens.
• Tepid oatmeal baths can help with the itching.
• Cool compresses.

WHEN TO CONTACT YOUR HEALTHCARE PROFESSIONAL

• Pus is oozing from sores.
• A fever goes away and comes back again.
• There is a skin infection from the scratching.
• There is vomiting.
• There is a stiff neck.

COMMON REMEDIES FOR CHICKENPOX

	*Antimonium crudum	Antimonium tart	Pulsatilla	Rhus tox	Sulphur
Symptoms	Irritable, doesn't want to be touched, talked about or even looked at. Pustular (yellow fluid) eruptions that itch or burn and are worse at night. The rash can be painful. White coated tongue.	Sleepy, much sleeping, drowsy when awake, irritable, whining and wants company. Sweaty, fussy and nauseated. If there's a cough, it will be rattling. Rash is mixed with vesicles (fluid-filled bumps) and pustules (pus-filled bumps). Rash may be delayed and is generally itchy.	Weepy, whiny and clingy. Thirstless, despite the fever. Symptoms are changeable and worse in the evenings and from warmth. Better fresh air. If rash goes to the pus stage and is yellow.	Restless and depressed. Itching of rash is extreme and not relieved by scratching and can burn after. Can feel like being pierced with hot needles. Worse from cold and at night. Better for warmth and a hot bath or shower.	Similar to Rhus tox. Rash is extremely bothersome and itchy. Burning sensation to vesicles. Sweaty, restless and irritable. Very thirsty and hungry and takes more than they can eat. Worse in the mid-morning and for any heat and bathing. Better in fresh air.

Dosing: Use the BLUE method. Observe and evaluate.

FIFTH DISEASE

Commonly known as "Slapped in the Face Disease," fifth disease is a viral illness caused by parvovirus B19, usually found in children between the ages of 5 and 15.
    Common symptoms include:

- low-grade fever

- rash doesn't itch or hurt

- cold-like symptoms such as a cough, sneezing, runny nose and sore throat may be present

- distinctive red cheeks rash, which may spread to the trunk of the body, arms, and legs

The incubation period (time between exposure to fifth's disease and the appearance of the first symptoms) is 4 to 12 days. Fifth disease is infectious during the early stages before the rash appears.

ADDITIONAL SUPPORT FOR FIFTH DISEASE

- Apply a cool or warm cloth to ease discomfort with fever – depending upon which helps the child feel better.
- As with any viral infection, recovery is fastest when a child gets abundant rest and drinks extra fluids.

WHEN TO CONTACT YOUR HEALTHCARE PROFESSIONAL

- A feverish, sick child is drinking less than usual or refusing drinks and has become lethargic.
- They have a fever of over 103°F (39.4 °C) that doesn't respond to treatment within 12 hours.
- A child is screaming and is obviously in pain, but you don't know where.
- The rash becomes infected.

IT'S AN EMERGENCY WHEN

- The child has a fever of 104°F (40 °C) for more than four hours.
- There is a lack of reaction and/or they appear listless or limp.
- The child has trouble breathing.

Remedies to consider:

- ***Ferrum phos:** Slow onset, low grade fever, with nosebleed.

- **Chamomilla:** Fever stage has flushes of heat in head and face, fiery red rash on face, burning, cold limbs with burning heat of face, perspiration is hot with fever. Behavior is key: irritable, whining, restlessness, wants many things, then refuses them. Aversion to touch but wants to be carried, very sensitive to pain.

- **Apis:** Chill stage of fever is worse from any warm coverings and better in open air and from uncovering. Heat stage of fever finds the child extremely drowsy with great thirst, barely any perspiration. Wants cool cloth on red cheeks, has a 'slapped' face look: swollen, shiny and feels stinging and hot (just like a bee sting would look and feel). Possibly with a sore throat, fear of being alone and possessive of the mother.

Dosing: Use the BLUE method.
Observe and evaluate.

HAND, FOOT AND MOUTH DISEASE

Hand, foot, and mouth disease (HFM) is a viral illness caused by the Coxsackie A16 virus that usually affects children ages six months to four years. It's a rash that looks like tiny red spots and/or water blisters on the hands and feet, and sometimes on the buttocks. Mouth sores may also be seen.

Common symptoms include:

- low-grade fever

- sore throat

- muscle aches

- general malaise or sleepiness

- reduced appetite

- drooling (due to painful swallowing)

The incubation period (time between exposure to HFM and the appearance of the first symptoms) is 4 to 12 days. For the most part, children with HFM are contagious during the first week of illness, but sometimes they can transmit the virus for days or weeks after symptoms have resolved. It is also important to note that adults may become infected and not develop any symptoms but can still spread the virus. So, it is important to observe basic hygiene – such as frequent hand-washing – when caring for a child with HFM to minimize the possibility of spreading the virus.

IT'S AN EMERGENCY WHEN

- The child has a fever of 104°F (40 °C).
- A baby is under three months old and has any rise in temperature.
- There is a lack of reaction and/or they appear listless or limp.
- The child has trouble breathing.

ADDITIONAL SUPPORT FOR HAND FOOT AND MOUTH DISEASE

- As with any viral infection, recovery is fastest when a child gets abundant rest and drinks extra fluids.
- Apply a cool or warm cloth to ease discomfort with fever – depending upon which helps the child feel better.

WHEN TO CONTACT YOUR HEALTHCARE PROFESSIONAL

- A feverish, sick child is drinking less than usual or refusing drinks and has become lethargic.
- A baby under six months old has a fever.
- An older baby has a fever of over 103°F (39.4 °C) that doesn't respond to treatment within 12 hours.
- The child is screaming and is obviously in pain, but you don't know where.
- The rash becomes infected.

Remedies to consider:

- **Mercurius:** Mouth sores can be very severe, and the child is very sensitive to hot and cold. May have a fever before getting the blisters and may alternate between getting too hot with perspiration and becoming chilled at night. Becoming too hot or too cold makes the person worse in general. There is a narrow range of comfortable temperatures with this remedy type. Blisters tend to be more painful at night. Tendency to drool or to have an excess of saliva in the mouth. The breath may be quite offensive with pus visible on the tonsils or elsewhere in the mouth.

- **Antimonium tart:** Chill stage of fever produces gooseflesh and icy cold skin. Heat stage of fever, one sees the child cling to those around and wants to be carried. Does not want to be touched or looked at. Thirstless despite a dry parched tongue. Sweat stage of fever is profuse, cold, clammy, or sticky. Dry, cracked, parched tongue with whitish discoloration in the center. Tongue tip and sides clean, moist, and red. May crave apples or apple juice.

- ***Borax:** Refuses to talk during fever. Desire for cold drinks and cold food during fever. Great heat and dryness of mouth with white ulcers. Tender, ulcers bleed on touch and when eating. Painful red blisters on tongue; sore mouth prevents infants from nursing. Fear of downward motion. Startle easily. Very sensitive to sudden noises.

Dosing: Use the **BLUE** method.
Observe and evaluate.

MEASLES

Measles is a highly contagious disease caused by the measles virus. It is characterized by the three "C's": cough, coryza, and conjunctivitis. A rash breaks out usually three to five days after symptoms begin. If you suspect measles, look for small spots like grains of sand (known as Koplik's spots) in the mouth and/or inside the cheeks.

Common symptoms include:

- high fever

- dry cough, runny nose and red watery eyes

- ear infection

- diarrhea

- Koplik Spots appear which are tiny white spots with bluish-white centers on a red background inside the mouth.

- flat red spots that appear on the face at the hairline and spread downward to the neck, trunk, arms, legs, and feet. Small raised bumps may also appear on top of the flat red spots.

Measles can last up to two weeks, and children should be carefully tended to throughout the illness to reduce the possibility of complications developing (infections of the airway, ears, eyes, etc.).

The incubation period (time between exposure to measles and the appearance of the first symptoms) is 8 to 12 days. Measles is infectious four days before and 5-10 days after a rash appears.

IT'S AN EMERGENCY WHEN

- The child has a fever of 104°F (40 °C) or above that lasts for more than four hours.
- A baby is under three months old and has any rise in temperature.
- There is a lack of reaction and/or they appear listless or limp.
- The child has trouble breathing.

ADDITIONAL SUPPORT FOR MEASLES

- Consider giving Vitamin A as a possible preventative or to make symptoms more mild. (A medium carrot contains 10,000 IU's of Vitamin A.) Consult with your healthcare provider for appropriate dosing.
- Keep a child with measles and sensitive eyes out of bright light, with curtains partially closed and lights dimmed.
- As with any viral infection, recovery is fastest when a child gets abundant rest and drinks extra fluids.
- Apply a cool or warm cloth to ease discomfort with fever – depending upon which helps the child feel better.

WHEN TO CONTACT YOUR HEALTHCARE PROFESSIONAL

- A feverish, sick child is drinking less than usual or refusing drinks and has become lethargic.
- A baby under six months old has a fever.
- An older baby has a fever of over 103°F (39.4 °C) that doesn't respond to treatment within 12 hours.
- The child is screaming and is obviously in pain, but you don't know where.
- The rash becomes infected.

COMMON REMEDIES FOR MEASLES

	Aconite	Apis	Belladonna	Bryonia
Symptoms	Useful at the beginning stages of measles—a high fever, dry barking cough, and red pink eye. Light sensitivity and hoarse voice. Skins burns and itches. Restless, anxious, and frightened. Joint pains and excessive sweating. Excessive thirst. Better open air. Worse cold and nighttime.	Rash is slow to come out, when it does it itches and stings. Face and eyelids are puffy and red. Affected parts (skin rash, glands, etc.) are puffy, itchy and sting. Children are extremely restless, anxious, and clingy and may cry out in their sleep. Generally thirstless. Cannot bear heat or pressure of any sort and they do not want to be touched. Have a high fever with scanty urine and feel better for cold and cool bathing.	Useful when there is sudden onset of a high fever, reddened face, and throbbing headache. Tends to be drowsy, a little delirious and have some difficulty falling or staying asleep. Not very thirsty. Redness and swelling in throat and inflamed tonsils. Feeling of lump in throat. Difficulty swallowing, especially liquids. Throat pain can be shooting or stinging especially while swallowing. Better from bed rest and warmth. Worse from drafts and motion.	Illness is slow to develop, the rash is slow to appear and may be accompanied by a bursting, frontal headache. Children are irritable and want to be alone, do not want to be disturbed or moved. Generally thirsty for large quantities of liquid and gulp it at frequent intervals. Worse from heat or movement of any sort.

	Euphrasia	Kali Bich	Pulsatilla
Symptoms	Measles with very sore, swollen, burning watery eyes that are sensitive to light. Nose runs also, but does not irritate the skin. There may be a harsh, dry cough, worse in the day and better when lying down. Headache better once the rash appears.	For later stages of measles where there is stubborn catarrh (excess mucus in nose or throat) which is stringy and ropy. With swollen glands and/or earache and deafness from catarrh in the eustachian tubes.	Cold symptoms are prominent and rash is slow to develop. Profuse tearing from the eyes. Minimal fever. Stuffy nose producing yellowish mucus, a gagging cough (most often dry at night and loose in the morning), and inflammation in the ears is common. Not much thirst. Strong desire for a lot of comfort and attention. Worse from warmth and stuffy rooms. Better in open air.

Dosing: Use the **BLUE** method. Observe and evaluate.

MUMPS

Mumps is a viral illness caused by a paramyxovirus. It is usually a mild childhood infection most known for the swelling of one or both of the salivary glands (in front of the ear and just above the angle of the jaw), which gives the person a hamster-cheeked appearance. The glands under the tongue and jaw may also swell.

Common symptoms include:

- fever
- headache
- nausea
- weakness
- reduced appetite
- swelling of one or both salivary glands
- swelling pains in the joints; in testes for boys

The incubation period (time between exposure to mumps and the appearance of the first symptoms) is 12-28 days. The contagious period starts a day or two before the swelling begins and will continue for about 5 days.

IT'S AN EMERGENCY WHEN

- The child has a fever of 104°F (40 °C) for more than four hours.
- A baby is under three months old and has any rise in temperature.
- There is a lack of reaction; the child is listless or limp.
- The child has abdominal pain.

ADDITIONAL SUPPORT FOR MUMPS

- If it is painful to open the mouth, give drinks through a straw (if age appropriate); otherwise use a baby bottle.
- Wrap a hot water bottle in a towel and let your child lie on it to soothe painful swellings.
- As with any viral infection, recovery is fastest when a child gets abundant rest and drinks extra fluids.
- Apply a cool or warm cloth to ease discomfort with fever – depending upon which helps the child feel better.

WHEN TO CONTACT YOUR HEALTHCARE PROFESSIONAL

- A feverish, sick child is drinking less than usual or refusing drinks and has become lethargic.
- A baby under six months old has a fever.
- An older baby has a fever of over 103°F (39.4 °C) that doesn't respond to treatment within 12 hours.
- The child is screaming and is obviously in pain, but you don't know where.
- The boy's testicles have become painful.

COMMON REMEDIES FOR MUMPS

	*Jaborandi	Mercurius	Lachesis	*Phytolacca
Symptoms	Mumps with exhaustion. Glands are swollen making swallowing and talking difficult. Profuse sweating and salivation (with a dry mouth). Breast, ovaries or testicles become painful. Generally thirsty, worse from cold and after sweating.	Glands swollen and painful, especially on right side. Pains shoot to ears and/or neck. May be accompanied by a runny nose, earache, sticky eyes, sore throat. Profuse, smelly perspiration and salivation. Metallic taste in mouth (may have mouth ulcers) and smelly breath. Tongue is swollen, coated and may show indents around the edges from the teeth. Generally, feels worse at night, from extremes of temperature (from heat and cold) and from sweating. Better from resting.	Left-sided mumps with glands that are very painful and sensitive to the slightest touch or pressure. Throat is very sore and is difficult to swallow anything except for hard foods like toast or chips. Children are much worse from heat and when they wake after sleeping.	Mumps with glands that are hard and swollen. Pains may spread to breasts, ovaries and testicles. Pains radiate to the ears on swallowing. Throat hurts, especially when sticking out the tongue. Tongue is red-tipped and breath smells. With copious sweating and salivation. Children are floppy and tearful. Better from cold drinks. Worse from hot drinks.

Dosing: Use the **BLUE** method. Observe and evaluate.

RUBELLA (GERMAN MEASLES)

Rubella, also known as German measles, is typically a mild viral infection that is short-lived. It is different from measles, though the two share some characteristics, including a red rash. The disease is spread through close contact or through the air.

The incubation period (time between exposure to rubella and the appearance of the first symptoms) is 14-21 days. Rubella is infectious five days before and seven days after the rash appears.

Common symptoms include:

- mild fever of 102 °F (38.8 °C) or lower

- pink rash and swollen, tender glands at the back of the neck or behind the ears

- rash starts on the face and then spreads to the neck, torso, arms, and legs and fades from the face as it moves to other parts of the body.

Important note: Avoid contact with pregnant women when your child has Rubella and notify pregnant women with whom you were in contact in the three-week period before the spots came out since the virus can cause serious problems in a developing fetus.

IT'S AN EMERGENCY WHEN

- The child has a fever of 104°F (40 °C) for more than four hours.
- A baby is under three months old and has any rise in temperature.
- There is a lack of reaction, the child is listless or limp.
- The child has trouble breathing.

ADDITIONAL SUPPORT FOR RUBELLA (GERMAN MEASLES)

- As with any viral infection, recovery is fastest when a child gets abundant rest and drinks extra fluids.
- Apply a cool or warm cloth to ease discomfort with fever – depending upon which helps the child feel better.

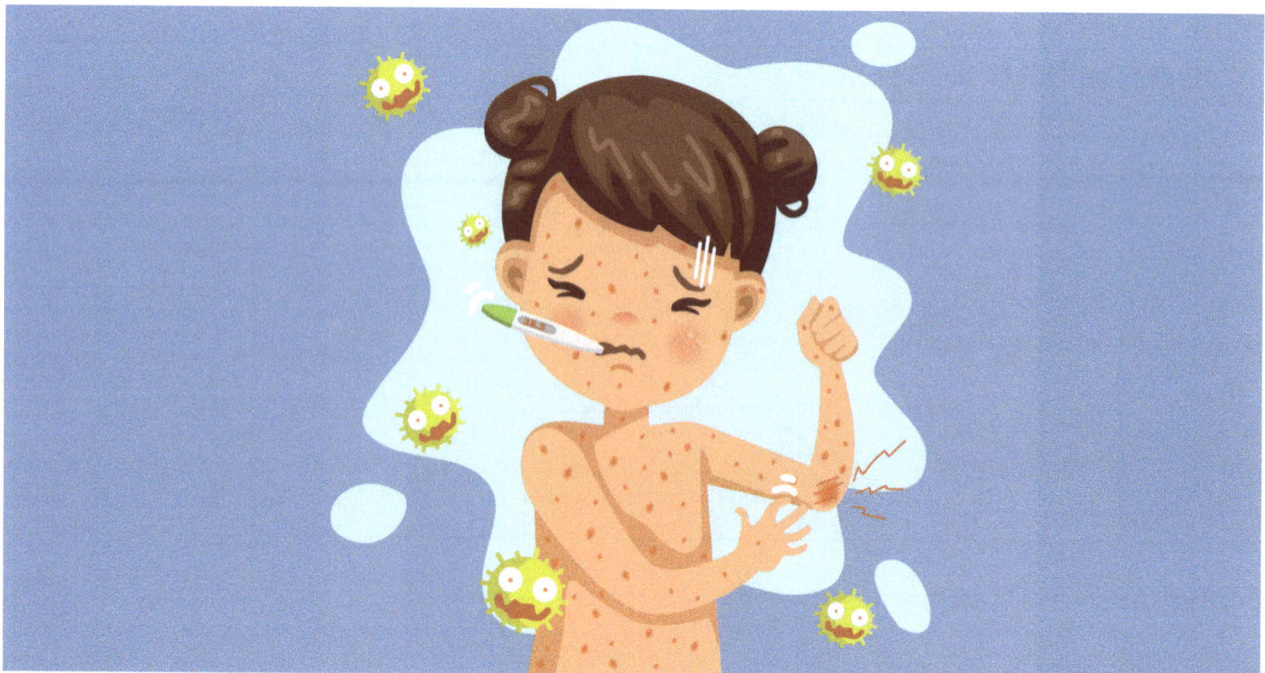

WHEN TO CONTACT YOUR HEALTHCARE PROFESSIONAL

- A feverish, sick child is drinking less than usual or refusing drinks and has become lethargic.
- A baby under six months old has a fever.
- An older baby has a fever of over 103°F (39.4 °C) that doesn't respond to treatment within 12 hours.
- The child is screaming and is obviously in pain, but you don't know where.
- The rash becomes infected.

COMMON REMEDIES FOR RUBELLA (GERMAN MEASLES)

	Aconite	Belladonna	*Coffea	Gelsemium	Pulsatilla
Symptoms	Most effective in the very first stage of illness. Sudden onset of a rash with a fever. Very thirsty.	Sudden onset of high fever with a flushed face and reddened lips. Hot head, but may have cold extremities. Fever is a dry heat, without perspiration. Skin is so hot it radiates heat. Strong and throbbing pulse. Temperature gets highest at night, causing the child to be agitated, sometimes delirious. Better from warmth.	Recommended when the child is overly excitable, extremely sensitive to pain, sleepless because of sensitivity to all noises. Desires ice and cold drinks.	Slow onset with fever and headache. Pains in back of head, spreading to forehead. Head feels heavy, vision blurred. Heaviness, drowsiness, and lack of thirst with chills. Trembling, weakness and dizziness. Heavy feeling in legs, drugged feeling. Head pain at the back of the neck. No thirst even though feverish.	Thirstless, clinging and weepy. Low fever and itchy skin. Eruptions are worse from heat. Eruptions itching with white or yellow discharge. Desires open air, but needs to be properly covered. Has a flushed face.

Dosing: Use the **BLUE** method. Observe and evaluate.

SCARLET FEVER

Scarlet fever is a highly infectious bacterial disease caused by the streptococcus bacteria. It often is associated with streptococcal infection of the throat, but can also be associated with streptococcal skin infections. Nowadays it is not very common, however, when it does crop up, it can swiftly move through neighborhoods, daycare centers, or schools.

The incubation period (time between exposure to scarlet fever and the appearance of the first symptoms) is 1-7 days. Scarlet fever is infectious for one to two weeks after the rash appears.

Common symptoms include:

- very red, sore throat with difficulty swallowing due to pain and swelling

- a day or two into the illness a rash, giving the skin a sandpaper-like texture, will appear

- after 5 days, the skin will peel where the rash was most intense

- swollen glands

- fever (101°F [38.3 °C] or higher) sometimes with chills

- headache and/or flu like body aches

- flushed face (though area around the mouth may be pale)

- tongue may be red, swollen and have a white strawberry like appearance (white coated with red spots)

- mild abdominal pain

IT'S AN EMERGENCY WHEN

- The child has a fever of 104°F (40 °C) for more than four hours.
- A baby is under three months old and has any rise in temperature.
- There is a lack of reaction; the child is listless or limp.

♥ ADDITIONAL SUPPORT FOR SCARLET FEVER

- Push fluids, especially if there is a fever, to prevent dehydration.
- If warm drinks feel better, make hot water with lemon and honey, which can be very soothing to a sore throat.
- If cold drinks feel better, fresh watermelon juice is soothing to a sore throat.
- Be sure the child gets plenty of rest.
- Apply a cool or warm cloth to ease discomfort with fever — depending upon which helps the child feel better.
- Discontinue products made from cow's milk during this condition, because milk and cheese can cause the body to produce more mucus, which raises the level of acidity in the system. (Goat's milk, rice milk, almond milk, or soy products may be substituted for cow's milk products.) Buy organic, when possible.
- The older child or adult can gargle with one teaspoon of **Calendula tincture** in one cup of warm water, three times a day.
- Adults and children over three years old can use lozenges that do not contain camphor, menthol, or eucalyptus. Instead choose blackcurrant pastilles, fruit cough drops, or lemon drops which are much less likely to interfere with the action of homeopathic remedies.
- Humidify the room.

The primary remedy to consider in cases of scarlet fever is **Belladonna**. Another remedy to consider is **Cantharis**. **Dosing:** Use the BLUE method. Observe and evaluate.

WHOOPING COUGH

See *Chapter 10—Throat and Chest* on *page 122*.

❓ WHAT'S THE FIRST REMEDY YOU THINK OF WHEN...

1. Your child usually wets the bed during the first part of their sleep.
2. Your child has a rash of itching and burning vesicles that is worse from anything warm including a bath.
3. Your child has a fiery red face, looking like they got slapped, with irritability and perspiration during the fever.
4. Your child has a low grade fever with a nosebleed.
5. Your child has painful sores in their mouth with excess salivation and a great sensitivity to both too hot or too cold.
6. Your child has measles that came on very slowly with a painful cough, great thirst and an irritable demeanor.
7. Your child has painful swollen glands with profuse smelly perspiration, metallic taste in the mouth and offensive breath.
8. Your child has hard and swollen glands where pain radiates to their ears when they swallow.
9. Your child has a sudden onset of high fever with a flushed face and red lips.
10. Your restless toddler keeps scratching, but nothing seems to relieve the itch of their chickenpox.

Answer key on page 324.

CHAPTER 22
Young Adults Ages 12–24

Being an adolescent is an exciting, adventuresome, chaotic, and stressful time. Aristotle stated, "The young are permanently in a state resembling intoxication." Teens are on a hormonal roller coaster. They can be calm and sweet one week, day, hour, or moment, and down in the dumps the next, easily agitated, impulsive, and on edge.

Each adolescent is different and has different needs. This is true even in the same family. The name of the game is patience, and support for who the adolescent is. It is good to remember that an adolescent's job is to find their own identity as they move from the safe boundaries of home to the big, wide, complicated world outside. They are trying to figure out how to negotiate their surroundings. Above all else, they need lots of acceptance, understanding, leisure time with their friends, enough sleep, and a good diet. Although boundaries are needed to gently temper the spirit, flexibility from time to time will go far in avoiding unhealthy rebellion. The best advice for dealing with most parenting issues is to "pick your battles."

A high school counselor once told a story about an underachieving student. He asked the student, "What would you like to be when you are an adult?" The reply was, "I want to be a snowboarder, dude." At this point, most adults would roll their eyes and proceed to tell the teen that this is unrealistic, not financially viable, etc. At this high school, however, the students learn quite quickly that whatever comes out of their mouth will be taken seriously. The counselor informed the student that a world-class snowboarder rides the back bowls of ski areas in the wild, so he would have to make a serious study of geology. It happened that this high school was in a town with a university that allowed high school students to take certain classes. The counselor helped the student sign up for a geology class and informed him that physical fitness is also required to be a top athlete. The student was enrolled in a local gym that was working with the high school to help teens be fit. This allowed the student to work out before or after school. This young man went on to be a photographer for Warren Miller Films, which films extreme snowboarding and skiing. He fulfilled his dreams. By receiving guidance without judgment, this adolescent became a success. It is a real gift to your adolescent to help them come into themselves, without judgment about who you think they should be—and to help them get the education and/or training needed to become a successful, fulfilled, and happy adult.

QUICK OVERVIEW OF THE ADOLESCENT BRAIN

The adolescent's awkwardness, both mental and physical, can be most annoying. The brain from ages twelve to twenty-five years of age is in a constant, intense state of rewiring and upgrading, so that transmissions can speed up to accommodate more conscious, sophisticated, and complicated ways of thinking. The brain is constantly redefining itself, so to speak. This is why adolescents can seem so spaced out and aloof at times. All it takes is some added stress, lack of sleep, or a social or emotional challenge to make the brain misfire, creating inconsistent, uncharacteristic, and sometimes foolish behavior.

Research shows that adolescents highly value rewards, giving little thought or attention to consequences. Cultural anthropologists have concluded that adolescents worldwide strongly desire thrills and uniqueness. And they are sometimes willing to take appalling risks to get them. Successful adaptation and flexibility are the names of the game for teens transitioning into the world they will face as adults. Some studies indicate that the adolescent brain reacts to peer rejection just as strongly as if there were a threat to their physical existence. This is why they can exhibit extreme reactions to social ups and downs.

Studies show that adolescents perform optimally when they get at least 9 ¼ hours of sleep each night. It makes sense, with all of the brain restructuring and hormones releasing, that adolescents need extra sleep. In one study, high school bell times were postponed, beginning at 9 AM. As a result, the teachers stated that their students were more alert, less moody, and better prepared to learn. Test scores improved, and there were fewer visits to the nurse's office. If your adolescent is not getting enough sleep during the week, allow them to catch up on the weekend. If there has been long term severe sleep deprivation, this will not be enough, but it can help somewhat toward reducing their stress.

Some of the adolescent's acute emotional and physiological woes can be addressed by choosing a well-indicated remedy. Any time the symptoms are not resolving, they need to seek the services of a professional homeopath and/or a professional counselor as well.

ACNE

See **Acne** in **Chapter 18—Skin** on **page 199**.

ANXIETY ABOUT SCHOOL PERFORMANCE

See **Performance Anxiety** in **Chapter 19—Mind and Emotions** on **page 221**.

TENSION HEADACHES

See **Headaches** in **Chapter 5—Head** on **page 71**.

HOMESICKNESS

Going off to summer camp, heading away to college, going for an overnight at a friend's house, moving to a new city, or just traveling for vacation are all exciting times where there is freedom from the routines, comfort or strictures of family life. However, for many it is uncomfortable being away from home, being on one's own and managing one's own life, even if it's just for one night. Sometimes it is too much change all at once; leaving all of one's friends, family, pets and support systems behind. It can often cause a complex series of feelings, emotions and reactions known as homesickness. The person can feel insecure or uncomfortable with where they are both physically and emotionally, and consequently want to return home. It is quite justified considering the enormous change of being in a family dynamic or with caretakers and now navigating a new environment with new responsibilities.

Homesickness is often hidden and can come in many guises. It can come in the form of recurring stomach aches, headaches, nervous tension or an inability to sleep. It can be demonstrated by the sudden development of panic attacks or the need to call home several times a day. It can also be as simple as a yearning or longing.

Most people don't want to admit that they are having these symptoms, so they develop strategies to hide them. It can show up as grief or sadness. Some students can become restless or anxious, confused and disoriented, while others may display petulance and anger or irritation and frustration.

Lastly, it can't be predicted. Some thrive greatly with the new found freedom, the new environment and the opportunity of making new friends, creating a new routine and starting fresh. But in people who experience homesickness, it isn't always obvious. Some become despondent, others have an inability to pay attention or take care of their basic needs while some may become averse to making friends so the feeling of loneliness then becomes overwhelming.

All the emotions and physical complaints of homesickness, when caught early, can be improved with a well-chosen homeopathic remedy.

Here is a short list of symptoms to look for:

	Cognitive	Behavioral	Emotional	Physical
Symptoms	• excessive preoccupation with thoughts of home • negative thoughts such as "I hate this place" • idealizing home • expressed feelings of inadequacy such as "Everyone else is fine, I'm the only one suffering"	• inability to concentrate • frequent bouts of crying • loss of appetite and insomnia • nightmares • not engaging in social life • not being able to develop a routine	• excessive sadness • loneliness • mood swings • anger • anxiety • overwhelm • unmotivated	• frequent, recurring headaches • nausea • diarrhea/constipation • excessive urination or urine retention • severe muscular tension including stomach ache • dizziness/vertigo

ADDITIONAL SUPPORT FOR HOMESICKNESS

- Join group activities.
- Get familiar with the new surroundings. If in college or a new town, explore and wander the surrounding area.
- Avoid social media where there is a constant comparison to others experiences that can create feelings of inadequacy.
- Seek the advice of a parent, good friend or professional counselor to talk through your feelings.
- Call home when needed.

WHEN TO CONTACT YOUR HEALTHCARE PROFESSIONAL

- Having active thoughts of suicide. Displaying suicidal behavior, such as taking unnecessary risks that could endanger oneself.
- Inability to sleep for three successive days.
- Excessive diarrhea, urination resulting in extreme weakness.
- Recurring headaches that impair one's ability to participate in life.

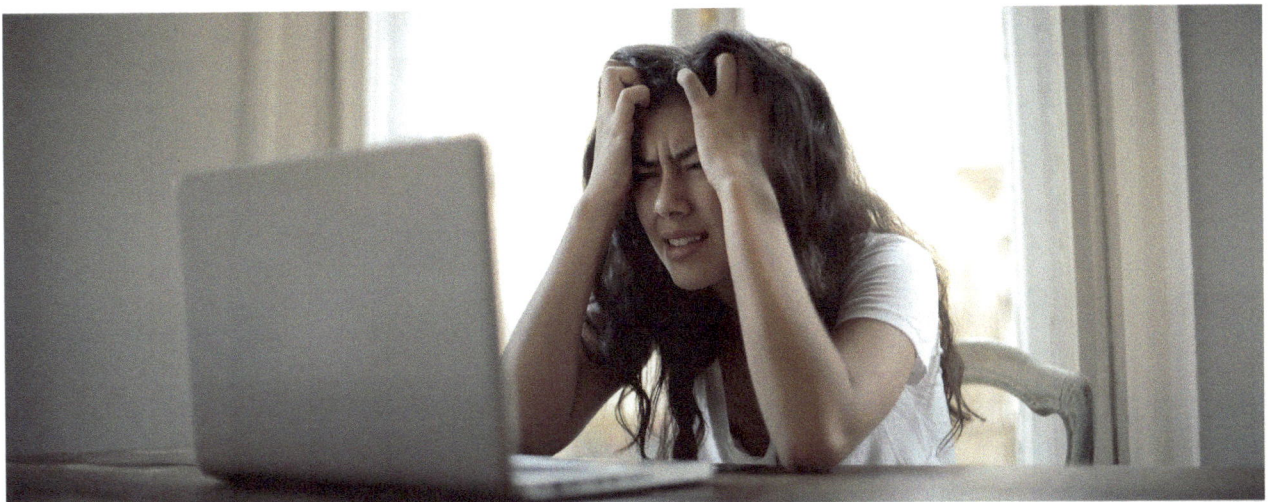

COMMON REMEDIES FOR HOMESICKNESS

	Arnica	*Aurum met	*Capsicum	Gelsemium	Ignatia	*Phosphoricum acidum	Pulsatilla
Onset	Shock or trauma from change in home life, especially going to college.	Despondency with a great sense of worthlessness.	Easily homesick, can't function outside of their routine.	A kind of stage fright because of the newness of the situation.	Rapid change of physical or mental condition.	Nervous exhaustion and debility. Homesickness related to change in environment.	Extreme feelings of loneliness, being forsaken, and weepy.
Symptoms	Nervous with muscle tension. Insatiable hunger. Sleepless and restless when overtired.	Oversensitive to noise. Hurried, burning in the stomach, constipation, rapid irregular pulse. Sleeplessness or sleep with frightful dreams.	Red cheeks, red hands, but cold to the touch. Chronic sleeplessness, inability to study. Bursting headaches, smarting in the throat.	Headache with a sensation of a band around the head. Muscular soreness around the neck. Dry cough. Diarrhea (cream colored). Urine retention. Heart palpitations.	Fainting, fevers, and headaches that feel like a nail is being driven into the skull. Involuntary sighing.	Mentally unfocused. Seem in shock, nauseous, distention of the belly, diarrhea (white and watery). Frequent profuse urination. Crushing headaches, dry cough from tickle, pimples on the skin. Loss of appetite.	Bad cold with thick or yellow discharge. Symptoms changeable and shifting. Chilly, but doesn't feel better from warmth.
Mood	Oversensitive. Indifferent. Inability to do continuous work. Sadness.	Longing, melancholy, sadness, depression, feelings of being forsaken. Despondent, peevish. Discontented.	Cross and unable to concentrate, obstinate and sullen. Desire to be alone, excessively peevish, easily offended.	Desire for quiet and to be left alone. Fearful, dullness, and tired. Fear of loss of control.	Agitated, overwhelmed and upset, can be hysterical. Disappointment, separation anxiety, grief, brooding, strong drive, emotional outbursts.	Longing, sad kind of resignation showing up as depression. Listless, overwhelmed, indifference.	Very sad, crying easily or simply tearful, fearful.
Indications	Person says, "I'm alright, there's nothing the matter with me."	Low-spirited, weakened memory, "lifeless". Suicidal disposition. Explosive fits of anger. Not making friends.	Constant complaining with a wish to go home. Tends towards chilliness.	Every exertion causes fatigue, trembling. Cannot get enough sleep. Desire for quiet and aversion to being disturbed.	Sigh a great deal and seem disconnected from what's going on around them. Insomnia from cares, tendency to "eat away" the stress.	Seems to have difficulty comprehending. Chilliness, profuse perspiration at night.	Feels all alone in the world. Seeks comfort and solace from others.
Worse	Least touch, motion, rest. Wine and damp cold.	In cold weather, when getting cold.	Open air, uncovering and drafts. Cold in general.	Warm, damp weather, fog, before a thunderstorm, excitement, 10 AM.	Stress, coffee, cold air, consolation.	Exertion, loss of vital fluids, sexual excess, from becoming cold.	Eating until full. Evening and nighttime.
Better	While lying down or lying with head low.	Night, motion, walking, walking slowly. Warmth.	While eating, from heat, continued motion and walking.	Bending forward, open air, continuous motion, stimulants, profuse urination, wine.	While eating and from a change of position.	From keeping warm, after sleep.	From consolation, touch, company, and sympathy. Open air, gentle motion.

Note: *Capsicum is not commonly found in a home remedy kit, however, it has homesickness as a keynote.
Dosing: Use the BLUE Method. Observe and evaluate.

MENSTRUAL CRAMPS — DYSMENORRHEA

See *Chapter 15—Female Issues* on *page 159.*

MONONUCLEOSIS

Mononucleosis is a virus that takes hold when there is stress, whether from peer pressure, scholastic pressure, or sports-performance pressure. It can also be brought on by indulging in a poor diet and lack of sleep. Some know it as the "kissing disease" as the virus can be spread via bodily fluids. Mononucleosis is also known as "glandular fever" because it can affect the tonsils and the glands in the armpits, abdomen, and groin. The glands become swollen and painful.

The symptoms a person may experience include a fever, sore throat, headaches, a swollen spleen, and sore, achy muscles. There is severe fatigue and weakness, and any task wipes them out. They can also suffer from a cough, shortness of breath, chest pains, or nosebleeds. A blood test may or may not confirm the diagnosis.

Homeopathy can help to reduce the discomfort, lessen complications, and shorten the duration of mononucleosis. Supportive measures sooner rather than later will help the person to recover more quickly and completely. Even though mononucleosis is an acute condition, there is a deeper root cause that needs to be addressed. So, in addition to giving the appropriate remedy, you will need to partner with your healthcare practitioner or naturopath to give the person support on a deeper level.

ADDITIONAL SUPPORT FOR MONONUCLEOSIS

- The person should recover good stamina and endurance before returning to school, work or sports, or be put back into any stressful situation. This can take from three weeks to two months.
- Keep the person on a healthy, light, nutritious diet.
- Avoid medications or alcohol as these can compromise the liver.
- Once the person is feeling better, take the opportunity to evaluate whether a lifestyle change may be needed to prevent future infections: Where is there too much pressure on the person? Do they have too much on their plate? Are they getting enough sleep? Are they making wise diet choices?

IT'S AN EMERGENCY WHEN

- The person develops a temperature over 103°F (39.4 °C).
- The person experiences swelling of the throat that is impeding their breathing.

WHEN TO CONTACT YOUR HEALTHCARE PROFESSIONAL

- The person is experiencing any fullness or discomfort on their left side. Sometimes the spleen can become painfully enlarged.
- The person has had a high fever for more than three days.

Glandular fever

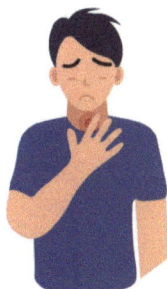

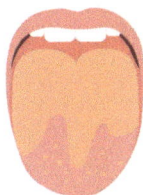

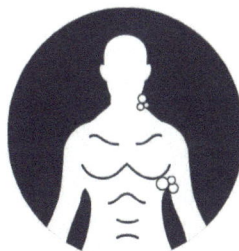

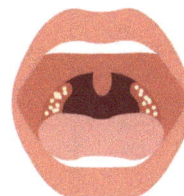

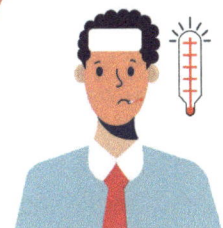

COMMON REMEDIES FOR MONONUCLEOSIS

	Apis	*Baptisia	Gelsemium	Mercurius	*Phytolacca
Symptoms	Swollen glands. If have a sore throat, it is constricted and inflamed, with sensation of a splinter. Pains are stinging and burning. Worse right side. Tongue, uvula, and throat are swollen. Tongue is fiery red and raw, and the mouth is dry. Throat is glassy red or purple.	Rapid onset with extreme exhaustion, fast deterioration and weakness. Body feels sore and bruised. Bed feels too hard. Breath and discharges smell foul. Has a heavy, numb head that feels too large. Heavy pain at the back of the head. Face, mouth, and tongue may be dark red or brown-red. May have an intensely sore, red throat, mouth sores, diarrhea, or vomiting.	Droopy, drowsy, and dizzy. Chilly and sensitive to cold. Great muscular weakness, heaviness, drowsiness, fatigue, soreness, and achiness all over. Teeth may chatter, even without chills. May have a dull headache in the back of the head, with stiffness and achiness in the neck and shoulders, and they may develop a sore throat.	Neck glands are swollen and tender. Breath smells bad and may have a metallic taste in their mouth. Excess saliva, and usually will have drooled a slimy, clear saliva on the pillow. Tongue may have a white or grey coating and is swollen so that it shows imprints of the teeth on the sides. Skin has a greyish look.	Throat is dark red or bluish-red. Feels hot, burning, raw, and too narrow. Much achiness at the root of the tongue and the soft palate. Sensation of a lump or red-hot ball in the throat. Pain comes and goes on the right, and shoots into the ear on swallowing. Thick, choking, stringy mucus that is greyish-white or yellow causing much hawking and clearing of the throat. Swollen, painful glands in neck and under the ears near jaw joints.
Mood	Very restless, but sleepy, and irritable when disturbed. May be weepy, but does not want to be touched.	Feels confused and dull. Can be restless. May have nightmares or delusions their limbs are double, scattered in pieces, or not connected to their body.	Indifferent to surroundings, dull, droopy, emotionally delicate or too tired to even be emotional, and want to be left alone.	Restless and nervous, constantly changing their mind.	Has very little interest in anything. Sensitive and restless.
Indications	May be swelling on the outside of the throat, and the face can look puffy. Skin feels sore and sensitive, as if bruised. Wants cold water to soothe the throat but are usually not thirsty.	May curl up tightly on one side. Eyes feel sore, with heavy eyelids. Look like they are drugged or drunk. Very thirsty and sleepy all the time. However, they can be restless.	Limbs feel very heavy and may be cold. Might say can't see or focus well. Often the tongue trembles when protruded. Face is hot and a dusky-red color. Appetite is low, with very little thirst. Weak, tired, and answers slowly.	May say their bones ache, they are weary and may tremble. Usually quite sweaty. Sensitive to heat and cold. Temperature may be unstable. Very thirsty for cold water but it does not satisfy their thirst.	Cannot swallow anything hot. Tip of tongue is fiery red, and may have a yellow patch down the center. Other joints besides jaw may be painful. Usually refuses food. Feels faint on rising, and greatly exhausted. May moan a lot.
Worse	Warmth, touch, heavy blankets, pressure, swallowing solid hot or sour food, on the right side, from 3-5 PM, after sleeping, or warm, stuffy room.	Around 6 PM, swallowing solids, open air, cold, heat with humidity, pressure, and on waking.	Overexcitement, strong emotions, spring, shock, damp weather, and around 10 AM.	Night, drafts, damp weather. Sweating, too much cold or heat, lying on the right side, warmth in bed, and warm drinks.	Cold damp weather, weather changes, hot drinks, touch, and pressure.
Better	Cool applications, cold liquids, cool air, motion, and light covering or being uncovered.	Drinking liquids.	Sweating, urinating, quiet and low-stress surroundings. Open air, reclining with head propped up, and continued motion, e.g., rocking.	Moderate, even temperatures, rest, lying on the stomach, and morning.	Warmth, cold drinks, rest, and lying on the stomach or left side.

Dosing: Use the **BLUE** Method. Observe and evaluate.

MOODINESS

Your adolescent may experience intense moodiness from time to time. Encourage your teen to let out whatever may be bothering them. To accomplish this, a safe environment without judgment is critical. Adolescents need guidance on how to deal with different emotional states. It is better to be in a state of acceptance, and not denial. Rudeness, verbal abuse, or violence should always be addressed and not accepted. If behavioral issues persist, consider connecting with a professional homeopath or counselor.

COMMON REMEDIES FOR MOODINESS

	Chamomilla	Ignatia	Natrum mur	Nux vomica	Pulsatilla
Onset	Ill effects of a bad temper.	Anxiety after a bout of rage, worry, fright, or humiliation. Also, after trauma or grief, shock, a strong reprimand, or if they are homesick.	Anger, disappointed or rejected love, fright or grief.	Too much mental exertion, anger, loss of sleep, tension, or stress.	Abandonment, grief or overwork.
Mood	Angry, impatient, abrupt, irritable, restless, oversensitive (especially to pain), easily offended, and snappy.	Nervous, excitable, introspective, easily frustrated, weepy, and tearful. Can have unpredictable reactions. Hysterically crying one moment, laughing the next, furious the next, distant or anxious or restless.	Sad and/or nervous. Has fears of being hurt or rejected, and gets easily discouraged. Are oversensitive and irritable, even irritated by sympathy.	Can be quite impatient, critical, angry, and oversensitive to just about everything. Hypersensitive to noise, odors, light, or touch. Overreacts to the slightest physical ailment.	Moods are quite changeable, even from hour to hour. Nervous, fidgety, sensitive, affectionate, timid, whiny, and clingy. Male may not be whiny, but can feel sorry for himself. Female can be both whiny and feel sorry for herself.
Indications	Moan and complain because they cannot have what they want. Otherwise, may be averse to talking, being spoken to, touched or to be looked at. Asks for something, gets it, and then doesn't want it, or complains about it.	Frequent sighing, yawning, grieves quietly. Does not want sympathy and may become antisocial.	Has a hard time sleeping, if in a state of grief. Has a hard time crying or expressing any strong emotion in front of others.	Time passes too slowly. May be driving themselves too hard.	Extreme ends of pain and pleasure. Can be easily persuaded and led by peers.
Worse	Cold, open air, wind, touch, night (especially around 9 PM), and anger.	Smelling tobacco, smoking, coffee, alcohol, touch, and consolation.	Just before or after menses, puberty, on awakening, and all day until sunset. Studying for long periods, sun, bright lights, violent emotions, especially anger, and around 10 AM.	Cold, touch, anger, motion, noise, odors, sunlight and morning.	Warm stuffy rooms, during menses, twilight and evening, sunlight, lying down, dehydration, excessive joy, and rich food.
Better	Rocking, cold applications, mild weather, and being engaged so they are not dwelling on their feelings.	Being left alone, eating, pressure, deep breathing. Warmth, but not intense heat.	Sleep, being still, low light or darkness. Fresh air, taking breaks, and being left alone.	Warmth, staying wrapped up, power napping, firm pressure, hot drinks, moist air, and lying or sitting.	Intake of liquids, walking in open air or any motion, cool, fresh air, cool applications, pressure, gentle massage, and erect posture.

Special dosing: Give chosen remedy once a day for three days. Observe and evaluate.

OSGOOD-SCHLATTER DISEASE

Osgood-Schlatter Disease is a condition caused by overuse and strain. It affects children, mostly boys, between the ages 10 to 15 after they've had a growth spurt and who are active in sports that involve running or jumping such as football, basketball, soccer, gymnastics, figure skating, or ballet. The chief characteristics are tenderness and soft tissue swelling found in one or both knees below the kneecap. Pain is worse from squatting, climbing, or extending the knee against resistance. The diagnosis is made by clinical examination. X-rays might be ordered to rule out other causes.

Treatment usually involves waiting for the growth spurt to resolve over a period of 6 to 18 months. During that time, the activities that worsen the condition must be closely monitored or stopped. The use of cold compresses, physical therapy, and pain management are standards of care. As an alternative or complementary approach, consider using homeopathy to address the inflammation and pain caused by this condition.

COMMON REMEDIES FOR OSGOOD-SCHLATTER'S DISEASE

	*Calcarea fluor	*Calcarea phos	Ruta	Silicea
Onset	Overexertion, overstraining and overstretching.	During rapid growth spurts.	Injury from damage or weakness.	Weakness in hips, legs or feet.
Symptoms	Knee swelling, overstrained joints or muscles.	Stiffness, especially after getting cold and wet, tendency for headaches if overworked.	Aching soreness, stiffness, parts feel broken, knees give way on stairs or on rising.	Headaches, cramping in calves and soles of feet, very smelly and sweaty feet.
Mood	Anxiety about health, sense of impending disaster. Fears of death, poverty, high places, and cancer.	Discontented for no reason, complaining and moaning, reserved, desire to travel, school phobias.	Dissatisfaction, defiant. Mind fogginess. Panic attacks when becoming hot, starting from sleep with the slightest touch. Fear of death.	Serious and proper, shy and timid, obstinate. Fears pins and pointed objects.
Indications	Sharp, darting or burning pains.	Stiffness, worse after rest. Growing pains.	Restlessness with frequent change of position, weakness in lower limbs.	Knee swelling, joint and limb weakness, limbs fall asleep easily.
Worse	Beginning motion, cold and damp.	Drafts, cold wind, cold damp or cold air, mental exertion, motions.	Pains worse when cold and wet, lying on painful side, motion.	Cold air, drafts, uncovering, touch.
Better	Continued motion, heat, warm applications.	Warmth, dry, lying down. Craves smoked meat.	Warmth, lying flat on back, continued motion.	Heat, warm rooms, rest, covering the head.

Additional remedies to consider: *Eupatorium perf** for sore, bone pains in the back and legs; *Guaiacum** for stinging and burning pains shooting up the leg from the ankle; and *Phosphoricum acidum** for pains at night that make the bones feel scraped.

Special dosing: Give chosen remedy once a day for a week. Observe and evaluate.

OVERINDULGENCE AND HANGOVERS

It is not uncommon for college students to overindulge in alcohol, sometimes on an alarmingly regular basis. Students should be educated before heading to college that alcohol poisoning is a severe life-threatening condition. A student should always be with one or more friends when socializing, especially if drinking is involved. If there is a family history of alcohol dependence, this is especially worrisome, as is overindulgence sufficiently high to end up in an emergency room.

When overindulgence does not produce severe disorientation, the young person may just wake up with a hangover. Classic symptoms are nausea, vomiting, headache and feeling very "sick." It is not life threatening, but very uncomfortable, and symptoms typically abate by late afternoon after the evening of drinking.

Alcohol poisoning, especially when the person can not stay conscious, is life threatening and an ER visit is essential.

*For more about **Alcohol Poisoning**, see **Chapter 4—First Aid** on **page 62**.*

IT'S AN EMERGENCY WHEN

- The person becomes so inebriated they cannot remain conscious and/or has had a seizure.
- The person has taken other recreational drugs along with alcohol (especially marijuana as this drug decreases the tendency to vomit, leaving more alcohol in the person's body which can then bring about alcohol poisoning).
- If the person is also using antidepressants, anti-anxiety or other medications, over the counter or prescription, and has become disorientated and incoherent.
- The person is vomiting profusely or is vomiting blood
- The person is experiencing slow or irregular breathing, i.e., gaps of more than eight seconds between breaths.
- The person has a low body temperature (less than 98.6°F or 37 °C).

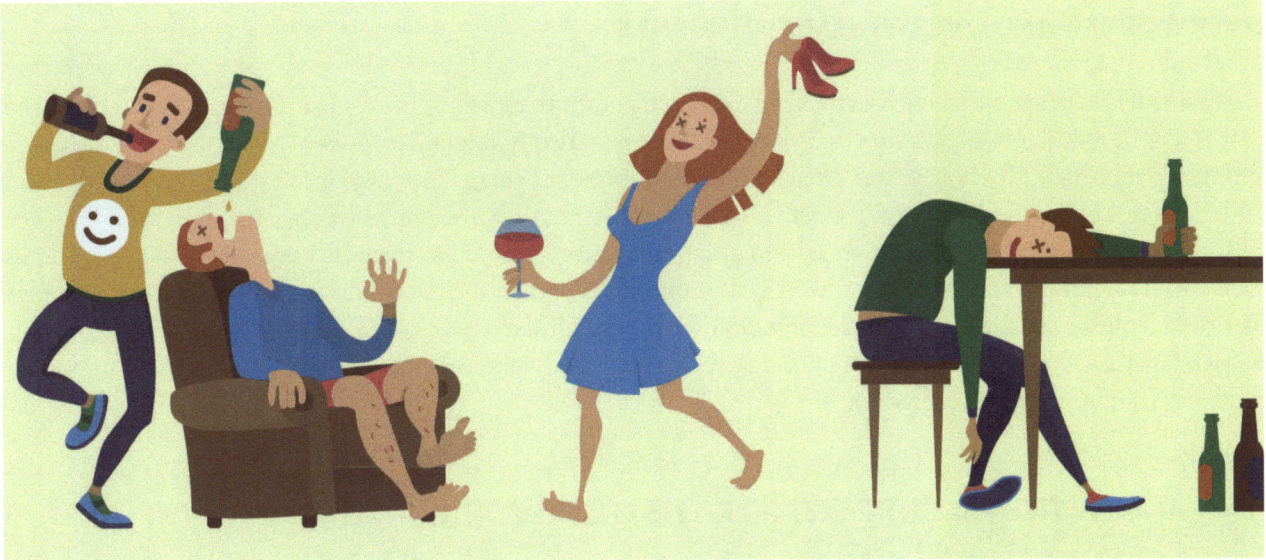

IDEAS FOR EDUCATING TEENS AROUND OVERINDULGENCE AND HANGOVERS

- Ask your adolescent to do their own research into alcohol (and drug) usage and effects of overindulgence. Then discuss their findings together. Share any family history of addiction and the nature of addictive drugs.
- Provide guidance on how to help them respond to peer pressure.
- Make sure to provide education around causes of alcohol poisoning (if they didn't find it in their research) especially about drinking too much in a short period of time, and how keeping number of drinks to a minimum is a better idea.
- If the person is going to drink, suggest they drink a glass of water for every alcoholic beverage they consume. This can help prevent dehydration that can occur from the diuretic effect of the alcohol and possibly avoid a hangover.
- Be adamant about never getting behind the wheel of a car or in the car with a driver who has been drinking.
- Strongly suggest they call for a ride home with the assurance that the parent will not "lecture" but simply get the young person home safely. Recommend calling a taxi or other car services rather than risk a fatal car accident.

WHEN TO CONTACT YOUR HEALTHCARE PROFESSIONAL

Alcohol and/or drug addiction are medical conditions, not a moral or behavioral issue. It is recommended that a person see a professional who specializes in addiction (especially if they have a family history of addiction) and experience any of the following:

- An inability to choose not to drink or use recreational drugs when socializing.
- Experiences cravings for alcohol and/or drugs when not using.
- Overindulges to the point of drunkenness or "high" each time they use.
- If use is happening early in the day.
- If use is interfering with their schoolwork or relationships.
- If they habitually use it in dangerous situations (driving a car, sports activities).
- If they habitually mix alcohol and other recreational drugs for the "effect."

THE remedy to consider for a hangover:

- **Nux vomica** is a powerful and effective anti-hangover remedy. Place one dose (a few pellets) of **Nux vomica** in a 16 ounce bottle of spring water. One sip is a dose. Shake vigorously before each dose. Typically, two to three sips spaced 15 minutes apart will reduce symptoms of a hangover.

OVERWORKED AND OVERWHELMED STUDENTS

There is truly no other era in life like the teen and young adult years of high school and college. It combines the best of ideas, enthusiasm, exploration, and vision with the remarkably vulnerable times of self-doubt, self-discovery and many important life choices. It is often a time when abundant energy is poured into rigorous educational and athletic programs, social agendas and creative arts. Schedules that are overfull, however, can take a toll.

Body changes and self-definition, social and group dynamics, and our electronically connected 24/7 world can each create their own type of stress for teens and young adults. When the relocation and newly assumed self-regulation of college are added to this, the potential for overwhelm, overwork, and despair increases. Fortunately, homeopathy can help. If the feelings persist despite the remedy choices provided, consider consulting with a professional homeopath or counselor.

ADDITIONAL SUPPORT FOR THE OVERWORKED AND OVERWHELMED

Teens and college students may not be familiar with the concept of self-care. Self-care involves regularly practiced activities and routines that reduce stress and maintain wellness. Good self-care supports better mood, energy and performance in school and extracurricular activities. This is especially important for those with full calendars and high expectations who may find it hard to take time to become aware of themselves.

- Sleep more: Numerous research studies have shown that many teens and young adults are sleep deprived, averaging only about six hours per night. Teens are biologically programmed to stay up late, and electronic devices can push that tendency even further. Combined with early morning class schedules, the lack of sleep alone can account for poor immune function, many types of body pain, depression, anxiety and moodiness. Just making time to sleep eight hours per night can help a person cope better with life's stressors and make a big difference in academic, creative, social and athletic performance.
- Check in with yourself regularly using The Stressor Life Scan Worksheet (see next page). Awareness of these symptoms can also help to select a well-matched homeopathic that can bring relief.

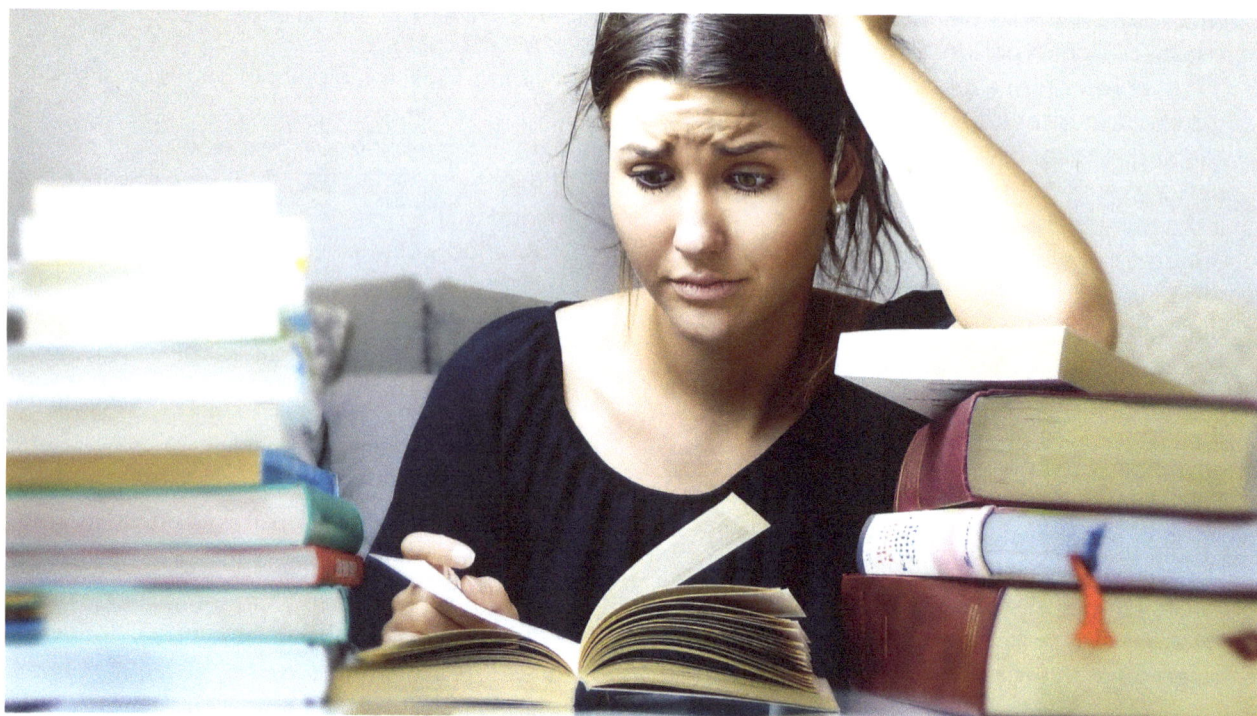

Stressor Life Scan Worksheet

1. Document your current symptoms first. Examples of each are provided below, but of course add others, not mentioned, that you may be experiencing:

    - **Physical symptoms**—examples include stomach discomfort, nausea, dizziness, frequent colds or other illnesses, an immune system that is not up to the task, increase in acne outbreaks and perspiration, body aches and tension, fast heartbeat or speedy pulse out of proportion to activity.
    - **Mental symptoms**—examples include anxious or racing thoughts, worried thoughts that prevent sleep, difficulty concentrating or remembering, reactive choices that show poor judgment, or a focus on negative circumstances.
    - **Emotional symptoms**—examples include moodiness, irritability, feelings of overwhelm, sense of loneliness or isolation, depression and unhappiness, or fearful anticipation of upcoming events.
    - **Behavioral symptoms**—examples include eating too much or too little, sleeping too much or too little, avoiding company of others to be alone, procrastinating or avoiding things, using recreational or prescription drugs to cope or relax. Behavioral symptoms can also include nervous habits such as twisting hair, biting nails, or pacing.

2. Then choose an action: For each stress symptom you wrote down, choose one specific action that you can take to possibly relieve the symptom. Some helpful examples might be journaling about it, or talking about it with someone you trust, exercising more to reduce your stress, making smarter choices for your health or giving yourself a long night of sleep. Again, add anything else you think might work for you.

Bonnie Thomas' book *Creative Coping Skills for Teens and Tweens*, and other books like it, offer suggestions, interventions and activities that can help put appropriate actions on the map for you. Find a resource you can count on, and turn to it often with your check in.

Stressor Life Scan Worksheet

My Current Stressors	1st Symptom	2nd Symptom	3rd Symptom
1. Physical Symptoms			
2. Action to take			
1. Mental Symptoms			
2. Action to take			
1. Emotional Symptoms			
2. Action to take			
1. Behavioral Symptoms			
2. Action to take			

WHEN TO CONTACT YOUR HEALTHCARE PROFESSIONAL

- Consult a professional homeopath and/or other licensed healthcare provider if symptoms are long-lasting and/or do not improve within a day or two after the administration of remedies.

COMMON REMEDIES FOR OVERWORKED/OVERWHELMED TEENS AND COLLEGE STUDENTS

	Argentum nit	Arnica	*Calcarea phos	*Cocculus	Nux vomica
Onset	Onset with anxiety before a test or other anticipated event.	Sore aching comes on quickly after overwork or injury, or within a day of exertion.	Onset with mental flatness after long periods of study.	Onset from a combination of physical and emotional stress.	Comes on after excessive lifestyle choices.
Symptoms	Overwhelmed, anxious. Impulsive emotions can lead to ill-considered action. Strong fears: being late, alone, in a crowd, fear of failing, heights, or claustrophobia. Loss of voice, hoarseness from nervous excitement. Headache. Trembling.	Aching, soreness in muscles and soft tissues. Bruising from an injury. Aching head after much studying, mental exertion, or after a blow to the head from athletics, falls, or car accident. Fatigue from overexertion.	Headaches in students, from mental exertion. Mental prostration after overwork. Pain in back or limbs, joints, tendons, ligaments, or muscles. Stiff pain in neck.	Dizziness, room spinning. Nausea and vomiting. Headache from being overwhelmed, overworked, burdened, and loss of sleep. Worry for others.	Nausea and vomiting. Waking 3-4 AM with clear mind, racing thoughts, sleeps again and wakes in morning feeling awful, or irritable. Chilly. Cramps, spasms. Headaches from study, loss of sleep, over-indulgence of alcohol, coffee.
Mood	Fearful, anxious. Cannot endure suspense. Feels hurried, restless.	Denial of the situation saying "I'm ok."	Loss of motivation. Can't perform as before. Dissatisfied, wants change. Frequent sighing.	Overly sensitive, feelings hurt easily. On edge from lack of sleep. Sensitive to grief.	Irritable, impatient, cranky. Strong willed, quarrelsome. Averse to wasting time, sense that time is moving fast.
Indications	Anxiety before social event, stage fright, exams, anxiety. Diarrhea from anxiety. Desire for sweets, or sweet and salty. Loud belching. Impotence from performance anxiety. Sore throat with sensation of splinter in throat.	Muscle soreness and tension from injury, overexertion, shock, fright, or trauma. Sore, bruised feeling, as if bed is too hard. Nightmares after an accident or injury. Hoarseness from overexertion of the voice.	Making mistakes due to mental prostration. Rapid growth spurts, growing pains. Jaw pain as wisdom teeth come in. Craving for smoked meats—bacon, ham, salt.	Ailments from loss of sleep. Ailments from too many responsibilities, caring for others. Motion sickness from car, boat, train, bus. Desire for beer during headache. Sensation of hollowness in the head or stomach.	Ailments from too much: hangover after alcohol, jitters after coffee, stomach ache from overeating or rich food. Sour stomach after eating. Ailments from loss of sleep. May crave coffee, energy drinks or other stimulants. Constipation with urging, but nothing passes.
Worse	Hot weather, warm room, after eating or drinking, before an exam or event.	Averse to being touched. Night, from motion, or becoming overheated.	From cold wet weather, catches cold easily. Rapid growth aggravates joint pain. Drinking coffee.	Thought or smell of food aggravates nausea. From touch.	Sensory input aggravates: smells, light, sound, touch. From motion, tight clothing around waist. Uncomfortable in cold weather and in open air.
Better	With company. From fresh air, cold drinks, cold food.	Being left alone. Feels better with open air, change of position.	Lying down.	Lying quiet in a warm room.	Feels better after loosening clothing. Heat. From rest and sleep.

Dosing: Use the **BLUE** Method. Observe and evaluate.

Also consider: *Kali phos 6X cell salt for ailments from over-studying, pulling all-nighters, general lack of sleep due to overwork and stress. Give four tablets up to four times a day for up to five days.

STRESS

See *Chapter 19—Mind and Emotions* starting on *page 227*.

RELATIONSHIP TURMOIL

For many people, high school and college can be a time of turmoil in relationships, with family, friends and love interests. Some may have already experienced stressful situations earlier in life, but for some it will be the first time. Both high school and college are much bigger than any previous school, and for some, meeting lots of new people can be stressful. The prospect of forming new relationships with people from different backgrounds and cultures can be quite scary and daunting, but it can also be exciting and invigorating. Emotions can range from pure fear, to trepidation, to anxious restlessness or just plain giddiness.

Temporary physical symptoms, such as headaches or diarrhea, may arise that actually stem from emotional feelings. It's the fear of the unknown and excitement about the news that can result in both highs and lows and all kinds of symptoms including sleeplessness. Sometimes people let you down, they are not who you thought they were, love relationships end, or people do not act according to your expectations. All this can be very distracting when trying to study or work. Thankfully, homeopathy can help to ease the turmoil.

ADDITIONAL SUPPORT FOR RELATIONSHIP TURMOIL

There's plenty a person can do to support oneself, a family member or a friend who is going through relationship turmoil. These may seem simple and obvious, but they are powerful and can greatly benefit someone who is suffering from emotional turmoil to help them feel like themselves again.

- Have a cup of nurturing hot tea.
- Give yourself a time out in a warm bath or shower.
- Get plenty of rest.
- Do repetitive and nurturing deep breathing exercises.
- Talk in confidence with a trusted friend, family member, counselor, therapist, or professional homeopath.
- Dance, run, do yoga or do any other physical activity you enjoy to activate a dopamine (pleasure hormone) response.
- Meditate every day, even if it's just for 5 minutes. Consider using a phone app such as Headspace, Calm or Insight Timer to get you started.

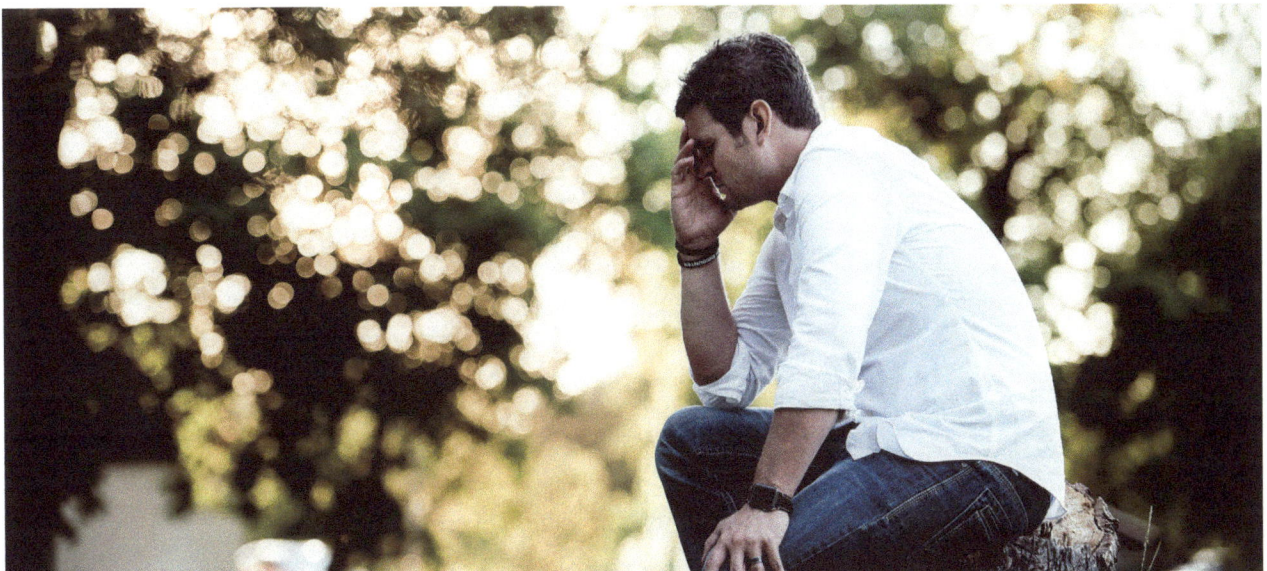

WHEN TO CONTACT YOUR HEALTHCARE PROFESSIONAL

• When there are disruptive thoughts or actions of self-harm (suicidal ideas, cutting, burning, unhealthy eating with food limiting or binging or purging, excessive use of drugs or alcohol, etc.) it is time to seek help. Know that you do not have to go through this alone, no matter what it seems like at the moment. Anyone can reach the Crisis Text HotLine by texting CONNECT to 741741 (www.crisistextline.org). Talk to a family member or friend. Connect with a respected religious leader. Schools have counseling support for students. Find out where help is available for you.

Sometimes, but not always, relationship turmoil may even result in a feeling of shock, or a shocking event may cause doubt and turmoil. It is important to know which homeopathic remedy to give if the person is in shock. There are two specific remedies for shock—**Aconite** and **Arnica**—and they are used in different situations, so it is good to familiarize yourself with the specific indications for each remedy:

• **Aconite:** The patient is very fearful, anxious, extremely reactive to pain, and inconsolable, with glassy eyes or dilated pupils; they are likely to be screaming, crying out, and trembling with terror and pain. **Note:** In a situation of relationship turmoil, also consider **Ignatia**.

• **Arnica:** The patient is stunned, irritable when offered help, exhausted, and uncooperative; they say they are fine, and don't want to be touched. They may complain of pain but will maintain that not much is wrong with them.

Special Dosing: Give chosen remedy every 15 minutes for an hour. Observe and evaluate.

Also consider **Bach Flower Rescue Remedy®**: This Bach Flower Essence reduces the effects of fright, shock, emotional trauma, grief, panic, hysteria, and fearfulness that cause trembling and loss of energy. It will restore a sense of balance, calm, and harmony. A dropperful of the liquid version can be taken directly from the bottle or put into water and sipped as needed. It is found in some drugstores, many health-food stores and online.

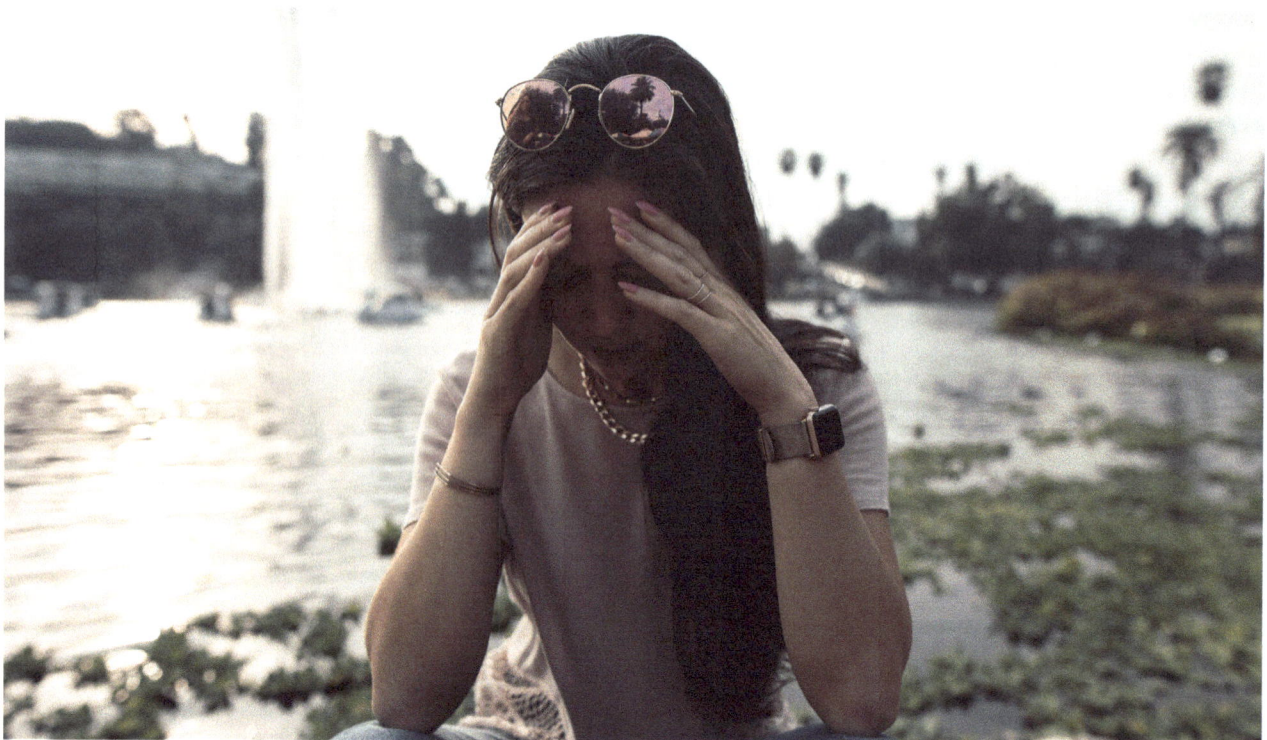

COMMON REMEDIES FOR RELATIONSHIP TURMOIL

	Arsenicum	*Calcarea phos	*Coffea	Ignatia	Lycopodium	Natrum mur	Phosphorus
Onset	Sudden great weakness, anxiety.	After bad news, lifting, over-study, grief, disappointed love, unpleasant news, getting wet.	Overstimulation.	Feeling forsaken, experiencing grief. Disappointed love, recent death of a loved one.	Ill effects from fear, fright, anger, anxiety.	Feeling forsaken, experiencing grief.	After putting out a lot of energy, now feel burned out.
Symptoms	Nervous, restless, chilly, weak, exhausted, trembling, burning pains, pale, puffy, drowsy. Restlessness.	Trembling, coldness or soreness in spots, on the vertex, eyeballs, tip of nose, fingers, etc. Ill effects of over study, too much sex, grief, disappointed love, unpleasant news.	Over-excitable and over-sensitive nerves, unable to sleep because of acute hearing. Emotions, even joyful or pleasant, produce symptoms.	Nervous, sighs a lot, moans, and is inconsolable, with changeable moods and contradictory symptoms.	Loss of self-confidence. Mistakes in spelling and writing. Indecision. Suspicious. Jealous of other's popularity.	Easily offended, hold grudges. Migraine with zig-zag vision. Craving salty foods.	Easily upset, over-sensitive, goes to sleep late. Excitable. Fearful about the future, indifferent and apathetic. Self-important. Wants sympathy.
Mood	Oversensitive, anxious, fastidious, fault-finding. Anguish and thinks they won't ever feel better. Fear of death from starvation or financial loss. Fear of being left alone, of self-harm.	Restless, fretful, forgetful, wants to go somewhere to some other place. Whining.	Ecstasy, full of ideas, impulsive, dramatic, sudden shifts from laughing to crying.	Alert, oversensitive, nervous. Highly emotional, moody, brooding. Silent and sad. Angry with themselves. Want to be alone. Irritable.	Confusion, melancholy, afraid to be alone, sensitive, fearful of meeting new people, does not want to do anything new yet does well at it.	Sad, nervous, fears of being hurt or rejected. Is easily discouraged. Does not want sympathy. Has a hard time crying or expressing any strong emotion in front of others.	Timid, weary of life, doesn't want to study or talk, laughs at serious things. Likes being center of attention and doesn't like when not.
Indications	Sensitive to disorder. Does not want to meet friends, feel they have offended their friends.	May also have skin problems, vertigo, migraine and rheumatic problems that come on after unrequited love.	Anxiety, faintness, hyperventilation, heart palpitations, restlessness, impatience.	Sighs, cries, or laughs when they should be serious. Changeable moods. Do not like to be contradicted.	Anticipate events with fear, often for long time before event. Envy people who seem to carry off any situation while they agonize for days.	Depression, palpitations and skin problems after disappointment in a relationship. Melancholic type.	Fearful, and wants lots of affection. May hold grudges. Swift temper.
Worse	Midnight, after midnight, cold, watery fruits, alcohol, tobacco, seashore, traveling.	Thinking about the problem. Exposure to weather changes, drafts, cold, dental issues, loss of fluids, fruits, ascending.	Every little noise keeps them awake. Touch, odors, cold wind. Emotions. Mental exertion. Night. Overeating, alcohol and narcotics.	Emotions; grief, anger, worry, fright, shock. After losing a valued relationship. Open air, cold air. Odors. Touch. Coffee. Tobacco. Yawning. Stooping. Walking, standing.	Pressure of clothes. Heat. Awakening. Wind. Indigestion. 4-8 PM. Wet, stormy weather. Milk. Vegetables, cabbage, beans, raw onions. Bread and pastry.	Consolation. Noise. Warm room. Lying down. Excessive heat.	Emotions, talking, touch, odors, cold, salt, sexual excess. Sudden change in weather, thunder and lightning, mental fatigue. Twilight.
Better	Hot applications, warm food and drinks, warm wraps. Motion, walking about, lying with head elevated, company, open air, sweating.	Alone. Warm dry weather. Lying down.	Lying. Sleep. Warmth.	Change of position. Urination. Alone. Pressure. Deep breathing. Swallowing. Eating. Warmth. Sour things.	Warm drinks and warm food. Cold applications. Motion. Urinating. After midnight.	Crying and being alone. Being at seashore.	Eating, sleep, washing face with cold water, massage, dark.

Dosing: Use the **BLUE** Method. Observe and evaluate.

TOP 20 REMEDIES FOR YOUR COLLEGE STUDENT'S REMEDY KIT[1]

A homeopathic remedy kit is a "must have" for your college student when it is time for them to leave the nest. Before they make the transition, take some time to review with them some of the challenges they will face and which remedies can help them navigate the stressors of daily life on campus. Going over this list together is a great way to prepare for the college experience.

- **Aconite:** First stage of illness; sudden onset with high fever, pale and chilly, worse cold dry wind. Great fear; ailments from sudden fright or shock.

- **Arnica:** Trauma; muscle injury, bruising, shock. First remedy after any accident or injury. Excellent after dental work.

- **Arsenicum:** Food poisoning. Anxiety with restlessness. Severe vomiting with exhaustion. Very chilly. Thirsty for small sips.

- **Bryonia:** Flu or bronchitis; slow onset with dry hacking cough, irritability with a desire to go home and lie in bed perfectly still, chilly, thirsty for large amounts of water infrequently.

- **Chamomilla:** Toothache; intolerable pain causing extreme irritability, worse at night, pain drives to despair, swollen gums with one cheek hot and red and the other cheek cold and pale.

- ***Cocculus:** Vertigo and motion sickness; nausea with vomiting, unsteady gait (as if drunk), feels the world is spinning, must lie down.

- **Gelsemium:** Flu; weakness and fatigue, slow onset with body aches, chills up and down the spine, frontal headache, low-grade fever with no thirst, worse any change of weather.

- **Hypericum:** Nerve pain; any wound, injury, or dental treatment that affects the nerves. Especially useful in spinal and eye injuries.

- **Ignatia:** Acute grief, hysterical reactions; involuntary tears, frequent sighing with a feeling of a lump in the throat from emotions.

- **Ledum:** Puncture wounds, wasp stings, or tick bites; the affected part feels cold with numbness, greatly sensitive to touch, and better from cold applications.

- **Magnesium phos:** Menstrual difficulties and colic; severe cramp-like abdominal pains, better from heat, pressure, and bending double.

- **Nux vomica:** Stomach flu and headaches. Symptoms come on from over-indulgence/toxicity. "THE hangover remedy." Very irritable, great mental and physical sensitivity.

- **Phosphorus:** Bleeding, nosebleeds, cuts, any excess bleeding with bright red blood. Also useful in bronchitis/pneumonia. Chilly, thirsty for cold drinks, need for and better from company and affection.

- **Pulsatilla:** Colds, bladder infections, and yeast infections. Changeable symptoms, thick bland yellow discharge. No thirst, clingy and tearful, craves open air.

- **Rhus tox:** Joint pains. Poison ivy. Pains worse on first motion and better after limbering up, worse cold wet weather, restlessness with the pains, better warm applications (the hotter the better).

- **Sepia:** Hormonal problems: PMS (premenstrual syndrome), postpartum depression, morning sickness, menopause. Irritability with aversion to loved ones. Strong desire for and better from dancing and exercise.

- **Silicea:** Abscesses in teeth or skin, wounds slow to heal, slow development of inflammation. Promotes drainage of abscesses, expulsion of splinters.

- **Staphysagria:** Lingering "cutting" pains after surgery or wounds. Also, bladder infection.

- **Sulphur:** Skin rashes and diarrhea. Heat, redness, burning, wakes at 5 AM. Desires sweets and spicy foods, worse from heat of the bed and bathing. Great for end stage colds and flus that won't completely resolve.

- ***Veratrum album:** Food poisoning and stomach flu; severe vomiting and diarrhea at the same time, very chilly with cold sweat on forehead and feeling of collapse.

Dosing: Good to start using the **BLUE** method. Observe and evaluate.

1   Excerpted from *Homeopathy Today* Autumn 2018—*The Ultimate College Care Package* by Loretta Butehorn, PhD CCH RSHom(NA) FSHom.

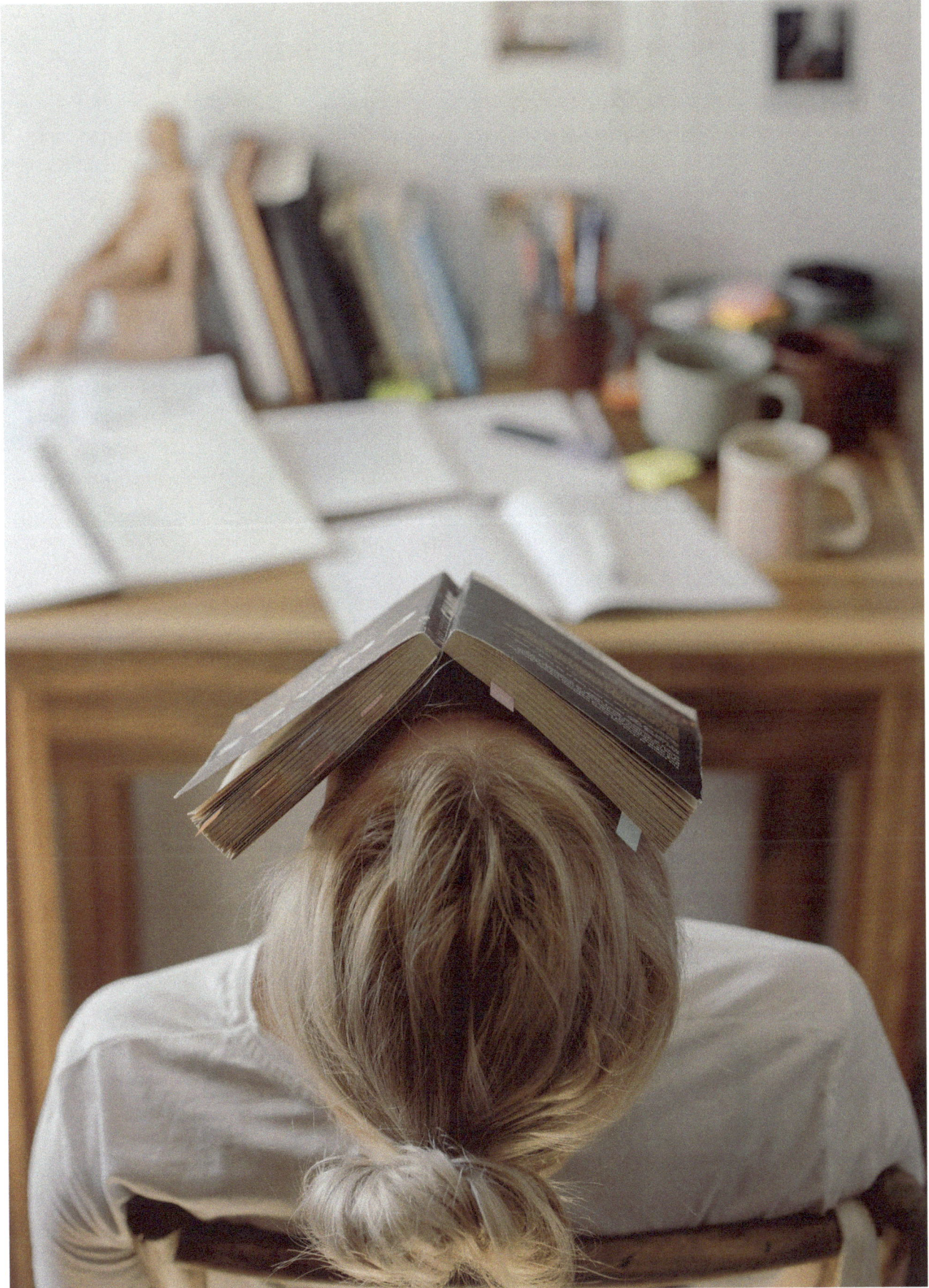

? WHAT'S THE FIRST REMEDY YOU THINK OF WHEN...

1. The person feels very alone in the world and is easily tearful and chilly with inability to get warm.
2. The student has swollen glands, bad breath, excess saliva with an alternation between hot and cold.
3. Your teen is sad, has fear of being rejected and irritated by your sympathy. They especially can't show strong emotions in front of others.
4. Your teen recently had a growth spurt and their knees feel stiff, worse from anything cold.
5. The person is irritable with a hangover.
6. The person is irritable, cranky and impatient with a strong desire to consume stimulants like alcohol, coffee and energy drinks.
7. The student has anxiety before a test, craves sweets and feels restless, hurried and anxious with diarrhea.
8. There is fright, shock, grief, hysteria, anxiety and/or fears causing trembling and a loss of energy.
9. There was a recent love relationship break-up and the person is incredibly emotional, inconsolable bordering on hysterical and moody.
10. The person suffers from indecision, has fears of doing new things (even though they are good at them), and agonizes for days before an event.

Answer key on page 324.

CHAPTER 23
Influenza

Homeopathy has a long track record of helping people with influenza. In 1918 the Spanish Flu was a pandemic in the U.S., and there existed no reliable medical treatment for the disease at the time. The flu claimed more lives than World War I. Yet, recoveries in the national homeopathic hospitals were common. There exist many papers and reports regarding the success and popularity of homeopathy in regard to treating the Spanish Flu. Statistics from Ohio show 24,000 reported cases of flu treated allopathically with a mortality rate of 28.2%; while 26,000 reported cases of flu treated homeopathically with a mortality rate of only 1.05%. Read on to learn about some homeopathic options for remediating flu-like symptoms.

INFLUENZA

Influenza, also called "the flu," is caused by many kinds of viruses. It may start out much like a cold with nasal discharge, low/medium fever, achy ears, sore throat, swollen glands, or coughing. But influenza is a much more severe infection than an upper respiratory infection (URI). It can also bring about aching in the muscles, joints and bones, fever, chills, loss of appetite, loss of taste or smell, exhaustion, nausea and vomiting, severe headaches, respiratory ailments, and a slow return of energy. A heavy cold may limit a person for a few days, but the flu can be debilitating, even fatal in a baby who is failing to thrive, someone who has a weakened immune system, or in a frail elderly person.

The flu used to occur mostly in winter or early spring but nowadays, people are reporting flu-like symptoms all year round. It is important to make sure that the person gets plenty of rest and a good diet while recovering. Otherwise, it is very easy to get sick again. The sooner treatment is started, the faster and more complete the recovery. Flu can cause exhaustion, depression, irritability, and lack of stamina for weeks if not properly addressed.

Since influenza is caused by a virus, homeopathy is a viable and effective option for treating one's flu-like symptoms.

IT'S AN EMERGENCY WHEN

- A child over three months old has a temperature over 103 °F (39.4 °C).
- If a child's temperature is very high with high-pitched crying or screaming, go to the hospital and give them a remedy on the way.
- A person is unresponsive, has trouble breathing or convulsions, or is listless or limp.
- A person is dehydrated from profuse vomiting or diarrhea and is not replenishing any fluids lost.

ADDITIONAL SUPPORT FOR FLU

- Get plenty of extra rest.
- Fluids need to be pushed to avoid dehydration, even if they only take a few sips at a time. Ice or frozen fruit bars or warm broths may feel good. A baby may refuse fluids but can suck on a clean towel soaked in water.
- Do not force the person to eat if they are not hungry. This gives the digestive system a rest and encourages the body to eliminate toxic wastes, aiding in recovery. If they ask for food, they should be given a light diet low in sugar and avoid stimulants such as cola or caffeinated tea. Mild herbal teas are OK. They should be kept on a nutritious diet for two to three days after the fever has broken.
- The face and forehead may be sponged with lukewarm water. Even though a person has a fever, they may be extremely chilly and feel they cannot bear to be uncovered. They can pile on the covers for chills and be kept lightly covered when the heat occurs. The room should be kept comfortably cool. They should be dressed in light clothing.
- The person should not go back to school or work until there is a complete return of health and they are sleeping well again. Too quick a return to life can cause a relapse, especially increased fatigue.

WHEN TO CONTACT YOUR HEALTHCARE PROFESSIONAL

- Usually a healthy baby will not get the flu unless it is a very strong strain. If a baby is failing to thrive or of low vitality, and you suspect that they have a flu, you must seek professional help. A child with low vitality or a compromised immune system may develop secondary complications such as ear or throat infections, bronchitis, or pneumonia. If in doubt, contact your healthcare provider.
- A baby under three months old and has any rise in temperature.
- The person has had a fever for more than three days.
- A rash appears on the body at the same time.
- The person is refusing to drink or keeps vomiting. Dehydration can lead to serious complications.
- If the fever is accompanied by swollen lymph glands and they are painful to touch. If children chronically have swollen neck glands, you should talk to their healthcare practitioner. If any swollen glands appear without fever, or if a child has persistent swollen glands and keeps getting the flu, viral infections, or a cough, you should also contact their healthcare practitioner.

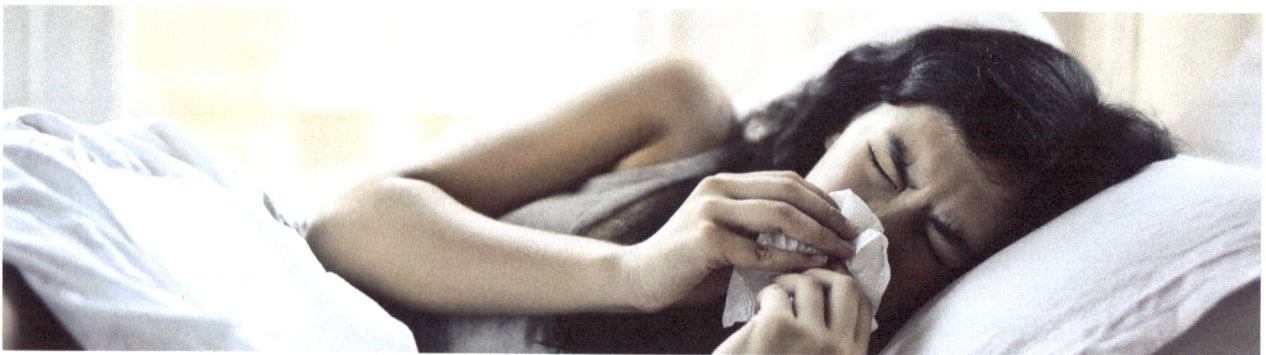

In addition to the remedies listed on the next page, a homeopathic remedy, commonly found over-the-counter in most health food stores and some supermarkets and drugstores, called **Oscillococcinum**®, has been shown to reduce the duration and severity of flu-like symptoms such as body aches, headache, fever, chills and fatigue when taken at the first sign of flu-like symptoms. Remember when choosing a remedy that the symptoms need to match the remedy picture. Appropriate for ages 2 and older.[1]

---

1   https://www.boironusahcp.com/clinical-studies-oscillococcinum.

COMMON REMEDIES FOR FLU

	Arsenicum	*Baptisia	Bryonia	*Eupatorium perf	Gelsemium	Phosphorus	Rhus tox
Onset	Getting chilled, wet weather, getting overheated, overexertion.	Rapid onset, with fast deterioration and high fever. From getting chilled in cold wind, autumn winds.	Slow onset, from getting chilled by a cold wind, especially in spring and autumn.	From exposure to icy coldness. Starts with intense thirst for cold drinks, followed by chills and fever.	Gradual onset, from damp, humid weather, shock, or fright. Common in spring.	Onset slow and steady. Ravenous hunger the night before onset. Getting drenched in rain.	Getting chilled and wet. Sitting on damp ground. Overexertion.
Symptoms	Burning pains relieved by heat. Very chilly, body cold, face hot, person may have high fever and feel achy. Strong thirst, but only takes constant small sips.	Sore, heavy, bruised feeling. Smelly sweat, mouth and stool. Profuse sweating. Face and tongue are a dusky red color. Intense thirst.	Long fever. Infrequent, but great thirst for cold drinks. Little discharge from nose. Achy all over body. Sore eyeballs. Cannot get comfortable.	Bones hurt so badly they feel broken. Muscles, limbs, and back are very achy. Skin feels sore. Head feels heavy, and eyes ache. Extremely weak.	Chills up and down spine. Feels weak, heavy, and drowsy. May be dizzy. Muscular soreness all over. Dull pain in head and eyes. Trembling.	Fever, chills, night sweats. Joints feel stiff. Burst of energy followed by weakness. Headache over one eye.	Extreme muscle aches and stiffness. Bruised and sore, with a constant desire to stretch and move. Extremely chilly.
Mood	Restless, anxious, irritable, fussy, over-sensitive, needy. Demanding. Desires company, but not to interact.	Dull, confused, drowsy, scattered, restless. May have nightmares.	Grumpy, fretful, intolerant of being disturbed or moved. Wants to just lie still in bed and be left alone, but is restless.	Restless with a lot of moaning. Any effort is just too much.	Indifferent to surroundings, dull, droopy, and emotionally delicate. Wants to be alone.	Needs attention and consolation. Affectionate, fearful, easily upset, irritable.	Anxious, weepy, helpless, mildly delirious, extremely restless.
Indications	Even though pains are burning, they want heat. Chilly with cold, sweat. Weak and tired, but restless.	Looks very ill, as if drugged or drunk. Eyelids heavy. Falls asleep while talking. Bed feels too hard. Yellow-brown coating of tongue.	Does not want to move, even the eyes. Mucous membranes and lips are dry, parched and cracked. Eyelids sore, red, and swollen. Frontal headache.	Chilly, but wants cold drinks. Bursting pain in back of head that can cause nausea.	Much sweat. Eyes ache and are droopy, making them look drunk. Cannot focus. Very little thirst, low appetite. Teeth chatter without chills.	At first, may not show how sick they are, then show their illness quickly. Effort difficult. Senses acute. Face is pale, then flushed.	Profuse sweating that relieves symptoms. Chills with any movement or uncovering. Hard, swollen, tender glands. Thirst for small amounts.
Worse	Physical exertion, after midnight, cold drinks, cold air, sight and smell of food.	Around 6 PM, waking, swallowing solids, open air, cold, heat with humidity, pressure.	Any movement or motion, 9 PM, touch, warmth, spring, autumn.	From 7-9 AM, autumn, winter, open air, movement, cold air, smell or sight of food.	Around 10 AM, over-excitement, strong emotions. Spring, shock, damp weather.	Change of weather, wind, thunderstorms, odors, lying on left side, light, morning, evening.	Cold and damp weather. Drafts, autumn, cold food or drinks, uncovering, lying still, night, first movement after rest.
Better	Warmth, hot food and drink, lying down, fresh air, company.	Drinking liquids.	Lying completely still, pressure, quiet, being left alone, pressure on the head for head pain. Cool air.	Sweating, lying still, loose clothing, conversation, staying indoors, hands and knees position when coughing.	Sweating, lying still, loose clothing, conversation, staying indoors, on hands and knees position when coughing.	Sleep, sympathy, low lights or dark, eating and drinking cold things, cool applications, open air.	Warm drinks and food, warmth, continued motion. Stretching, changing positions, massage.

Dosing: If the onset is fast, use the ORANGE method. If the symptoms have come on slowly and are not severe, use the BLUE method. Observe and evaluate.

Note: Especially with flu-like symptoms, today's uncomfortable symptoms can be helped with a remedy, but then tomorrow may present with different symptom(s) that need to be addressed with a different remedy. You may have chosen the right remedy yesterday but the person may have moved on to needing a related or different remedy today.

FEVERS

See **Chapter 5—Head** starting on **page 69**.

COUGHS

See **Chapter 10—Throat and Chest** starting on **page 115**.

RECOVERING FROM THE FLU

Because of the inflammatory response of the body to fight a flu virus, a person can experience such things as lingering fatigue, lethargy, slow mental activity, difficulty concentrating, and sleep changes.

WHEN TO CONTACT YOUR HEALTHCARE PROFESSIONAL

- If there has been no improvement after 48 hours.

Remedies to consider:

- **Gelsemium:** The person just cannot seem to turn the corner and regain their energy. They will be completely exhausted with a wiped-out expression on their face. The appetite is low and they have very little thirst. They have great muscular weakness, answer slowly, and want to be left alone. Many times, they feel lightheaded and may have a headache. There may be a sticky perspiration on the skin.
    Worse from: overexcitement, strong emotions, spring, shock, damp weather, and around 10 AM.
    Better from: sweating, urinating, quiet surroundings, open air, reclining with the head propped up, and continued motion, e.g., rocking.

- ***Phosphoricum acidum:** This remedy is given for weakness and exhaustion. The person just cannot seem to get their energy back. They look pale with dark circles under their eyes. They are very sweaty and chilly. There is a lack of appetite, but a desire for fruit and other light, refreshing foods. They are indifferent, quiet, easily overwhelmed, mildly irritable, cannot concentrate, and uncommunicative or answer with a minimal amount of words.
    Worse from: severe, acute illnesses, after eating, rising after long periods of sleep, any exertion, and walking.
    Better from: naps (but not long periods of sleep), fruit and other light, refreshing foods.

Dosing: Use the **BLUE** method.
Observe and evaluate.

WHAT'S THE FIRST REMEDY YOU THINK OF WHEN...

1. The person is weak during the flu.
2. The person is still weak after the flu.
3. The child is restless, chilly and only drinking small sips at a time.
4. The flu came on quickly with a high fever and was chilled in a cold wind.
5. The bones hurt so badly they feel broken during a flu-like illness.
6. There is extreme muscle aches and stiffness with a frequent need to move and stretch.
7. The person is dull, droopy, wants to be alone and has little thirst.
8. The flu includes night sweats with fever and chills and headache over one eye.
9. The person is achy all over, has sore eyeballs, and prefers to not move anything.
10. You think you may be coming down with something like a flu.

Answer key on page 325.

CHAPTER 24
Travel Related

When embarking on a journey, whether it's a leisurely vacation or a business trip, maintaining good health and well-being is paramount. In such instances, homeopathic remedies emerge as invaluable companions, offering a natural and gentle approach to addressing various health concerns encountered while traveling. With their compact size, ease of use, and minimal risk of adverse effects, homeopathic remedies prove to be convenient and reliable allies, providing relief from common travel-related ailments such as motion sickness, jet lag, digestive issues, and minor injuries. Their versatility and effectiveness make them indispensable additions to any traveler's toolkit, ensuring a smoother and more enjoyable experience while exploring the world.

TRAVELING ABROAD

It is essential to be informed about prevalent health conditions in countries you will be visiting. Before traveling, please visit the website www.tripprep.com.

MOTION SICKNESS FROM BOATING, FLYING, AND DRIVING

Motion sickness typically originates in the inner ear, bringing about headache, dizziness, and/or nausea. The body's balancing mechanisms can be disturbed by rapid acceleration, unusual movement, and confusing visual input, as from riding in a car or boat. Breathing petroleum fumes, smoke, or poor ventilation may also incite or aggravate motion sickness. If the queasy person is at the back of a boat, get them to the front, so they are not inhaling petroleum fumes. If they are below deck, bring them into the open air above deck.

A motion-sick person is usually sweaty, anxious, and pale. Often weak, they may be lethargic, or be hyperventilating or salivating. Encourage them to take slow, deep, rhythmic breaths. This will bring in much-needed oxygen and help calm the nausea. Chewing on ginger candy will often alleviate nausea as well.

- **Seasickness:** the motion of a boat or ship riding through the water – sliding up, over, and down waves –disturbs the balance of the inner ear, causing discomfort that may result in such common symptoms as nausea, vomiting, headache, excessive salivation or perspiration, and dizziness.

- **Air sickness:** also called flight sickness, this is another form of motion sickness. Because air travel involves both horizontal and vertical movement, your brain receives conflicting messages, causing symptoms similar to seasickness.

- **Car sickness:** yet another form of motion sickness, car sickness can arise when the motion of the vehicle stresses the eyes and upsets the inner ear's balance, creating queasiness, headache, anxiety, nausea, and vomiting. For those prone to car sickness, a good rule of thumb is not to read while riding in a car. Often riding in the front seat, with plenty of fresh air from an open window, will alleviate car sickness.

COMMON REMEDIES FOR MOTION SICKNESS

	*Cocculus	Nux Vomica	*Petroleum	Sepia	*Tabacum
Onset	From riding in cars, boats, or planes. Ailments from lack of sleep.	From riding in cars, boats, or planes. Ailments from anger or overindulgence.	From riding in cars, boats, or planes.	From riding in cars, boats or planes. Ailments during menses or hormonal changes.	From riding in cars, boats, or planes.
Symptoms	Anxiety with nausea. Vertigo with vomiting. Headache with vertigo. Nausea from vertigo.	Vertigo. Constant nausea. Splitting headache. Buzzing in ears. Retching, gagging, desire to vomit but can't.	Vertigo. Headache. Nausea with salivation. Vomiting.	Faintness during nausea. Vomiting with nausea. Empty feeling in pit of stomach. Flushes of heat during nausea. Headache on left side.	Headache with nausea. Vertigo. Cold perspiration. Deathly nauseated. Violent vomiting with motion.
Mood	Anxious and fearful.	Irritable and impatient.	Irritable and quarrelsome.	Weepy and irritable. Irritable to family or husband.	Despondent. Wretched.
Indications	Dry or metallic taste in mouth. Numbness, insensibility of body parts.	Chilly. Constipation or diarrhea. Hiccups.	Chilly, faint, pale, sweaty. Dry, cracking skin.	Cold hands and feet. Hormonal conditions. Craves sour/vinegar.	Extreme paleness. Icy, cold skin. Headache feels like a band around head.
Worse	Lack of sleep. Noise, smell of food. Rising up. Coffee.	Thought of food and/or alcohol. Anger. Tobacco smoke.	Smell of gasoline. Cool fresh air. Dampness. Rising and sitting.	Before or during menses. Thought of food.	Warmth. Opening their eyes. Tobacco smoke. Thought of food.
Better	Lying down. Closing eyes. Being still. Open air.	Lying down. After vomiting. Warmth.	Eating. Rest. Lying down.	Exercise, activity. Being left alone.	Fresh cool air. Eyes closed. Quiet, dark environs. Uncovering abdomen.

Special dosing: Give chosen remedy before embarking, then give on an as needed basis. Observe and evaluate.

TRAVEL VACCINATIONS AND MEDICATIONS

When traveling to any foreign country, know what vaccines may be required long before you go. To find out what's suggested, go to www.nc.cdc.gov/travel.

The following information will be helpful if you or anyone in your family will be traveling abroad:

- Malaria tablets are recommended by travel doctors for mosquito-infested areas. The herbal tincture Spilanthes is another more natural and effective option that is suggested for an anti-malarial, but it must be taken three times per day and may cause your tongue to tingle.

- A yellow fever vaccine is required for visiting many tropical or developing countries. Sometimes you also may need to have a vaccine if you're traveling from a country where yellow fever exists. For instance, if you flew from Colombia to Brazil, you might be asked for a certificate showing that you had been vaccinated against yellow fever. However, if you went to Brazil from the United States, the yellow fever vaccine would not be required.

Some insurance companies will insist on certain vaccines before issuing travel coverage. It's worth getting information from your healthcare practitioner or internet searches to find out what each country requires. Be informed before you and your family leave on your journey. Check, also, to see if certain allergies, such as an allergy to eggs, makes certain vaccines inadvisable for you or family members: you may be able to obtain an exemption from your physician or an infectious disease specialist.

Some people opt to take homeopathic remedies instead to preventively educate their immune system (also known as homeoprophylaxis) prior to encountering infectious diseases (this would only be an option if the country you are visiting isn't requiring a vaccine card). Taking remedies made from the potentized (extremely low concentration) disease material or vaccine material is possible through some professional homeopaths. These remedies do not have any dangerous side effects, but they may only protect the person for a limited amount of time. Hence, some homeopaths may recommend a repetition of the remedy while traveling.

If you do get a vaccine, consult with your healthcare practitioner and consider taking *Thuja, two pellets before and after the vaccination. Immediately after receiving the vaccine, give **Ledum**, which will reduce soreness at the puncture site. Neither remedy will interfere with the efficacy of the vaccine. If you have a severe general reaction to any vaccine, give one dose of *Thuja 200c (or 30c if that's what you have on hand) and call your healthcare practitioner at once.

If you do need to get vaccines, it's better to get one at a time, rather than several at once. This is less of a burden on your immune system.

Please make an informed decision on getting vaccines for traveling by visiting the following websites:

- www.tripprep.com
- www.thinktwice.com
- www.NVIC.org

A helpful book to have in your personal library is *The Savvy Traveler's Guide to Homeopathy and Natural Medicine: Tips to Stay Healthy Wherever You Go* by Judyth Reichenberg-Ullman and Robert Ullman. It's also available as an ebook so you can travel with it on your chosen device.

ILLNESS FROM DRINKING CONTAMINATED WATER

Contamination can be present in city water, well water, or fresh water such as lakes, streams, and rivers. Contaminated water may contain pesticides, metals, toxins produced by bacteria, and microbes or parasites. Consuming it can cause such gastrointestinal problems as diarrhea, nausea, vomiting, and dehydration as well as severe intestinal or stomach aches.

Check the safety of water in the area where you're traveling by logging into www.mappingmegan.com/travelers-guide-to-safe-tap-water. You can also check with management at the hotel (or other quarters) where you will be staying. Higher quality lodgings will often provide their guests with bottled water for excursions. If you'd rather be safe than sorry, consider purchasing and carrying with you a LifeStraw bottle and filter (www.lifestraw.com) that provides water filtration and purification from unsafe water taken from anywhere and making it safe to drink.

If you do drink contaminated water and are suffering from its effects with diarrhea and/or vomiting, it is imperative to keep hydrated with pure or filtered water. Fresh, pulp-free watermelon juice mixed with water is a quick and natural way to replenish electrolytes. You may also use 10 tablets of **Bioplasma cell salt**, a combination of Schuessler's twelve tissue salts, dissolved in bottled water and sipped as needed.

After a heavy loss of fluids from diarrhea and/or vomiting, improvement will be gradual. If the person has no appetite, encourage them to eat just a little, or drink miso soup, chicken broth or beef broth. If their symptoms have been severe, some young children may be too frightened to eat for fear of vomiting. If someone is weak, exhausted, and can't seem to get their energy back, **China** is often needed.

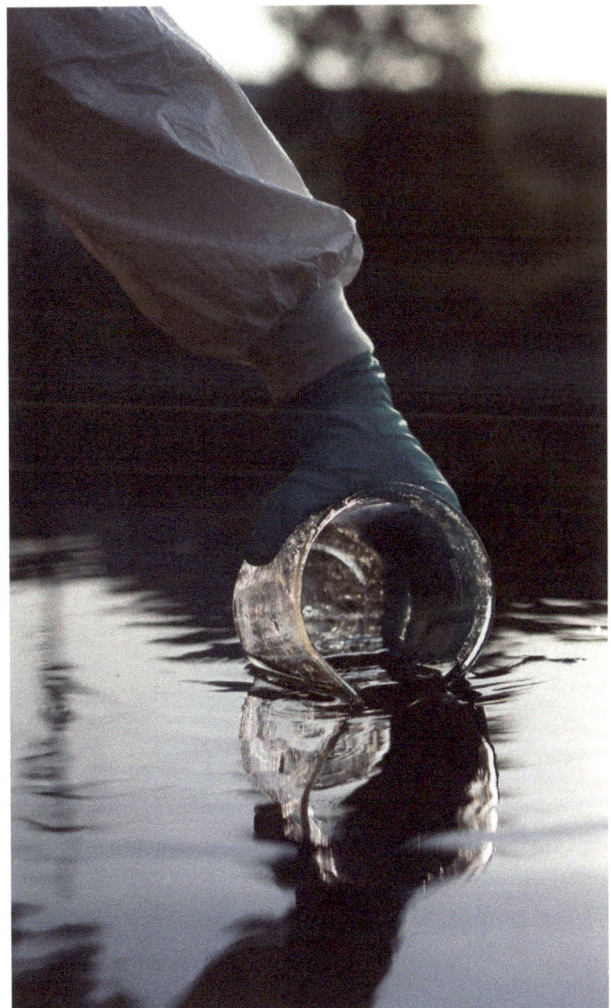

COMMON REMEDIES FOR ILLNESS FROM CONTAMINATED WATER

	Argentum nit	Arsenicum	China
Onset	Drinking contaminated water.	Drinking contaminated water (or having had contaminated ice cubes in a beverage).	Drinking contaminated water.
Symptoms	Vomiting. Full of thick mucus, sour or bitter taste. Burning, constriction in stomach, with pains radiating into all parts of abdominal cavity. Diarrhea. Noisy, watery, green stools looking like chopped spinach or flakes of green.	May have vomiting and diarrhea simultaneously, making them feel temporarily better. Retching after eating or drinking, especially ice-cold water. Vomit burns the throat. After vomiting subsides, wants small amounts of food often. Diarrhea is very watery, burning, slimy, brown, yellow, or black stools that may contain undigested food. Has foul-smelling stools in small quantities, that burn the anus. Cramping in the abdomen.	Vomiting. Frequent, sour-smelling vomit of undigested food. Sore and cold feeling in stomach. Hiccups, abdominal rumbling, and thirst for cold water. Diarrhea. Painless during evacuation, but can have gas pains making them bend over. Pale stools are acidic, profuse, frothy looking with undigested food. Can be involuntary. Much sweating.
Mood	Anxious and fidgety.	Anxious, restless, exhausted, but cannot lie still and has enough energy to be demanding. May fear they are going to die.	Irritable, nervous, oversensitive to touch.
Indications	Vomiting, preceded by loud belching. Severe bloating with loud passing of gas. Diarrhea. Abdominal rumbling, much bloating. Stools passed with much gas and an offensive smell.	Vomiting. Burning and rawness in pit of stomach. Abdomen is sensitive to touch. Diarrhea with great weakness after stool. Chilly, but wants sips of water to wet mouth. Might refuse water for fear of vomiting and cannot bear the thought of food.	Vomiting. Very swollen, painful abdomen with lots of gas and belching, which gives no relief when passed. Weakened state from loss of fluid from diarrhea and vomiting. May feel faint or have ringing in the ears. Persists after vomiting or diarrhea has ceased, due to dehydration.
Worse	Heat, too much excitement, and eating too much chocolate or sweets.	Midnight, around 2 AM, cold food or drinks, getting chilled, cold.	Drafts, noise, nighttime, and after eating.
Better	Fresh air, motion, passing gas, and burping.	Heat and warm applications to the abdomen.	Quiet, rest, firm pressure, bending double, warmth, and gently moving the limbs.

Other remedies to consider: **Nux vomica, Phosphorus** and ***Podophyllum.***
Dosing: Use the ORANGE method, then as things improve move to the BLUE method. Observe and evaluate.

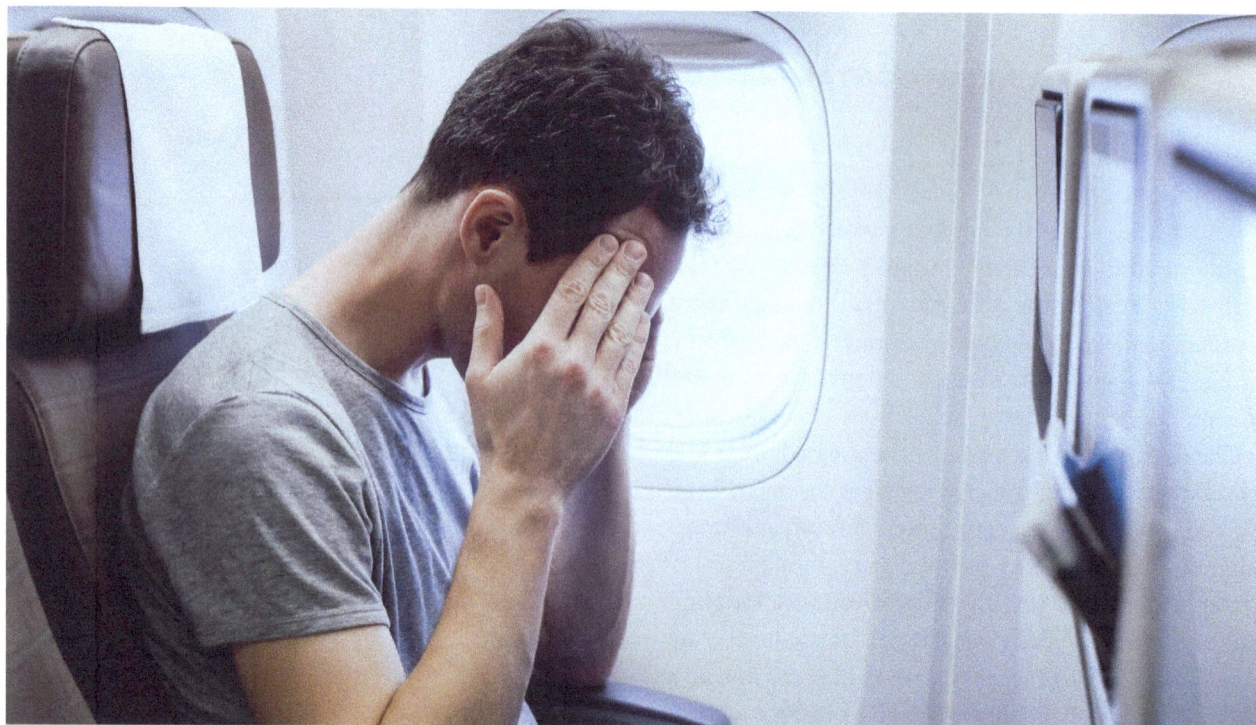

💡 HANDY TIPS FOR TRAVEL IN DEVELOPING AND TROPICAL COUNTRIES

- When brushing your teeth, do not rinse your mouth with tap water. Use bottled or activated charcoal-filtered water instead.
- When showering or bathing, keep your mouth closed and avoid inhaling or ingesting any of the water.
- Do not take ice in your drinks unless you can be assured it is made with filtered or purified water.
- Never ever eat food from a street vendor.
- Do not eat salads or any fresh fruit without a peel, as it may have been washed in unfiltered water.
- Avoid any dairy products, including ice cream, that does not come with a sealed wrapper out of a freezer.
- Be careful not to overexert in a hot climate. If you get overheated, sponge yourself down with cool or tepid water—cold drinks or a cold shower may provide too much of a shock to your system.
- Rabies runs rampant in some countries. If you are bitten by an animal, seek immediate medical advice.
- It is sensible in hot climates to avoid drinking any water other than bottled or filtered water.
- For snakebites and suspected poisonous insect or spider bites, **seek medical help immediately**. If possible, capture the critter, take a picture of it, or write down the details of what it looked like. Stay calm and try to keep the person calm, keeping the bitten part below the level of the heart, and applying an ice pack to slow the spread of venom. **Ledum** can be given for the puncture wound. Also, consider **Apis** if the bite is red, hot, and swollen and there's a desire to put cold on it. For snakebites, the appropriate remedy depends on the nature of the venom and its effects upon the blood or nervous system – and that is beyond the scope of this book. For more information, see **Bites and Stings** in **Chapter 18-Skin** starting on **page 208.**
- If you are near the ocean, do not swim alone (especially at night). Know how to look for riptides and how to swim parallel to shore to escape one. Unless you are able to test the depth and temperature before swimming, check with locals about these and other conditions, such as hidden rocks, dangerous tides, and murky waters that give cover to predators. Make sure to avoid swimming with a full stomach to prevent cramping. Use a naturally made sunscreen or wear a coverup to avoid sunburn.

FLYING-RELATED CONDITIONS

AIRSICKNESS

See **Motion Sickness from Boating, Flying and Driving** earlier in this chapter on **page 285**.

EAR PAIN AND POPPING

Ear pain during takeoff and landing can be excruciating. As the plane climbs to the higher altitude, air pressure in the cabin drops, causing the pressure in the ear canal to drop as well. When pressure in the canal becomes less than the pressure in the middle ear, the eardrum bulges outward—and there is considerable pain unless you manage to equalize the pressure. When you land, the opposite happens: pressure in the ear canal increases and the eardrum is pushed inward.

If you're traveling with an infant, be sure to breastfeed or bottle-feed your baby on takeoff and landing, since sucking will relieve the pressure. For toddlers, give them a lollypop to suck on to encourage swallowing, or have them chew a piece of dried apricot, dates or mango as a substitute for the action of chewing gum. Teach older children to swallow hard or yawn frequently. Chewing gum can also be an aid in reducing pressure on the eardrum.

If a remedy is needed, the main remedy to give is **Silicea** if there is a feeling of stoppage in the ear and better when yawning or swallowing. If this doesn't help, try one dose of **Chamomilla** if ears feel painful and stopped up, or **Pulsatilla** if ears feel plugged with noises in the ear or *****Rosa damascena** for a feeling of a blocked eustachian tube.

Dosing: Use the ORANGE method to start. Observe and evaluate. If the remedies fail to act, know that this discomfort should subside within 24-48 hours. If not, consult your healthcare provider.

DEEP VEIN THROMBOSIS

Deep Vein Thrombosis (DVT) tends to happen in people over 50 or those confined to sitting during very long flights. A blood clot forms in a deep vein, usually in the upper leg or calf, although clotting can occur anywhere in the body. It typically occurs in one leg only, producing swelling, inflammation with redness, heat, and sharp, cramping pains. The risk of developing a clot is increased if you've recently given birth or had surgery or cancer treatment, if you are on estrogen-based contraceptives or hormone replacement treatment, if your mobility is limited by a cast, or if you have a catheter in a large vein.

To help prevent clot formation, it is best to get up and move about the cabin often to keep your blood moving. Some other suggestions include moving your legs frequently, extending your legs as far as you can and extending and flexing your ankles. Some airlines suggest pulling your knee to your chest and holding it there for 15 seconds, repeat this 10 times, then do the next knee. Search the internet for "exercises for a long haul flight" to see some useful videos and articles.

If you believe you are a candidate for a blood clot in your leg owing to your personal or family history, order ***Hamamelis virginica 30c** and take two pellets before the flight. If there is swelling, inflammation, or pain during the flight, you can repeat the dose, as needed. If any symptoms persist after the flight, you can also repeat the dose, as needed. As soon as symptoms start to subside, no further doses will be needed. Do not take any more than four doses after the flight. If the remedy fails to act, consult your healthcare provider.

If you're on blood thinner medication, it is advisable to connect with your prescribing health care provider to discuss your travel plans.

FEAR OF FLYING

Fear in general can induce feelings of dread, anxiety, distress, panic, or terror. It can even cause a histamine reaction that produces welts on the skin (hives). If being afraid of flying escalates into a phobia — a deep-seated, chronically ingrained fear — you should consult a mental health professional.

Homeopathy, hypnosis, and EFT (Emotional Freedom Technique) have been shown to be effective for the treatment of phobias.

First Remedies to consider:

- **Aconite:** for fear of flying on airplanes or for the after-effects from fright. There is sheer terror with a rapid pulse and profuse perspiration. The person is very fearful, anxious, easily startled, restless, panicked, and extremely reactive to pain. They are also likely to be inconsolable, with dilated pupils, and possibly screaming and crying out with fear. They are afraid of crowds and death because they are sure they are going to die.

- **Argentum Nit:** for fear of flying on airplanes, fear of heights, fear of being unable to escape once the door is closed on the plane, claustrophobia, or general fear of losing control. The person is anxious, nervous, easily excitable, trembling, timid, and impulsive. They have a sense that time is going by too slowly, and they want everybody to hurry up. They may pace up and down in a panic, or talk fast in a childish way. In their anxiety, they can get frequent watery and smelly diarrhea.

- **Gelsemium:** for fear of flying because they anticipate mechanical problems with the plane, issues with the pilot, etc. Even though they are anxious and fearful, their reactions become slowed, with great weakness, confusion, exhaustion, and trembling. They become dull, heavy, sluggish, and sometimes dizzy, with stuttering or diarrhea. While their head may ache in the forehead and/or at the back of the head, droopy eyelids give them a drowsy look. Bending forward while sitting or lying down with the head slightly elevated can be helpful. They also need air, so open the overhead air vent all the way.

Other remedies to consider: **Arsenicum, Calcarea carb, Phosphorus**.

Dosing: Use the ORANGE method to start. Observe and evaluate.

JET LAG

Jet lag is the result of traveling rapidly across time zones, which can disrupt the body's circadian rhythms, also known as the body's clock.

Sleep disturbances or insomnia, lethargy and fatigue, a heavy, aching head, irritability, confusion, difficulty focusing, loss of appetite, a dizzy, unsettled feeling, and sometimes diarrhea or constipation – all may result from jet lag. To minimize the effects of jet lag, make sure to drink plenty of water while in the air (flying can dry out the skin and mucous membranes) and avoid drinking alcohol. A cocktail or glass of wine may make you feel better temporarily but will only dehydrate you further and make you feel worse later on.

Remedies to consider:

- **Arnica:** can be taken as a preventative before and/or after the flight. Take one dose of a 30c potency every four hours if the flight is longer than four hours. **Arnica** is particularly indicated if you feel very sore, almost beat-up, after the flight.

- **Belladonna:** take only if there is a hot, heavy feeling in the body. The face may be flushed. Take one dose every four hours, on an as-needed basis, depending on how long the flight is.

- ***Cocculus:** take if there is a worn out and spacey feeling after loss of sleep. Weak legs. May have nausea at the sight or smell of food.

- **Gelsemium:** take if there is extreme physical tiredness, with a heavy feeling in all the limbs. Take one dose every four hours and repeat if the flight is longer than four hours.

- **Nux vomica:** take if after arriving at your destination, you fall asleep but wake up miserable. Chilly with constipation and muscle cramps. Craving alcohol and coffee.

ILL EFFECTS OF AIR-CONDITIONING

Sitting in a cold draft, such as from the plane's air conditioning system, can take a toll, resulting in symptoms ranging from earaches, headaches and colds to hives to facial paralysis (also known as Bell's palsy), not to mention a stiff neck and shoulders.

The first remedy to consider is **Aconite**. If this doesn't have any effect after several doses, try ***Causticum**, particularly for any paralytic symptoms. For itching, hive-like eruptions from the cold air, try **Rhus tox** or ***Dulcamara**.

Remember to turn off the air or at least position the nozzle so the current does not blow directly on you, especially if you are sensitive to drafts. Also, covering up can help shield you from the air conditioning.

ALTITUDE SICKNESS OR MOUNTAIN SICKNESS

Altitude sickness, also known as mountain sickness, is an acute illness that occurs for those not used to being in higher altitudes. It typically occurs around 8,000 feet—or 2,400 meters—or higher above sea level. Hikers, skiers, adventurers, and travelers to higher altitudes can experience it no matter how good a shape they are in.

Symptoms may include dizziness or light-headedness, nausea and vomiting, headaches, fatigue, loss of appetite, and shortness of breath on even the slightest exertion.

Most instances of altitude sickness are mild and resolve quickly, typically in a few days, once your body adjusts to the higher altitude. Some tourist places expect visitors to experience issues with the higher altitudes and offer oxygen assistance. Do your research before going to any high altitude location so you can be prepared. If you are anemic, have lung or respiratory issues, or are taking medications that lower your blood pressure, consult with your healthcare provider before making a trip to a higher altitude.

COMMON REMEDIES FOR ALTITUDE AND MOUNTAIN SICKNESS

	Arnica	Calcarea carb	Carbo veg
Onset	Ailments from high altitudes. Ailments from ascending.	Ailments from high altitudes. Ailments from ascending.	Ailments from high altitudes. Ailments from ascending.
Symptoms	Headache. Anxiety with vertigo. Difficulty breathing.	Vertigo. Headache. Oppression in chest. Difficulty breathing.	Headache. Difficulty breathing. Fainting. Bloating and indigestion.
Mood	Irritable and averse to company. Says "I am well," when they're actually sick.	Anxious and worried about their recovery. Obstinate.	Indifferent and apathetic. Can be irritable at their family.
Indications	Any trauma to the body. Jet lag. Nosebleeds.	Fear of heights. Even slight ascending causes problems. Out of shape.	Desire for fresh air and/or to be fanned. Frequent burping. Collapse.
Worse	Exertion. Touch. Being approached. Damp cold.	Ascending. Cold, wet weather. Exertion. Looking down from high places.	Being covered. Lying flat. Rich foods. Cold night air.
Better	Lying with head lower. Being outstretched.	Lying down. Breathing fresh air.	Being fanned. Sitting upright. Belching. Elevating feet.

Other remedies to consider: **Belladonna, *Coca** or **Gelsemium**.
Special dosing instructions: Give chosen remedy before arriving at the high altitude then repeat as needed for symptoms.

? WHAT'S THE FIRST REMEDY YOU THINK OF WHEN...

1. The traveler is experiencing buzzing in the ears, constant nausea with a splitting headache.
2. After a mountain climb, a headache develops with bloating and indigestion.
3. After an overseas flight, the passenger is experiencing extreme tiredness or lethargy with a heavy feeling in the limbs.
4. A passenger has a fear of flying, claustrophobia and has been pacing up and down the aisles during the flight.
5. Drinking water causes both vomiting and diarrhea leaving a burning sensation in the throat and anus.
6. You have tried everything (besides taking a remedy) to relieve the ear popping and pain.
7. A passenger in a car experiencing motion sickness has become extremely pale with a headache that is described as feeling like a band around the head.
8. Vomiting is very sour smelling and consists of undigested food from drinking water that may have been contaminated.
9. Catching a chill from the air blowing on you during an airplane flight, you have a stiff neck and shoulders and the beginning of an ear infection.
10. You have the feeling that you have mountain sickness from climbing that morning due to a headache, bloody nose and vertigo.

Answer key on page 325.

CHAPTER 25
Surgery Considerations

The prospect of having surgery can be quite scary for most of us. Emotions may range from giddiness, to anxiety and trepidation, to pure fear. Homeopathy can be very helpful before, during, and after surgery for easing emotional distress, allaying pain, reducing risk of infection, and speeding recovery. Some remedies have an affinity for various tissues in the body and can support recovery from various types of surgery. Homeopathic remedies can be used to recover from the effects of anesthesia, reduce bleeding, help with incision wounds, and assist the person in regaining their stamina post-surgery. Remedies will not interfere with pain or other conventional medications but may, in fact, allow a reduction in their dosage.

BEFORE SURGERY

Everyone can benefit from homeopathic support before surgery. If the person is experiencing anger, fear, anxiety, or weeping, it may be useful to select a remedy from the following chart:

COMMON REMEDIES FOR BEFORE SURGERY

	Aconite	Arsenicum	*Coffea	Gelsemium	Ignatia	Nux vomica	Phosphorus
Symptoms and Indications	Anxiety and panic attacks, often with a fear they will die. Very restless, feels better with company. Heat and flushing to the face, thirsty for cold drinks, cold extremities, pupils constricted.	Anxious and prone to panic attacks, with the fear they may die. Feel chilly. May have burning stomach pain with their anxiety and/or diarrhea with burning pain. May be thirsty and take small, frequent sips of liquid.	Anxiety is experienced as inability to sleep, with uncontrollable thoughts and a racing mind. May experience a headache and general weakness.	Fearful, though presents as timid and reserved. May have weakness, forgetfulness, and difficulty thinking. Also trembling from anticipation, sticky perspiration, chills alternating with heat, and a worn-out expression.	May be an element of grief around the surgery. Easily hurt feelings, sighs a lot, and averse to consolation. May experience perspiration only on the face, coughing fits, or back spasms.	Feeling angry. Easily offended and irritable. Can be chilly, sensitive to light and noise. May have stomach cramps and/or insomnia.	Anxious when alone and better around company. Hungry and thirsty and feel better after eating. Sympathetic and easily reassured.

Another remedy to consider for fear of anesthesia is *Aethusa.

Dosing: Give one dose of the chosen remedy the night before the surgery. If needed, another dose can be given the morning of surgery.

THE DAY OF AND AFTER SURGERY

Homeopathy can make a profound difference during the first 24 hours following surgery. Consider using homeopathic support for adverse reactions to anesthesia (see section in this chapter) and for physical trauma and shock related to surgery.

ADVERSE REACTIONS TO ANESTHESIA

Some people may experience adverse reactions to anesthesia after surgery, such as nausea or vomiting, disorientation, and dizziness or difficulty walking for more than a few hours after waking from anesthesia.

Remedies to consider:

- **Phosphorus:** for anesthesia reactions, especially if there is vomiting. The person is fearful and complains a lot, yet is sweet-natured, seeks affection, and craves ice-cold drinks. As people needing **Phosphorus** tend to be chemically sensitive, they can have difficulties coming out of anesthesia. **Phosphorus** speeds the process of regaining full consciousness and feeling grounded once again. This remedy can be given before surgery if the person has previously experienced vomiting from anesthesia after surgery. It can also stave off possible post-op hemorrhaging.

- **Nux vomica:** if there is constant nausea with violent, but ineffectual, retching and possibly a feeling of faintness. Those needing **Nux vomica** have a hard time vomiting, but when they succeed their vomit is sour-smelling and can be full of bile or bitter mucus. Their stomach and intestines feel bruised and sore, with cramping, gas, sour and bitter belching, and dryness of the mouth. They are chilly and are often constipated. These persons tend to be driven and may be angry, irritable, nervous, and spiteful or, at the other extreme, very sensitive and easily offended. Sleepy during the day, they have a hard time falling asleep at night.

- **Ipecac:** for constant and unyielding nausea that is incapacitating and not relieved by vomiting. They may have a terrible headache with their nausea, be unable to stand the smell of food, have increased salivation, and experience horrible cutting and cramping pains. Their face is flushed and may be hot on one side.

Dosing: Start with the ORANGE method and gradually move to the BLUE method as symptoms improve. Observe and evaluate.

THE DAY AFTER SURGERY

Homeopathy can be extremely helpful during the recuperative phase following surgery by addressing the deep shock to the system and trauma to the body, and by speeding repair of injured tissue.

Two primary post-surgery remedies to give are **Arnica** and **Calendula: Arnica** for pain, bruising and soreness following any surgery and **Calendula** for healing surgical wounds. You can give one dose of each twice a day for one week following surgery. It's best not to combine the remedies but to take them separately, allowing one hour or more between them.

Following is a brief overview of remedies for healing from specific types of surgeries. *Also consult the chart in this section,* **Common Remedies for Post-Surgery.**

General note: IF the remedy **Silicea** is indicated AND the person had a foreign object surgically implanted into the body, it is suggested to wait 6 months or more to dose it. This is because **Silicea** has an affinity for pushing foreign objects out of the body, such as a splinter. The jury is out among some homeopaths whether it really is an issue or not but to be on the safe side, consider looking for another remedy for the current symptoms.

- Abdominal or Pelvic Surgery: *****Bellis per** or **Staphysagria.** Consider *****Bismuth** if there is intense vertigo, with nausea and vomiting, especially of fluids. There may also be attacks of violent epigastric pain.

- Amputation: **Hypericum**

- Appendectomy: **Rhus tox**

- Breast Surgery:
  - ***Phytolacc**a: this remedy has an affinity for the breast. Someone needing ***Phytolacca** may have a history of fibrocystic breasts, mastitis, or mammary abscesses, with breasts that are hot, swollen, hard, and extremely painful. They may feel worse at night and from cold, damp weather, even developing lumps in the breast with each wet, cold spell.
  - ***Hamamelis**: a remedy for slow, steady, passive hemorrhages, ***Hamamelis** has an affinity for the chest walls. This is a remedy to consider when a breast must be removed in whole or in part. There is a sense of bruised soreness throughout the body.
  - ***Bellis per**: a remedy to consider, in addition to **Arnica**, after plastic surgery on the breast or where there is an injury to the breast.

- Bunion Surgery: **Bryonia, Ruta, *Symphytum**

- Cesarean Section: **Arnica, *Bellis per**

- Circumcision: **Staphysagria, Arnica**

- Dental Surgery:
  *See also **Chapter 9—Mouth and Teeth** on **page 105.***
  - **Hypericum:** for shooting pains from nerve involvement
  - **Ruta:** for deep bone pains, or if the jaw is sore from overstretching
  - **Staphysagria:** oral surgery often requires an incision and suturing. This remedy will help ease any pain from that part of the operation
  - If a dental implant has been inserted, consider a course of ***Symphytum** and ***Calcarea phos** to help regenerate bone in the jaw, following the recommendations for orthopedic surgery

- Eye Surgery: **Aconite** (following eye surgery, use a low potency, such as 6c daily, for up to a week)

- Gallbladder Surgery: **Lycopodium**

- Gastrectomy: ***Raphanus sativus** for incarcerated gas

- Hemorrhoid Surgery: ***Aesculus, Staphysagria**

- Laparoscopic Surgery: **Ledum, Hypericum**

- Orthopedic Surgery:
  - **Arnica:** in cases of broken bones, this remedy should be given first, preferably in 200c, to minimize shock and swelling of surrounding tissue from trauma.
  - ***Eupatorium perf:** affinity to the bones, with bruising and acute intense pain from fractures. Intense pain, the bone feels as if it is broken, and the pain is worse with motion. **Do not give *Eupatorium perf before a broken bone is set.**
  - ***Symphytum:** this remedy is to be used only AFTER a broken bone is set. It facilitates a strong union of the break, speeds healing of the fracture of the bone, and reduces pain. **Like *Eupatorium perf, DO NOT GIVE BEFORE a broken bone is set, as it will facilitate union of the bone.** The pain can be severe. With ***Symphytum**, the pains persist long after the injury. May also be used for phantom limb pain after amputation.
  - ***Calcarea phos:** usually follows ***Symphytum** to ensure proper mineralization of the healing fracture.
  - **Ruta:** this remedy is indicated for any surgery involving primarily the cartilage, such as arthroscopic surgery on the knees.

- Plastic Surgery: **Arnica** internally and **Calendula ointment** externally

- Prostate Surgery: **Staphysagria**

- Spine or Coccyx Surgery: **Hypericum**

- Surgery for Bullet/Stab Wounds: **Staphysagria**

- Tonsillectomy/Adenoidectomy: **Rhus tox, *Phytolacca**

- Varicose Veins Surgery: **Ledum, *Hamamelis**

COMMON REMEDIES FOR POST-SURGERY

	Arnica	*Bellis per	Bryonia	Calendula	Hypericum	Ledum	Ruta
Symptoms and Indications	For post-operative recovery. It absorbs blood in the soft tissue and assists with reducing inflammation. May feel sore and constantly change position to feel comfortable. May not want to be approached or touched and may insist that nothing is wrong. Useful for both the trauma and shock associated with surgery.	Recuperation after surgery on the trunk of the body. May feel sore and bruised. Can help person recover from incision, bruising, and bleeding under the skin. Continues the work of **Arnica** to completely clear the bruising and other healing tissue.	For healing of bones and cartilage. Sharp, stitching pain, worse from any slight motion and is better from lying on the painful side. May feel irritable and prefer to be alone. Dry mouth with great thirst.	Very helpful for wounds and incisions related to surgery. Controls bleeding, prevents infection, and promotes healing. Can be applied topically or taken internally. (Note: if also using topically, area must be cleaned thoroughly before application since **Calendula** helps the skin heal rapidly)	Trauma or injury to nerve-rich areas, especially crushing, puncture or lacerations. For head, toes, teeth, spine, fingers. Also, for after laparoscopic surgery. For sharp, shooting, nerve-like pains.	For puncture wounds and after laparoscopic surgery. Feels better with cold and worse with heat. Wound can feel cold with purple bruising and swelling.	For injury to the connective tissue, tendons and periosteum (the membrane that covers the outer surface of the bones.) Very stiff, easily fatigued, and worse from exertion. Injuries from twisting motion and/or chronic overuse. Stiff and bruised. Affected area may be weak and lame. Specific for knee surgery involving tendons and ligaments.

Dosing: After surgery, give one dose of the indicated remedy and observe and evaluate. If symptoms persist, use the BLUE method. Continue to observe and evaluate.

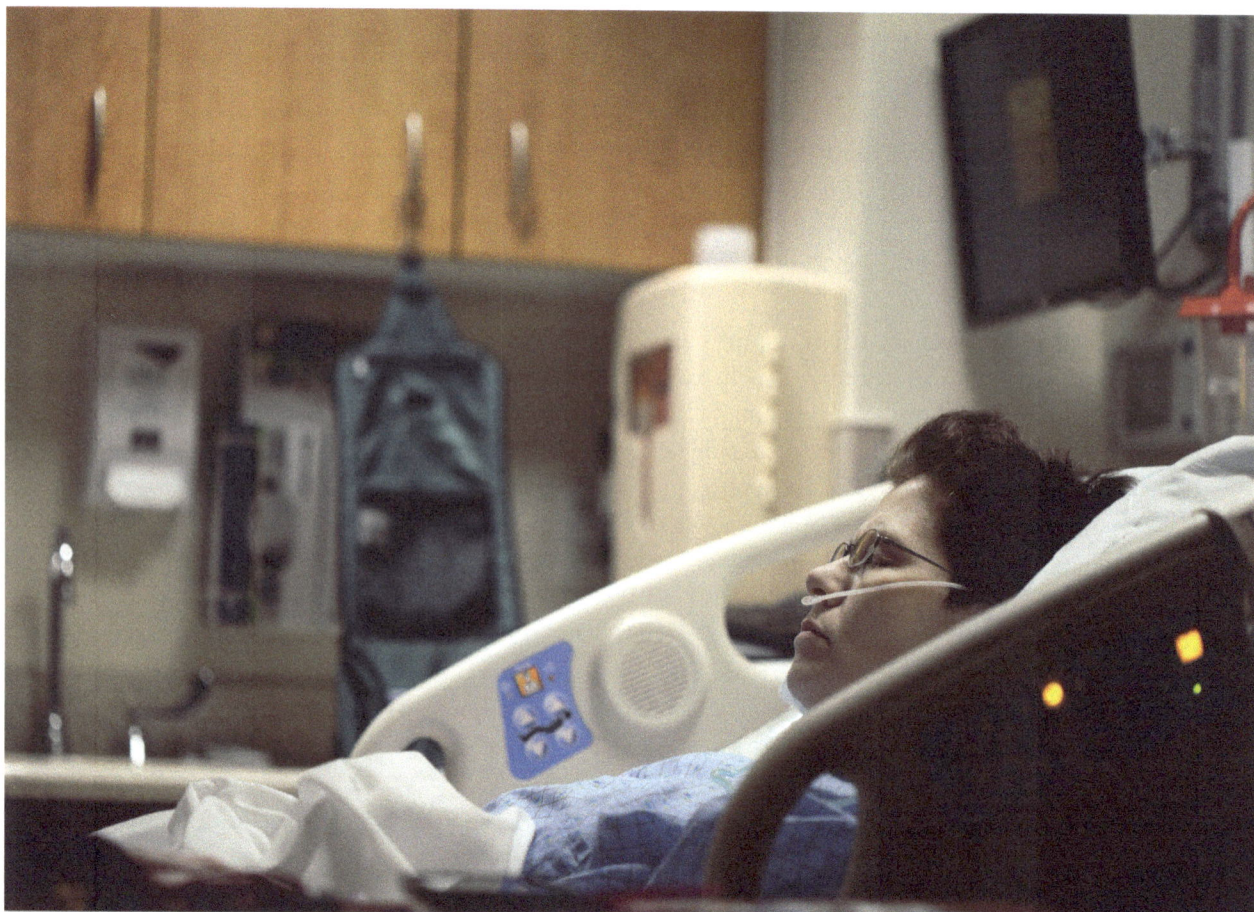

RECUPERATING AFTER SURGERY

Homeopathy can be extremely helpful in getting people back into the swing of life—the way it was before the surgery. Think of homeopathic remedies for shock, post-operative depression, weakness, and prolonged prostration.

WHEN TO CONTACT YOUR HEALTHCARE PROFESSIONAL OR SURGEON

- You feel that someone is not recovering from surgery in a timely manner.
- Depression or negativity persists for more than a few days, consider consulting with a professional homeopath.

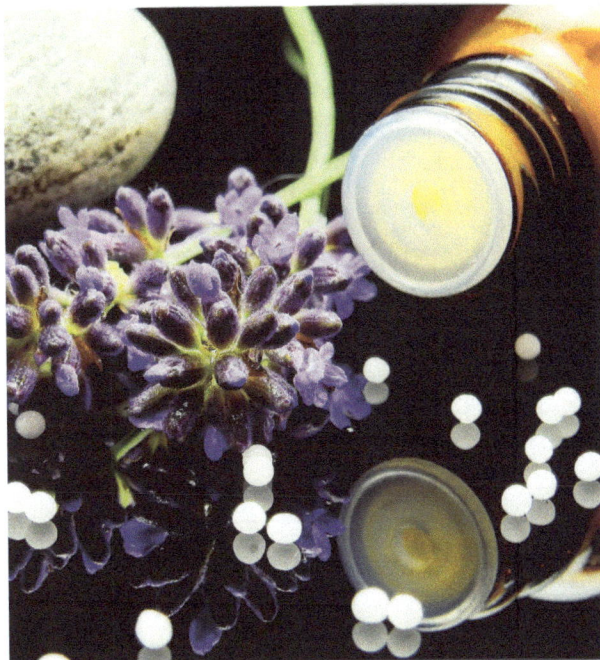

COMMON REMEDIES FOR RECUPERATING AFTER SURGERY

	Aconite	Arnica	Carbo veg	China	Pulsatilla	Staphysagria
Symptoms and Indications	Very fearful, anxious, extremely reactive to pain. Inconsolable, with glassy eyes or dilated pupils. Likely to be screaming, crying out, and trembling with terror or pain.	Stunned, irritable when offered help, exhausted, and uncooperative. Say that they are fine, and don't want to be touched. May complain of pain, but will maintain that not much is wrong with them.	Debilitated and collapsed, both physically and mentally. Indifferent, apathetic, and irritable. Feels cold, but doesn't want to be covered up. Desire for open air or to be fanned.	Debilitated and in a collapsed state, but contrary to **Carbo veg**, they are aggravated by drafts of air. Moody and sarcastic. May have abdominal bloating with burping and gas. May have night sweat and difficulty sleeping.	Sadness after surgery. May weep frequently and feel much better with consolation. Warm and aggravated by heat. Thirstless despite having a dry mouth.	From the trauma of the surgical knife. Person is acutely aware of the incision, feels indignation toward the surgeon or family, or has been very angry since the operation. Post-surgical depression or negativity.

Special dosing: Give the chosen remedy once a day until improvement begins. After three days, consider another remedy if not better.

A note about Bach Flower Rescue Remedy®: This flower essence reduces the effects of fright, shock, emotional trauma, grief, fearfulness, and panic or hysteria. It will restore a sense of balance, calm, and harmony. It's found in some drug stores, health food stores and online in various styles: liquid (contains some alcohol), pastilles, pillules, gum, etc. **Bach Flower Rescue Remedy®** was invented by an English homeopath and comprises five different flower essences. It is acceptable to give alongside homeopathic remedies.

POST-SURGICAL BLEEDING

If bleeding persists following surgery, consider using one of the remedies below or **Calendula**.

*See also the section in this chapter on **How to Care for a Surgical Incision** on **page 299**.*

IT'S AN EMERGENCY WHEN

- Bleeding from anywhere that is severe or persistent.

COMMON REMEDIES FOR POST-SURGICAL BLEEDING

	China	*Crotalus	Ipecac	Lachesis	*Millefolium	Phosphorus
Symptoms and Indications	If person is experiencing symptoms as a result of loss of fluids, such as blood loss, vomiting, and/or diarrhea. May feel irritable and sensitive, does not like to be touched, has a bitter taste in their mouth, has night sweats and insomnia.	Widespread bleeding from any orifice, even tears or sweat. Blood tends to be dark and unclotted. Good for retinal hemorrhage or gastro-intestinal bleeding.	Tendency for hemorrhage with nausea and/or headache. Consider for a uterine hemorrhage with bright red uncoagulated blood.	Thin, dark, almost black blood. Great exhaustion. Much bleeding from small wounds. Flushes of heat. Wound may have purplish discoloration. Tense and nervous, both physically and mentally. May talk a lot. Good for a retinal hemorrhage.	Profuse bright-red blood. Blood is very thin. Wound feels bruised, but not much pain. Bleeding may include a copious mucus discharge. Keep the person resting, as bleeding will start again upon exertion. Especially helpful after a tonsillectomy or nosebleed. May be moaning and spacey.	Bright-red, thin, constant, slow-streaming blood. Persistent bleeding of even small wounds. The wound tends to break open and bleed again. One of the most common remedies for bleeding that persists after surgery. Especially helpful for extensive bleeding after tooth extraction.

Dosing: Use the ORANGE method. Observe and evaluate.

BLEEDING FROM THE MOUTH

After getting the bleeding to stop, you can spray on diluted **Calendula tincture**. This solution can be used three times a day until the wound is healed.

*For more info, see **Chapter 9—Mouth and Teeth: Blows to the Mouth, Lips, Jaw and Teeth** starting on page 106.*

BLEEDING FROM THE NOSE

After getting the bleeding to stop, the blood vessels in the nose are in a fragile state. Some people may keep getting bloody noses.

Put a small dab of **Calendula cream or ointment** on a cotton swab and apply to the inside septum of the nose three times a day. The septum of the nose is the bone and cartilage that divide the nasal cavity of the nose in half. You can purchase **Calendula cream or ointment** at a health food store, some drug stores or online.

*For more on **Nosebleeds**, see **Chapter 8—Nose** on page 99.*

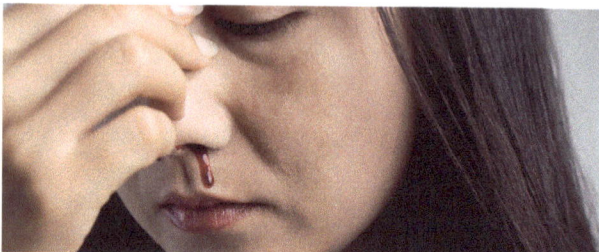

CATHETER REMOVAL PAIN AND DISCOMFORT

Give one dose of **Staphysagria**. Repeat only if the pain returns.

DIFFICULTY URINATING OR DEFECATING AFTER SURGERY

*Causticum** is helpful if surgery has resulted in difficulties passing urine owing to weakening or paralysis of the muscles of expulsion. *Causticum** can act as a homeopathic catheter, assisting the person with the return of urination following surgery. It can also help if the opposite has happened, namely, that the urinary sphincter has become paralyzed, leading to involuntary urination. Give one dose hourly until the person urinates.

Nux vomica can be useful if the person experiences constipation as a result of pain medication. Give one dose up to three times a day. Stop once the bowels begin to move, repeat if they stop again.

*Raphanus sativus** is indicated for the colicky pain of incarcerated gas that often follows abdominal surgery. The bowels may move but no gas passes, and the abdomen swells, grows hard, and is painful from pressure. Give one dose three to four times a day until the gas is released.

HOW TO CARE FOR A SURGICAL INCISION WOUNDS

🏥 IT'S AN EMERGENCY WHEN

- Wounds that become severely infected will exhibit pus-filled pockets, extreme redness, swelling, and tenderness. In a case of severe infection, there will be red streaks running up the extremities toward the heart, and there may or may not be a fever present. If this is the case, dial 911 or take the person to the nearest emergency room.

Staphysagria is the primary remedy for incision wounds, helping them to heal quickly and properly. The incision may be unusually painful, sensitive to the touch, and itchy; there may also be an emotional state of feeling wounded or humiliated, or anger or indignation towards the surgeon for being cut.

💚 ADDITIONAL SUPPORT FOR INCISION WOUND CARE:

- Allow a wound to bleed for a short time. This cleanses the wound and activates lymphocytes (immune cells that produce antibodies).
- Wash the wound well with warm, mild-soapy water.
- When the wound is clean, apply a solution of **Hypercal**, a combination of **Hypericum tincture**, which heals damaged nerves, and **Calendula tincture**, which repairs damaged skin. This combination is invaluable when applied topically (see instructions for making **Hypercal** below); it not only brings about rapid healing but helps prevent scarring and reduces pain. You can obtain these tinctures at any health-food store, natural pharmacy or online. It is very important, however, not to use them full-strength, because they will sting.
- When the wound is no longer oozing, you may use Vitamin E oil or **Calendula cream** or **ointment** to prevent scarring. (**Calendula gel** should be used only after the wound has scabbed over as it will sting an open wound.) The cell salt ***Calcarea fluor 6x** is also helpful in treating surgical scars.
- Even with great care, some wounds may become slightly inflamed and swollen, with redness around the margins. If this is the case – and especially if pus has developed – you can give a dose of **Hepar sulph**, three times a day for three to five days. (The exception is if there are surgical stitches, in which case **Hepar sulph** should not be used until these are due to be removed.)

> **How to Make Hypercal Solution**
> *Make **Hypercal** by putting five drops each of **Calendula tincture** AND **Hypericum tincture** to a ¼ cup of spring water, distilled water, or fresh water that has been boiled and cooled. The wound must be clean before applying this solution. Alternatively, you may use a solution of only **Calendula tincture**, prepared in the same way as the **Hypercal**. Apply a sterile piece of gauze or a bandage dampened with a solution of either **Hypercal** OR **Calendula tincture**. It is important to keep the gauze moist to prevent it from sticking to the wound. The dressing should be changed once a day. **Calendula** tincture helps to prevent scarring and keeps pus from forming. It prohibits germs from thriving, but does not kill them. That is why it is important to clean the wound first.*

Important note: Never put **Arnica cream, gel,** or **tincture,** on an open wound: these are to be applied ONLY to unbroken skin.

Dosing: Give once daily until the incision begins to heal.

BEDSORES

Bedsores, also known as pressure sores or decubitus ulcers, can occur in those who are bed- or wheelchair-bound for any length of time. Prolonged pressure on the skin, especially over bony areas such as the heels, ankles, tailbone, and hips, gradually breaks down both the skin and underlying tissues.

Most surgeries today presume minimal recuperation time; the impetus is definitely to get patients out of bed and into rehab activities as quickly as possible. The kind of situation that gives rise to bedsores is more likely to occur with people requiring long-term nursing, such as the elderly infirm or paralyzed patients. Poor nutrition, smoking, and impaired blood flow, as from diabetes or vascular disease, also increase one's vulnerability. For someone at risk, bedsores can develop within hours or days.

Bedsores, like many diseases, have stages of development.

Stage 1: The skin, typically over a bony prominence, is pink or red but intact; it does not blanch (turn white) when touched. (It may be hard to see the beginnings of a bedsore on dark skin.)

Stage 2: There is some loss of epidermis and a shallow red/pink wound but no sloughing (separation of dead tissue from living tissue). There may be a blister over the ulcer.

Stage 3: The ulcer has penetrated both the epidermis and the dermis into subcutaneous fat; deeper layers, like muscle and bone are not yet exposed.

Stage 4: The ulcer has penetrated through all subcutaneous tissue, exposing tendon, muscle, or bone.

WHEN TO CONTACT YOUR HEALTHCARE PROFESSIONAL

- If a bedsore becomes infected, there may be fever and chills, considerable pain and heat at the site, along with swelling, a foul smell, and possibly oozing pus.
- You may be able to care for Stage 1 or Stage 2 bedsores, but deeper ulcers require wound specialists, proprietary dressings, debridement (the removal of dead tissue), and possibly surgery.
- Be aware that bedsores can have serious complications, including cellulitis (infection of soft tissue) and bone and joint infections. Bedsores can turn gangrenous, often fairly rapidly, which may require amputation. They can even turn cancerous.

ADDITIONAL SUPPORT FOR BEDSORES

- Changing body position frequently is the best way to prevent bedsores, though this may require help. A useful rule of thumb is to shift one's weight at least once an hour. If you're in a wheelchair and have enough upper body strength, try doing wheelchair pushups to move the pressure points around.
- It's also helpful to use special cushions or mattresses (low air pressure, sheepskin bed pad, etc.) to relieve the pressure. If you have an adjustable bed, elevate the head no more than 30 degrees to reduce the likelihood of sliding down in bed, which causes the shearing of tissue over bone and friction from skin rubbing against clothing, two more ways in which fragile tissue can be injured.
- Be sure to keep the skin dry and clean, as it becomes much more vulnerable if moistened by urine and stool, or even perspiration. A developing bedsore may be cleansed with sterile saline solution and very gently patted dry. In areas where pressure sores might develop, use moisture barrier creams to protect the skin. Check regularly for changes in skin color or sensations like tenderness, warmth, or coldness.
- A nutritious diet and staying well hydrated are vitally important. Bedsores are more likely to develop in someone who is malnourished. They are also more likely to develop in smokers, and nicotine will slow their healing.

COMMON REMEDIES FOR BEDSORES

	Apis	Arnica	*Fluoricum acidum	*Petroleum	*Secale	Silicea	*Sulphuricum acidum
Symptoms and Indications	Rosy pink bedsores, burning sensation and pain, especially upon touching the spot. Desire to be uncovered to reduce burning and pain.	Sores on areas of scanty muscular tissue, especially over sacrum and hips. Sores form early and progress rapidly. Black and blue spots on skin. Change from side to side in bed searching for soft place to rest, complaining the bed is too hard. May complain area is itching.	Obstinate ulcerations and bedsores, especially on parts that don't perspire such as ankles. Sweat may excoriate the skin and cause an ulcer to develop. Ulcers can have blisters, copious discharge, red, inflamed edges that are hard and glassy. Skin tends to break down near bone or cartilage. Itching around edges.	The slightest scratch makes the skin suppurate. Skin is cracked, extremely sensitive, clothing painful. Ulceration of the legs and feet, originating in blisters; feet are tender and bathed in a foul moisture. Deep ulcers with stinging pain and raised edges. Pus scanty, acrid corroding, watery and blood-stained. Violent itching.	Sores over the sacral area, commonly in people with paralytic diseases. There are pricking sensations, numbness in the limbs with progressive ascending paraplegia. Prominent is a burning sensation though the skin may feel cold to touch. Marked aversion to heat and being covered.	Inflammations tend to fester ending in suppuration or refusing to heal. Ulcers may have sensations of coldness, be painfully sensitive, particularly on the feet and toes. Hard ulcers with reddened surrounding flesh, corroding pus and offensive smell. The pus can be bloody.	Bruises easily, sore black and blue spots that seemingly last forever. Gangrene develops from injuries, including bruises, especially in the elderly. Old, indolent ulcers that easily ooze dark blood. Stinging, burning pain in ulcers, with thin yellow or bloody discharge. Putrid ulcers on legs.
Worse	Warm room, heat of bed.	Touch.	Warmth.	From cold in winter. Touch of clothes.	Affected parts covered.	Cold, drafts. Touch, pressure.	Open air, cold. Excessive heat or cold.
Better	Cool air.	Damp cold air.	Cold.	In summer. Warm air, dry weather.	Oddly, the sensation of numbness is better by rubbing. Burning sensation better by cold applications and uncovering.	Warmth.	Warmth or moderate temperature.

Dosing: Use the BLUE method. Observe and evaluate. If the bedsore is growing larger or the ulceration deepening, call your healthcare provider for a referral to specialized wound care practitioners.

ADHESIONS AND SCARRING

Consider *Graphites 6c once daily for two to three weeks, if there is concern about the formation of adhesions or scarring from an incision. Another remedy if scars form, especially keloids, or adhesions have already formed, is *Thiosinaminum 12c.

WEANING OFF PAIN MEDICATION

For some who have been dependent on pain medications, it can be very challenging to stop using them. To help with the cravings, consider taking one dose of **Nux vomica**, dissolved in a 16-ounce water bottle, with one sip given as frequently as needed for any symptoms of withdrawal or as cravings for the medication are experienced. One bottle treated with the remedy can be used per day as needed.

? WHAT'S THE FIRST REMEDY YOU THINK OF WHEN...

1. The person has just had surgery.
2. The person is having a panic attack the night before their surgery.
3. There's vomiting after the anesthesia.
4. Someone needs healing from a surgical wound.
5. There is plastic surgery on the breast.
6. The bone is set and ready to heal after orthopedic surgery.
7. The person just had orthopedic surgery.
8. You want to support a person mentally or emotionally who is recuperating from surgery.
9. The person isn't passing urine or defecating after surgery.
10. There is any type of incision wound.
11. There is inflammation and pus discharging from a wound.
12. Someone is dependent on pain medications and wants to get off them.

Answer key on page 325.

Chapter 26
Homeopathy for Pets and Plants

One of the many beautiful and mysterious things about homeopathy is that it is not concerned with size, weight, or even species. Homeopathy supports the vitality of any living entity—be it a human, animal, plant, tree, or even our soil.

This chapter will provide you with the opportunity to broaden your study of homeopathy to now include the pets, plants, gardens, and wildlife around you. It can also be used for growing seasonal vegetables, so you know you are eating healthy!

Homeopathy for Pets

What kind of pets benefit from homeopathy?

All animals can benefit from homeopathy. Homeopathy is used with cats, dogs, horses, rabbits, chickens, goats, sheep, ducks, wildlife, and more. In many cases, the remedies and the dosing we use for people are the same as for animals and plants.

How do you know what to give your pets?

For animals, as with people, we look for the totality of symptoms. If you observe your pet when they are healthy, you will get a "baseline" for their typical behaviors. So when they are unwell, your continued observations will be incredibly helpful for choosing a homeopathic remedy for the different, new, and specific conditions and symptoms.

How do you go about finding the totality of symptoms with your pet?

As you approach taking your pet's case, do your best to set aside the tendency to humanize your pet's emotions and mental state. Focus on what you can observe that is different from your pet's normal/regular behavior or their baseline.

Similar to, yet a little different from, the CLAMS case-taking introduced in *Chapter 2—Taking the Case and Giving the Remedy* starting on *page 25*—you will focus on the five areas that aggregate to the totality of symptoms for your pet. These areas can be used to establish your pet's baseline as well as for identifying specifics for remedy choices when they are unwell or when you feel they are in need of a remedy.

If you're just looking to establish your pet's baseline, then your symptom picture will be broader than if there is something that needs to be resolved, such as a wound, bee or insect bite, diarrhea, skin eruptions, behavior, etc. **Take the example case of a dog named Hann, who was recently stung by a bee;** consider the following five areas for each condition or symptom:

1. LOCATION and SENSATION

Where is the symptom located and what do you observe? In the example of Hann, the dog, where is the bee sting and what does it look like? Is it red and swollen? Warm or cool to the touch? Any discharge? Does touching the area aggravate?

Observation sample: Front right paw, one sting only, large bump, feels hard, red skin under fur, feels hot. No discharge from the wound and no apparent stinger remains in the wound.

2. CAUSE

When did it occur or begin? Make note of the event that initiated a change in your pet. This may be simple: the bee sting occurred when your pet was in the yard, noting the date and time. Sometimes there are emotional reasons for a symptom, such as the owners went away for the weekend and the pet sitter reported your pet appeared upset or forlorn. It's helpful to note the place, date, and time of the event in case the symptom is more serious or repeats, such as in cases of skin rashes, behavioral challenges, etc.

Observation sample: August 1 mid-morning—Hann was sniffing the allium plants that are loaded with bees. He yelped and returned to the house licking his front right paw. He was restless and walking around in circles while we attempted to take a closer look at the paw.

3. TIME and FREQUENCY

What is the time and frequency of the symptom? In the case of a bee sting, this may be a single event but in other cases, you may identify a symptom that occurs regularly at a specific time of day such as in the evening, mid-day, or morning. Perhaps the symptom occurs hourly, daily, monthly, yearly, or upon the specific occurrence of an event. Very often the frequency leads us to identify events, routines, and seasons that trigger an animal's symptom(s) or condition. This is also a wonderful question to ask when working on resolving behavioral challenges in your pets.

Observation sample: This was a single event.

4. MODALITIES

What things or circumstances make the symptom or condition better or worse? Cold or hot applications, getting bathed, laying on a soft or hard surface, time of day or season, weather such as shade, heat, cold, rain, etc.

Some other modality examples may include:

- appetite and food preferences

- thirst

- preference for exercise/movement

- sensitivity to pressure or touch

- sensitivity to light, darkness, and noise

Observation example: After applying a cold cloth, Hann stopped licking the bee sting. The swelling and heat remained.

5. MOOD AND BEHAVIOR

What is your pet's mood and behavior? It can be a challenge for many of us to observe objectively our pet's mental and emotional symptoms. Below are some examples of pet behaviors to assist you with your assessment.

a. licking one or more areas of the body

b. unusual barking or other sounds

c. trembling

d. pacing

e. unusual stillness

f. pressing head against a wall or surface

g. pressing the back end of the body against a wall or surface

h. panting

i. unusual sweating

j. picking or chewing on one or more areas of the body

k. avoiding eye contact

l. avoiding touch

m. constantly looking at you and moving close

n. constantly looking at you and staying at a distance

o. reacting to noise

p. reacting to color

q. reacting to smell

r. reacting to touch

s. reacting to an animal's approach

t. reacting to people (may only react to a particular gender)

u. changes in eating

v. changes in drinking

w. possessiveness of food or toys

x. head shaking, bobbing, or other continuous body movement

y. biting into the air

z. pawing the ground

Observation example: Hann's mood was anxious, observed by his pacing and licking of his wound.

At this point, you have a list of symptoms and the unique characteristics of the symptoms. You have created a profile of your pet's current state!

It is time to consider some remedies. Let's start with the remedy given for the bee sting example.

Hann was given **Apis 30C** for three doses at 20-minute intervals. **Apis** is created from the honeybee. The symptoms that point us to this remedy are not simply because it was a bee sting but because of the characteristics of the sting; red with heat, burning, and swelling. An interesting emotional characteristic the dog displayed was anxiety and moving or "buzzing" around. This emotional characteristic also points us to **Apis**.

Read more about **Apis** *and other remedies for bee stings in* **Chapter 18—Skin** *starting on* **page 208**.

Remedy Dosing for Pets

Deciding on dosing frequency is similar to human dosing but will vary based on an animal's vitality and circumstances. Remember, observation and evaluation are key to deciding how much and how frequently to give a dose. Review **How Often to Give A Dose** in **Chapter 2** starting on **page 34**.

Understand that the dose size itself does not vary based on the animal's species or size. What's most important is for the remedy to reach the mucous membranes of the animal. Review **Special Dosing Instructions for Infants, Young Children or Pets** in **Chapter 2** on **page 35**.

How do I give my animal a remedy?

There are many views regarding how to provide remedies. The following guidelines work well and provide positive results when working with animals:

- Homeopathic remedies come in tiny white pellets or in liquid form. Either form can be placed directly into your pet's cheek or into their water bowl or bucket.

- Remedies can be dispensed into a small bathroom-size paper cup, or onto a spoon before giving the dose.

- Drop the remedy straight from a cup or spoon into your pet's cheek. Avoid the use of metal spoons or bowls.

- If your pet tends to spit out the pellets, then you can crush the pellets between two spoons creating a dissolvable powder that can then be placed into the pet's mouth to melt.

You may use a syringe to provide a dose directly into your pet's mouth especially if you have multiple animals in your home. One to two teaspoons is sufficient to ensure your animal has received a dose of the remedy.

If you want to add the remedy to their water, instead place one pellet in 8 oz of water. It is effective for animals (and plants). One dose consists of one session of drinking so once they get some into their mouths and they are finished drinking, take up the water dish and only put that one back down if another dose is needed. When finished with that bowl, thoroughly clean the dish with warm water and soap and dry with a clean cloth. A dry pellet dose needs to melt in a clean mouth on the pet's gums so the remedy should not be hidden in a treat or in food.

ADDITIONAL GENERAL GUIDELINES FOR DOSING

- Try not to handle the remedies any more than you need to and if you do, make sure your hands are clean and washed with a gentle soap that doesn't contain chemicals or strong astringents or herbs.

- Avoid pouring unused but handled remedies back into the bottle or vial to avoid contamination or inactivation.

- When giving an animal a remedy, have them avoid food or non-remedy water for 30 minutes.

- While working with remedies, protect your animal from exposure to strong odors including perfumes, essential oils (such as peppermint, eucalyptus, camphor, tea tree oil, tiger balm), or strong-smelling chemicals.

- Check labels of other products such as sprays, shampoo, liniments, treats, etc., as these substances may interfere with the action of the remedy if used in close proximity to dosing.

HOME USAGE AND SUPPORTING YOUR PETS HOLISTICALLY

Homeopathy is used with animals of all kinds for constitutional care, as a preventative and in non-emergency occurrences. It is also highly effective for animals with behavioral challenges and traumas. It is wonderful for animals that have suffered abuse and is used in many animal shelters since it is a gentle, effective, and affordable solution for organizations and people adopting animals that need ongoing care and support.

If this chapter is inspiring you to start using homeopathy for your pets, please note that it doesn't replace conventional care provided by a veterinarian. It's also important to note that when you have successfully resolved an observed symptom, it may not have eradicated an underlying problem that is identified by your pet's healthcare provider. Therefore, make sure to keep track of what remedies you have used and for what ailment, and provide that information to your veterinarian when you arrange a healthcare visit. Homeopathy works well with conventional care. Working together with your veterinarian will best serve your animal's overall well-being.

IT'S AN EMERGENCY WHEN

- Your pet was bitten by a snake or attacked by another animal.
- Your pet is unusually lethargic and unable to stand up or walk.
- Your pet has eaten something poisonous or has an unusually high fever.
- If your pet seems to be in a lot of pain or discomfort preventing them from bowel movement, urination, eating, drinking, or moving.
- If your pet has a head trauma, broken or torn a bone, ligament, etc.
- If your pet has an eye injury beyond a minor exterior scratch or abrasion.
- If your pet shows any sign of choking or a possible obstruction in their airway.

WHEN TO CONTACT A VETERINARIAN

- If your pet has frequent diarrhea or vomiting and is at risk for becoming dehydrated.
- If your pet has sudden stools that are bloody, excessive, watery.
- If your pet has a cough that does not quickly resolve or reoccurs.
- If your pet has a fever, vomiting, unusual sweating or panting.
- If your pet has unusual skin eruptions, abscesses or growths that do not quickly resolve or reoccur.
- If your pet has any eye injury or a complaint such as allergies that does not quickly resolve or reoccurs.
- If your pet has been in the presence of another animal identified as sick and/or unusual symptoms arise.
- Your cat is hiding and not coming out to eat, drink or socialize for longer than usual.

Behavioral Challenges

In behavioral and trauma cases, it is recommended to consult with a homeopathic professional for further guidance and training. Below are some examples of remedies that are helpful in such cases. We find great success for animals, especially in cases such as food aggression, a fear of being alone or separated from a person or another pet, or a fear of strangers, a particular gender, a venue, storms, specific noises or movement. The beauty of these remedies are that, if the remedy is well-suited, they work to improve not only the mental and emotional states of your pet but any physical symptoms as well!

We have delineated the remedy charts into three specific behavioral areas: aggressiveness, anxiety and fear, and grief.

COMMON REMEDIES FOR BEHAVIORAL ISSUES—AGGRESSIVENESS

	Lycopodium	Nux Vomica	*Stramonium
General Description	Aggression when cornered, kenneled or other animal or human are in their space, food, etc. Tends to be protective, greedy or pushy but when challenged will back down. Digestive disturbances that are caused by the emotional state. Aggression as a protective mechanism and tends to have remorse after they bite or are aggressive. In rescue situations where there is food aggression or animal feels overcrowded. Fear or anxiety around unfamiliar objects, animals and strangers. Anxious when unable to see their companion animal or human. Lack of self confidence, jealousy and may be very apprehensive or suspicious.	For aggressive behavior. Appears tense, alert. Wants to be in charge, defiant and overly sensitive. The alpha animal. Habit of kicking, growling or biting. Irritable, angry, stubborn, mischievous, indifferent, and jealous. Anger from correction. May frighten easily as they are constantly tense and reactive. Has a tendency to overeat, digestive complaints from over indulging. May be food aggressive and will not back down when challenged. Can be seen as lazy and irritable when asked to do anything simply because it doesn't want to do or has overeaten and doesn't feel well. May have a destructive nature and habits.	Aggression from a trauma or bad experience. From fear. A biting habit with a sense of remorse or guilt. Frightens very easily and will be terrified by anything related to the trauma or event, especially in the evening. Eyes may have a dilated fearful look caused by trauma or bad experience. Highly impacted by bright lights. Pushy, jealous, highly vocal, very insecure. Fear of enclosed places and water. May have a destructive nature and habits but you will feel a remorse in them unlike the destructive nature of **Nux vomica**.
Modalities	Worse when cornered in a room, stall, crate, or challenged, jealous.	Chilly and better by warmth, and aggravation after eating and from correction. Worse from noise, bright lights, crowds.	Animal tends to be worse in dark areas, when alone, from touch, or motion. Dislikes very cold water. Worse bright lights.
Physical Differential	Digestive complaints, overeating or food aggression.	Sensitive to stimuli such as change of routine, light, noise, and odors. May bark and growl.	Eyes are dilated and glassy. May have incessant barking, growling, etc.
Emotional Differential	Tends to be aggressive, the alpha, and possessive of their owner or herd.	Aggressive and jealous and may appear tense with dominant behavior.	Very hyperactive. Fear of water, dark and shadows. Sensitive to light, night terror-like symptoms. Rage is sudden and uncontrollable yet shows signs of remorse after the rage. Has a tendency to try to escape the terror.

COMMON REMEDIES FOR BEHAVIORAL ISSUES—ANXIETY AND FEAR

	Aconite	Argentum nit	Arsenicum	Gelsemium	Phosphorus
General Description	Anxiety. Often used in rescue situations, trauma. Tend to have a shocked, worried or startled look in their eyes. Startle easily. Useful when there is anxiety, anger or other unusual anxious behavior from a fright. May be a recent or past stressful experience that continues to be triggered by similar conditions or events. Behavior may be heightened in crowds, enclosed spaces, evening, bad weather. Other possible causes: an outdoor accident especially during a storm or rain; witnessing or involved in a fight or altercation with another animal or human; negative experience during a visit with a healthcare provider, groomer, or kennel stay; transportation loading accident; car accident; crating; thunderstorms; etc.	Anxious, fearful. Appears hurried, impulsive and may have irrational behavior. May have a fear of enclosed spaces, heights, strangers. Tends to be very active, intelligent, stubborn and desires to please owner. Very helpful for anticipatory anxiety in animals that are in competitions, agility, etc.	Anxiety and fear of being alone. May be a bit wary, insecure, nervous, frightens easily. Not interested in cuddling. For when a new animal or baby is introduced into the home and the existing animal begins to display signs of anxiety. Over grooming, bald or hot spots from chewing. Be a fussy eater and wants the security of being close to owner. Bothered by a change of routine and the hierarchy in the household May have fear of unfamiliar objects. General nature is gentle, reserved, timid, restless with possible pacing and talking especially in the evening. Helpful for separation anxiety. Also consider **Pulsatilla, Ignatia, Aconite.**	Anxious, with trembling. Anticipatory nerves with diarrhea or loose stools. Diarrhea from fright, shock, emotional excitement. A sensitive nature, timid or bashful. May tremble, be physically and emotionally weak or indifferent. For animals that tremble and hide during thunderstorms or loud events. Also consider **Phosphorus** and **Aconite**.	Affectionate, easily excitable. React to sudden changes in weather, environment, noises, smells. Highly sensitive and love energy of others—both animals and humans. Fearful and anxious, fear of water, and vehicles approaching. Spooks easily. Open and friendly. Very active and may easily overextend themselves. May jump up, nip or rough play with people or other animals as difficult to control their energy. Fun loving nature with lots of energy. Anxiety with excitement during thunderstorms or when left alone. Great remedy for spooked and bolting animals.
Modalities	Worse by dry cold winds, evening, and at night. Better in the open air.	Worse by warmth in any form, at night, after eating, from stress. Better by fresh air and in the cold weather.	Worse in the evening. Chilly and worse by cold. From exercise. Cold wet weather. Better by heat, warmth and company.	Worse in storms, damp weather, rain. Loud noises, excitement, exercise or activity. Better by open air, cold air, sweating and urinating.	Worse bright lights, noise, smells, cold, before and during thunderstorms, change of weather, emotional disturbance, touch. Better by warmth, eating, after rest, exercise, and open air.
Physical Differential	Symptoms appear suddenly although they may be caused by a past similar event. Fright with diarrhea.	Tends to be high energy and alert. May see trembling, diarrhea and gas. Photophobia.	Tends to be well groomed, tidy. May have diarrhea. Dry, scaly skin.	May look tired, weary, trembling. Diarrhea with frequent urination.	Very thirsty and hungry. Typically is lean and bright eyed.
Emotional Differential	Tends to react to every touch and sound. Tends to be light sensitive.	Tends to be impulsive, unpredictable and dislikes uncertainty.	Restless, sensitive to disorder or confusion. Nervous, pacing.	Quiet from fear, reserved, timid. Fatigue and weakness.	Very sensitive and reactive to many things yet very enthusiastic to participate in life.

COMMON REMEDIES FOR BEHAVIORAL ISSUES—GRIEF

	*Cocculus	Ignatia	Natrum mur	Pulsatilla
General Description	Wonderful remedy for motion-sickness and travel-sickness. (Also consider Pulsatilla). Helpful for grief in birthing where mother loses a baby and shows signs of grief, worry and looking for the baby. Typically a quiet disposition (also consider **Ignatia**).	For grief and often used in rescue situations. Typically an affectionate animal, may be vocal or "whiny." Sensitive to reprimands. For homesickness. Grief can be from a change of home, loss of a person or another pet. For separation anxiety such as when the owner is gone for extended periods of time, pets are separated for extended periods of time, animals within a herd are separated, loss of mother or baby in an animal birthing scenario. May see anger with anxiety but root cause is typically grief of some kind. Mood tends to be variable—between pining, anger, affectionate. (Also consider **Natrum mur, *Cocculus**)	Often used for rescue situations, long standing or multiple griefs, moves, trauma. Look wary or detached, often off on their own with distance between themselves, owners and other animals. Quiet, reserved and in severe cases of grief, both low appetite and thirst, eyes and body language may look defeated. Sensitive to reprimands. Emotionally and physically shutdown by grief and disappointment which may be seen as laziness. May see irritation and anger. Mood tends to be variable—between anger, irritation, distant or shutdown. When this remedy is well suited and given to an animal, we see a lightness and energy return as if a weight has been removed. Multiple doses are often given. (Also consider **Ignatia** for grief)	Affectionate, stay close to owner or other animals for reassurance and company. Tends to have a fear of crowds, enclosed spaces. Gentle nature, timid and insecure. Can also be clingy, whiny and very dependent on the owners. Constantly check back in with the owner or alpha before going too far away from their group. Like to be the center of attention and will attempt to be in your lap. Can become indifferent or sulky when do not get the attention they want. Moods are variable between affectionate, restless, sulky.
Modalities	Worse by travel, lack of sleep, touch, emotional upset, heat of the sun. Better laying down.	Worse in morning, open air, after eating. Better by eating, changing position or movement.	Worse by heat, noise, from too much attention, from exercise, mid-morning. Better by open air, gentle motion, sweating, rest, gentle massage of back.	Worse from heat, humidity, in the evening. Better by open air, gentle movement or exercise, massage and attention.
Physical Differential	Weakness in back legs, appears dizzy or off balance. In extreme cases signs of paralysis. Eyes may be droopy or just look tired.	Moves around a lot and is unable to find a comfortable place to rest.	Physically fatigued. Will not be especially hungry or thirsty. May have dry skin.	Looks friendly, laid back, heavier set, ready to receive or pounce for affection.
Emotional Differential	Nervousness. Great difficulty sleeping, getting comfortable but fatigued.	Irritable and difficult to please or calm. Has a look of anxiety, confusion, or fear in the eyes.	Reserved and will tend to go off on its own. A dull look of distrust or sadness in eyes although very sensitive to everything going on around them. Tend to absorb any sadness around them.	Changeable moods, sweet and engaging, calm, sometimes jealous but not aggressive. A little excitable at times and can be easily hurt from reprimands but quickly come back from it looking for affection.

Abscesses

Abscesses are very common in animals, and homeopathy is a wonderful option to consider. An abscess can be any swollen tissue with an accumulation of pus, including ulcers, cysts, boils, or other infections. Abscesses of the mouth from an injury or dental challenge, or skin, are common and can benefit from a well-suited remedy. The remedies are also very successful in abscesses located in the lower extremities, such as the feet or hoof, due to surface injury, exposure to damp weather, poor footing, after a procedure, etc.

COMMON REMEDIES FOR ABSCESSES

	*Calc sulph	Hepar sulph	Mercurius	Silicea
General Symptoms	Teeth, skin, foot, internal abscesses. Remedy assists with infection. Will bring an abscess to resolution and promote discharge.	Teeth, skin, foot, internal abscesses. Remedy assists with infection. Will bring an abscess to resolution and promote discharge.	All types of abscesses and other chronic skin conditions. Slow to heal or to come to a head. The animal tends to have a poor resistance to infection overall.	All types of abscesses and other chronic skin conditions. Slow to heal or slow to come to a head. May help with drainage and expulsion of foreign bodies through the skin. Also helpful for ringworm, fungal infections.
Modalities	Worse change of weather. Better in the open air, desire to be carried or comforted.	Chilly and aggravated by cold. The abscess is painful at the slightest touch.	Worse at night, wet damp weather, warmth of rug. Better by rest, tend to see symptoms on the right side of the body.	Abscess appears to cause only minimal pain. Chilly and wants to be warm or inside.
Physical Differentials	Lumpy yellow discharge. The animal tends to sweat easily.	Yellow discharge, offensive odor. Tends to sweat easily. Abscess tends to have significant inflammation or redness of the surrounding area.	An important indicator is the foul-smelling green discharge (sometimes bloody).	May see a little clear or slightly milky discharge, but no pain on touch. Symptoms are minimal or weak as the animal's immune system appears weakened. May see brittle hair, nails, and the animal's coat lacks luster or doesn't grow well with the change of seasons.
Emotional Differentials	Strong personality, bossy, irritable, whiny.	Anxious, and possibly irritable, May act out or have angry outbursts toward people or other animals.	Irritable but closed. Will present as depressed or withdrawn but may sense a quiet irritability or suspicion when approaching.	Animal tends to be quiet, and reserved. May lack self-confidence, anxious by noise.

Skin Issues

Skin conditions are increasingly common in our animals and can leave us feeling very frustrated after countless food and product changes produce minimal results. Seasonal allergies and vague environmental allergies are also on the rise in our pets. The remedies below are just a few to consider. In many cases your pet's skin conditions and allergies may be long standing, as far back as immediately following their birth. In such a case, consulting with a homeopathic vet for a constitutional remedy is advisable in order to see the best results.

COMMON REMEDIES FOR SKIN ISSUES

	Apis	Arsenicum	Ledum	Rhus tox	Silicea	Sulphur	*Urtica
General Description	Rashes, bites, welts, and stings of insects or unknown origin. Often have much redness and inflammation resembling bee stings. Can be any lesion, bite, or skin irritation that looks like one or multiple bee stings.	Lice, mange. Intense itchiness without or with only small eruptions. Eczema with dry skin and intense burning and itching.	Fleas, mites, lice, mange, ticks, insect, or snake bites.	Seasonal allergic reactions such as hives, sweet itch, plants such as poison ivy, grass, and chemically treated lawns and fields.	Itchiness, dry, brittle, or dry-looking coat. Cracked nails.	Allergy-based skin problems, dandruff, and scaling. Lice, mange, thrush, bacterial skin infections.	Seasonal allergic reactions such as hives, sweet itch, plants such as poison ivy, grass, chemically treated lawns and fields. Allergic reactions to foods. Very helpful in first-degree burns. Allergic reaction to shellfish.
Modalities	Burning pain, welts that resemble a bee sting. Better by cold, movement.	Itching worse by scratching. Worse midnight to 2 AM, on exertion, cold, wet weather. Better by heat and warmth and company. Tend to lack an appetite.	Worse from heat. Better by cold application or cold bath.	Worse after lying down. By cold water or bathing. Better by continuous motion and heat. Skin will be better with very warm water.	Chilly, worse by cold.	Worse by heat, wet weather, bathing. Better by dry weather if not too hot. Better by motion and eating.	Worse cold, aggravated by cool moist air, touch, and marked exertion. Worse by seasonal changes or sudden weather from warm to damp and cold. Better by rest.
Physical Differential	Welts, fluid production sometimes in areas of joints from a reaction to the environment or medicine. Usually feel some heat in the areas even if can't see redness due to hair and coat.	Typically, thin-looking, coat and skin dry, flaky, lackluster.	Skin greatly inflamed and swollen. Better with cold applications. Stiff-looking walk or gait.	Typically, lean animals. Itchy, may also notice cracking of joints, and overall stiffness after laying down, and will be better after moving around a bit.	Doesn't grow well or healthy. Slow to heal.	Looks unkept no matter how much grooming, unhealthy-looking coat, and skin. Bad odor from the coat.	Violent itching, burning.
Emotional Differential	Restless, noisy, irritable, angry, short-tempered. May be hard to please or calm.	Wants security. Anxious and restless.	Irritable, may seem touchy.	Restless and friendly but may be timid. May have the reputation of appearing to have a sense of humor and play tricks, hide things, etc. on owners or other animals. Always in motion.	Animal tends to be quiet, and reserved, may lack self-confidence, anxious by noise.	Tend to be lazy and easily distracted.	N/A

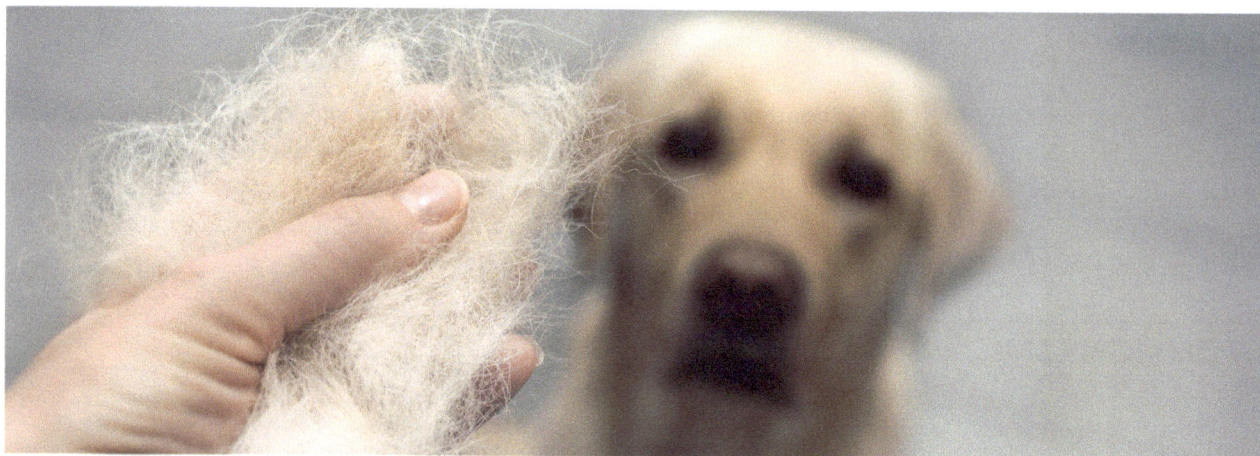

Hair Loss

Hair loss in pets, similar to in people, can be caused by allergies, medications, environmental factors; it is also often associated with stress. We don't always consider our animal's emotional state. Many things stress our animals, such as a change of routine, loss of an owner or another pet, addition to the family such as a newborn, visitors to the home, boarding, vet and groomer visits, etc.

Two common remedies for hair loss:

1. **Arsenicum**: this is a great remedy for hair loss in animals where you see hair loss and excessive self-grooming or where animals pull their hair or feathers out. They feel cold and thirsty but only for small amounts and tend to lack an appetite. This is typically a tidy pet in their grooming, litter box habits, etc. They remain close by, but don't wish to be snuggled or touched. They tend to be irritable, restless, anxious and are pacing. This remedy is very common when there is a change in routine in the home or herd, such as when people or animals are removed or introduced into the home, like a new baby.

2. **Silicea**: another great remedy for hair loss in which the skin and hair may lack luster and grow slowly. Look for poor stamina and any conditions that weaken the immune system. They tend to be chilly and seek warmth. The animal tends to become ill from the slightest weather changes and may lack vitality. They are quiet and reserved, may lack self-confidence, and feel anxious from noise.

Eye Issues

Eye complaints are abundant in our animals, including complaints from injuries, allergies, or conjunctivitis. Applying the classical principles of homeopathy, when looking at an eye complaint, we pay special attention to the discharge consistency, color, timing. When does the discharge occur? Time of day? After a meal? Change of environment, etc. We are also concerned with any discoloration within or around the eye, such as cloudiness, visible tears, dilation, etc. When an animal is experiencing pain or discomfort with an eye complaint, you often will see them scratch at the eye with a paw, rub along the ground, or blink excessively.

Eye complaints can be very serious, and a veterinarian should initially be consulted and informed of any homeopathic remedies provided to alleviate symptoms. With that said, we have seen many success stories using homeopathy for eye conditions that have been otherwise unresolved!

Homeopathic remedies are an excellent tool to use for your pets. At this point, you recognize many of the same remedies are used for multiple complaints. Remember, you will see your best results when you select a remedy that matches your pet at the physical, emotional and mental level. Pay attention if you keep seeing a remedy show up for the various symptoms your pet experiences!

COMMON REMEDIES FOR EYE ISSUES

	Aconite	*Allium cepa	Hepar sulph	Mercurius	*Sabadilla	Silicea	Sulphur
General Description	Acute conjunctivitis with great sensitivity to light. Susceptible to sickness from sudden storms with eye or other symptoms.	Allergy symptoms. Helpful when allergies involve the upper respiratory system especially the eyes.	Conjunctivitis infection with a fair amount of yellowish discharge.	Conjunctivitis Infection.	Seasonal acute allergy symptoms.	Infection of tear ducts or blocked tear ducts, styes. Slow healing, chronic eye ulcers.	Conjunctivitis infection.
Modalities	Symptoms appear suddenly, very often from a cold dry wind.	Worse in the evening, springtime, indoor dusty conditions. Aggravated by a warm room or application. Better in the open air.	Worse touch, dry cold winds, cool air, least draft. Better by warmth, damp weather, and after feeding.	Worse at night (sunset to sunrise). Wet damp weather. Worse in extremes of hot or cold.	Worse cold weather, cold air, drinking cold water. Better by warmth or covering. Thirstless.	Worse by cold air and weather, dampness, full moon. Better by warmth, summer covering, or rest.	Worse by heat, wet weather, bathing, standing around. Better by dry weather if not too hot. Better by motion and eating.
Physical Differential	Eyes will be red, with swollen lids and excess tears. Only one eye may be impacted.	Profuse watery irritating nasal discharge, sneezing. Watery eye discharge. Dry hacking cough.	Some kind of pus with a tinge of yellow and red with inflamed lids and eyes. A low pain threshold.	Green discharge, swollen, red sore looking eyes. Appears to be burning as the animal will rub their eyes on something for relief.	Watery thin irritating nasal and eye discharge with violent sneezing and inflamed eyelids. May have coughing or choking-like symptoms. May notice rubbing of eyes or nose with feet or on the surface for relief.	Chronic mild yet stubborn symptoms may come and go or take a long time to heal. History of skin, hair, and teeth challenges.	Redness, inflammation, and irritation of the margins of the lids.
Emotional Differential	Animals tend to react to every touch and sound. Tend to be light sensitive.	N/A	Anxious, and possibly irritable. May act out or have angry outbursts toward people or other animals.	Irritable but closed. Will present as depressed or withdrawn but may sense a quiet irritability or suspicion when approaching.	Nervous timid nature, easily startled, agitated.	Quiet, and reserved, may lack self-confidence, anxious by noise.	Can appear to be lazy and easily distracted.

Coughs*

> ***Important Note:*** Coughs can often be a key symptom in more serious conditions. If a cough does not quickly and permanently dissipate, the animal should be brought to a veterinarian for evaluation.

Our animals can be impacted by allergies, inactivity, weather changes, simple colds, etc. The remedies below are a few common ones to consider for a pet's cough.

Aconite: think of **Aconite** as the first remedy when a cough comes on suddenly, especially after being outside; for a sudden cold or respiratory issues after exposure to dry cold air. This remedy is very helpful for outdoor animals preventatively before a sudden temperature drop. The eyes may be red and tearing or they simply have clear to white nasal discharge, possibly a slight cough or congestion. They tend to react to every touch and sound and also tend to be sensitive to light.

Bryonia: for a dry cough and upper respiratory complaints. The animal is worse from touch and better with large quantities of water. The cough is worse eating, worse motion and worse in a warm room or enclosure. There is a desire to sit very still and not move. They tend to be irritable and standoffish.

Pulsatilla: for upper respiratory complaints with a dry cough in the evening and at night and a loose cough in the morning with copious mucus. The animal is clingy and seeks attention. They tend to be worse in the heat and sun and also worse while indoors but better in the cool outdoors. They desire to be touched and reassured. There may be a bland and yellowish-green nasal and eye discharge with congestion in the nasal passages. They tend to be timid yet seek attention.

Digestive Complaints

Many pets experience digestive complaints from a dietary change, too many snacks, or a stressor such as boarding, change of venue, etc. Homeopathic remedies are a gentle way to address stomach upsets and strengthen your pet's overall digestion and bowels.

MOST COMMON REMEDIES FOR DIARRHEA/COLITIS

	*Aloe	Arsenicum	Lycopodium	Nux vomica	*Podophyllum
General Description	Colitis related to diet, worms, ulcers, and medications. Helpful for digestive side effects from medicine. Also consider **Nux Vomica.**	Colitis is accompanied by nausea and vomiting. Stomach ulcers, watery foul diarrhea (may see blood) with collapse or weakness. Helpful in cases of suspect food or foraging on toxic plants. Also consider **Nux Vomica.**	Colitis is related to the mental and emotional state of the animal such as anxiety and confidence challenges. Helpful for low-grade chronic colitis.	Helpful in cases of suspect food or foraging on toxic plants. Also in cases of overindulgence in meals, treats, grass, etc. Also consider **Arsenicum.**	Long-standing diarrhea especially in the morning.
Modalities	Worse early morning, in the summertime, heat, hot damp weather, from eating. Better in cold weather, open air, passing gas.	Worse midnight to 2 AM, on exertion, cold, wet weather. Better by heat, warmth and company.	Generally worse in the morning or 3 PM to 8 PM, more right-sided symptoms, or right to left. Worse from the heat of the sun.	Worse after feeding, typically flatulence after with grumbling of the gut.	Worse especially in the morning and with heat. Worse touch and motion.
Physical Differential	Groaning while going to the bathroom. Takes multiple attempts to pass stool. May have an explosive or jelly-like stool. Gurgling of the gut is common.	Will be a tidy pet, grooming, litter box, etc. Watery diarrhea is often related to emotions. May find the animal walking during diarrhea.	Stool begins hard and constipated, then turns soft or liquid. Will eat very little before filling yet may be food aggressive and rush to and through their meals. Stomach may appear bloated and foul gas is common.	Slimy diarrhea alternating with constipation. May pass small amounts which temporarily relieves the urging only to attempt to pass more soon after.	Cause is often diet related, gushes out effortlessly, green, and watery.
Emotional Differential	Irritable.	Wants security and is anxious. Tends to be restless, especially in the evening.	Anxious and low self-confidence. Dislikes being cornered or enclosed.	Aggressive and may appear tense, dominant behavior.	Appears detached and depressed.

Joints and Arthritis

Our pets experience joint and tissue inflammation, aging, and pain very similar to us. Many of our homeopathic remedies can ease these symptoms and improve their overall health and vitality. Some examples below reflect remedies that have an affinity for the musculo-skeletal system of various animals and can be used even in long standing chronic challenges.

MOST COMMON REMEDIES FOR JOINTS AND ARTHRITIS

	*Calc Fluor	*Causticum	*Manganum	Rhus tox	Ruta
General Description	Affinity for the hips, and lower limbs, very often bone on bone. Bone degeneration, enlargement of joints of lower limbs. Helpful for arthritic symptoms and fibrous growths.	Deformed joints, slow progressive paralysis.	Chronic arthritis, joints sore to touch, swollen. Significant bone pain. Progressive weakness to hind limbs.	Affinity for the neck and back. Helpful for shoulders, large joints, hind-end stiffness injuries, and arthritic symptoms.	Affinity for the smaller joints. Helpful for connective tissue, tendons, sprains, ankles, and feet. Helpful for injuries, back pain, and arthritic symptoms.
Modalities	Worse resting, changes of weather. Better heat, warmth, covering up, and motion.	Chilly, worse from the cold winds. Prefer and better in cloudy, wet, or rainy weather.	Worse cold, wet weather, dampness, change of weather, at night. Better in the open air, after lying down.	Worse after lying down or standing too long without exercise. Worse damp, cold weather. Better dry, warm weather. Better by continuous motion, heat.	Worse damp, cold weather. Worse by motion. Better by lying down, massage, and heat. Better dry, warm weather.
Physical Differential	Sometimes compared to **Ruta** for fibrous growth after injuries.	Tends to be right-sided symptoms. Contractures of muscles and tendons.	Swollen painful joints. May see animal stumbling.	Marked restlessness and better by continued motion.	In the comparison of **Rhus tox**—marked restlessness BUT worse by motion, and better lying down.
Emotional Differential	Anxious.	Quiet, stiff looking. Conditions arising after long-standing grief.	N/A	Restless and friendly but may be timid. May have the reputation of a jokester. Always in movement.	Anxious, irritable, rigid.

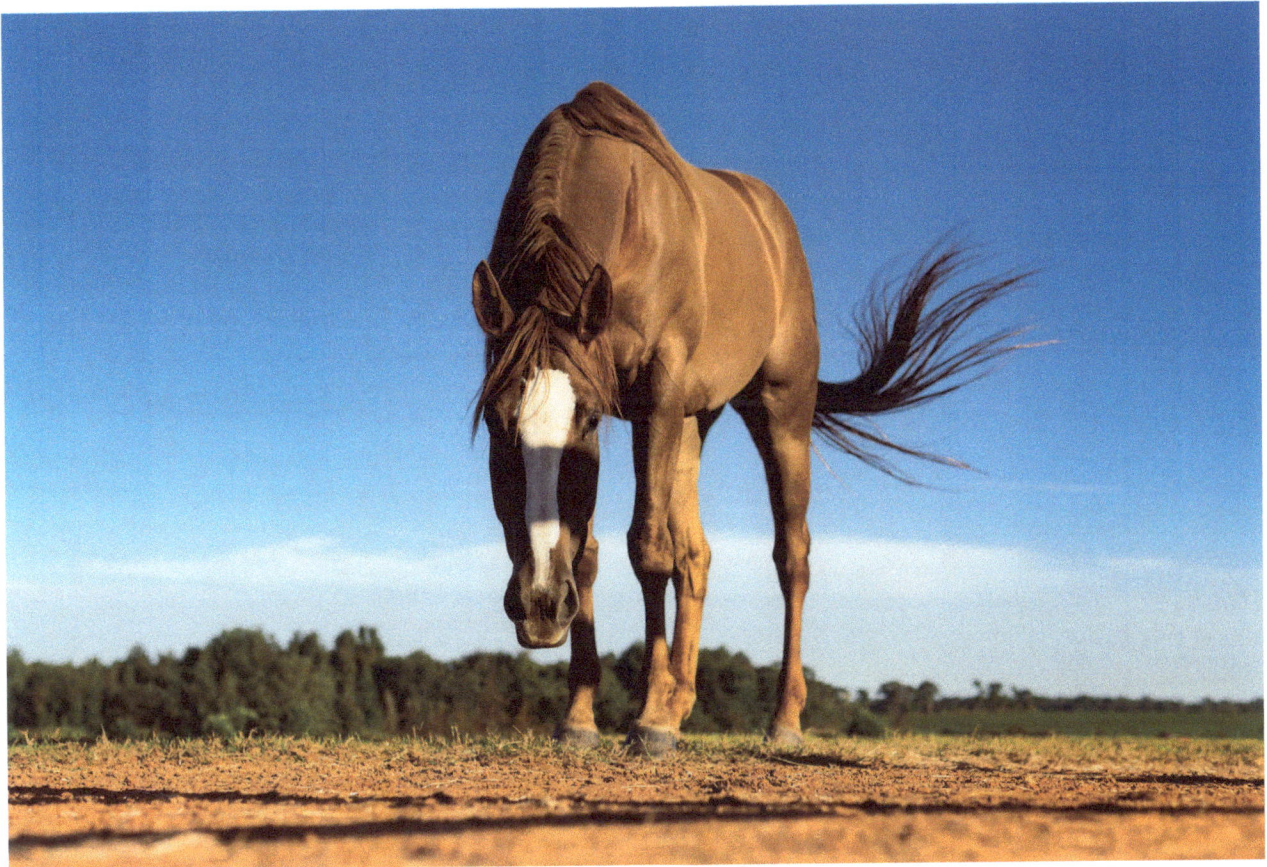

Injuries and Abrasions

Homeopathic remedies truly shine for non-emergency injuries for all of our pets. Injuries from simple cuts, bruising and abrasions, sprains, paw pad injuries to an extra long hiking adventure, rough play and countless sports type injuries. Remember, homeopathy isn't limited to one animal species, so for those in wildlife rehab and rescue consider these remedies when you only have limited access or time with any animal!

COMMON REMEDIES FOR INJURIES AND ABRASIONS

	Arnica	*Bellis per	Calendula	Hypericum	Ledum	*Symphytum
General Description	Blunt trauma, consequences of emotional trauma. Consider pairing with **Hepar sulph** for concussions. Assists with brain healing and mental fogginess.	Injuries to deeper tissue, trauma to the pelvic region, lower back, and soles of feet. For muscles and the muscular fibers of blood vessels.	Promotes wound healing. Make sure the wound is very clean before dosing as it will close it quickly. Do not use if you want drainage of the wound. For eye injuries with subsequent infection. Works as an antiseptic.	Puncture wounds, paw and tail injuries involving the nerves. Relieves nerve pain and promotes nerve regrowth. Especially helpful for lower limbs, spinal injuries, tooth pain, and concussions. Sharp shooting pain.	Bites and stings of insects often with much inflammation. (tics and others) Puncture wounds, eye injuries.	Trauma to eye and orbit (also consider Arnica). Fracture, bone spurs. For pain and improved reunion of bone.
Modalities	Worse touch, cold, at rest, after too much exercise, damp weather. Better by warmth, lying down, and gentle motion.	Worse on the left side, in cold weather, before storms. Better by continued motion, local cold compress.	Worse damp weather.	Worse in cold air and damp weather. Avoids touch and tends to be worse while moving.	Chilly but better by local cold application. Worse from heat.	Worse by touch.
Physical Differential	Bruising, muscles, restless.	Bruising, soft tissue, especially helpful for injuries, soreness of the bottom of an animal's foot.	N/A	Sharp shooting pains, punctures, twitching.	Puncture wounds, with much swelling and inflammation. Body or limb stiffness, fever.	Helpful for all bones in body.
Emotional Differential	Dull and disconnected.	N/A	N/A	Watch your pet's movements and verbal cues such as a sudden physical movement followed by a yelp.	Irritable from discomfort.	N/A

There are other remedies with common uses for your pet. See the chart that follows:

OTHER USES OF COMMON REMEDIES

	Arnica	Arsenicum	Hypericum	Nux vomica	Staphysagria	*Symphytum
General Description	For pain and inflammation, bruising and tissue swelling. Promotes healing.	Good remedy for end-of-life care.	Nerves, pain relief, and promotes regrowth. Dental surgery, injuries of the spine.	Remedy for after anesthesia. For inflammation of connective tissue after surgeries. Natural detox for the liver from medications.	Promotes healing of incisions, sutures, preventing scarring.	For the healing of fractures and bone damage including dental. For eye injuries that involve blunt objects, and bone pain after surgery.
Modalities	Worse by touch, cold, at rest, too much exercise, damp weather. Better by warmth, lying down, and gentle motion.	Worse midnight to 2 AM, on exertion, cold, wet weather. Better by heat, warmth and company.	Sharp shooting pain. Worse in cold air and damp weather. Avoids touch and tends to be worse while moving,	Chilly. Aggravation after eating. Better by warmth.	Constant scratching of the incision.	Worse touch.
Physical Differential	Bruising, muscles, restless.	Urinates in odd places. Paces, restlessness, finicky eating, or loss of appetite. Small water intake.	Sharp shooting pains, punctures, with twitching.	Sharp pains, back pains.	Agitated animals after surgery.	All bones in the body.
Emotional Differential	Dull and disconnected.	Seeks security and is anxious. Restless, especially in the evening.	Watch your pet's movements and verbal cues such as a sudden physical movement followed by a yelp.	Aggressive and may appear tense with dominant behavior.	Irritable but still sweet and timid type.	N/A

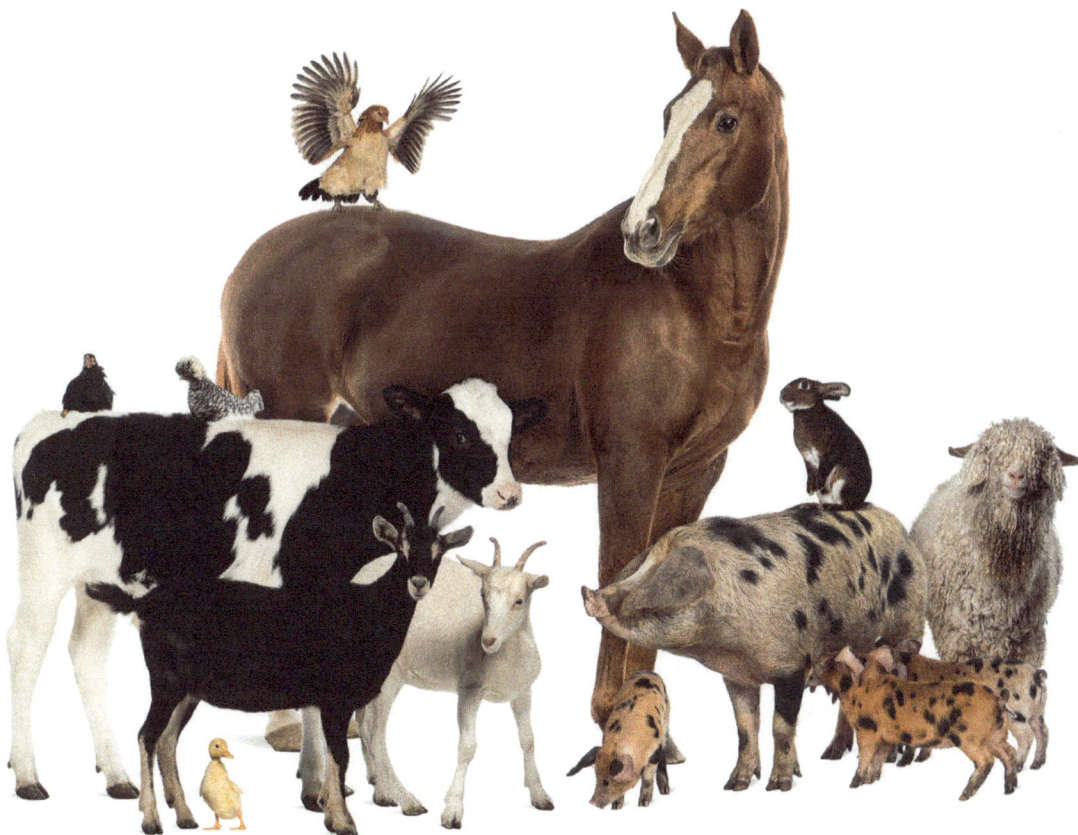

What is Agrohomeopathy?

Agrohomeopathy is a unique area within homeopathy used to support trees, plants, soil, and agricultural resources. It is an inexpensive, chemical-free, non-toxic method strengthening a plant, allowing it to reach its optimum health and to reduce—and sometimes eliminate—its susceptibility to pests and diseases.

Agrohomeopathy uses the same homeopathic remedies described in this book. To reiterate, these remedies are made from natural sources such as minerals and plants and are harvested in a sustainable, environmentally-friendly way.

Why use Agrohomeopathy?

The incorporation of agrohomeopathy into our homes, yards, and farms will bring both amazing short and long-term benefits.

Agrohomeopathy can be used in place of pesticides and herbicides, and the remedies will build up the tree and plant's ability to resist pests and diseases. Currently, in the application of conventional herbicides and pesticides, we are typically spraying to kill the weed, plant, or pest. In agrohomeopathy, the goal is to build the plant's resistance and vitality so that the diseases and pests they are prone to and suffer from will be deterred, if not eliminated.

Homeopathic remedies are applied in very low doses following one of the core principles of homeopathy, less is more. The homeopathic remedies disbursed into the environment are harmless, allowing our plants, soils, and surrounding waters to remain safe for human and animal consumption.

You will not find a better non-toxic means to a healthier garden and environment! In addition, with our climate changes, homeopathy has become a wonderful resource to assist our plants with sudden shifts in weather, such as frost, drought, wind damage, and more.

How can you use agrohomeopathy in your home and gardens?

Similar to homeopathy for people, in agrohomeopathy we apply the same three core principles of homeopathy; (1) less is more, (2) totality of symptoms, and (3) like cures like. We only need to view our gardens and land as the living beings they truly are, and to observe them from a homeopathic perspective to provide the remedies needed that will bring the environment into a state of balance.

There are endless ways to use homeopathy in your gardens and on your land. Think about how you might want to assist your garden. Do you want to fertilize, improve a plant's health, increase flower and fruit yield, heal a damaged tree or branch, deter insects or wildlife, stop powdery mildew, pear rust, tomato blight, leaf spot? Perhaps you would like to aid in regrowth when transplanting or dividing your plants? Possibly, you would like to improve your soil?

How do you know what to give your plants, trees, or soil?

In Agrohomeopathy, we are looking for the totality of symptoms, just like in humans.

Take a few minutes to observe your plant and collect information about how your plant looks: the color and texture of its leaves, branches and surrounding soil, its response to watering, sun, and shade, and how it responds to your local weather.

Focus on these FOUR areas when collecting the totality of symptoms, for your plants, trees, and soil.

1. **Condition or circumstance to resolve:** In many cases we are simply looking to assist our plant or tree with the healing process after neglect, a change of location, temperature, sunlight, or a wound or weather damage. In other cases, it may be more complicated, we may not even know what the condition is! It is okay if you are not sure of the condition! Similar to homeopathy for people and animals, we are not solely focused on the name of the condition or disease. We are focused on observing the symptoms. Note any visible fungus or mildew. Look at the leaf, stem and bark of the plant or tree. For each of these areas, make note of strange patterns, textures, growths, and color changes. Pay attention to the insects, on or near the plant, tree, or soil even if you aren't looking to deter them. Don't

forget to look at the underside of the leaves. Look at the entire plant or tree from top to bottom. This information will guide you to a remedy that is well suited for the entire plant.

2. **Location:** Where do you observe the issue—on the leaf stem, roots, whole plant, lower leaves, upper leaves, flowers, fruit, soil, etc.?

3. **Cause:** Event(s) that initiated a change in the plant, tree, or soil: weather changes, transplanting, accidents, soil depletion, plant or tree additions to the area, etc.

4. **Modalities:** Things or circumstances that make the plant, tree, or soil better or worse: time of day or season, location, shade, heat, cold, rain, etc.

Once you observe your plant, tree, or soil and create a profile of the condition or circumstance, it is time to find the remedy profile that is the best match, following the homeopathic principle of "like cures like."

How do you prepare and apply homeopathic remedies to your plants?

Homeopathic remedies are typically given to plants, trees, or soil by adding the remedy pellets to water. Typically, we use **30C** for most conditions and **6X** for homeopathic fertilizer options.

Place **one pellet per cup of water** in a clean glass or plastic container designated for homeopathic solutions. It is not recommended to use the same garden sprayers or containers with homeopathic remedies and other kinds of applications such as biodynamics, herbicides, or pesticides.

Shake, or stir with a wooden or plastic spoon. Avoid metal and gardening equipment used for chemical applications.

Water the base of the plant or tree to ensure the solution reaches the root system. There is no need to apply it to the leaves, unless there is a pest infestation or to deter a pest from nibbling. If you are spraying the leaves, make sure to do so when it is not too wet or sunny to avoid further leaf damage. Avoid spraying leaves if there is already a fungus or mildew challenge.

How do you store homeopathic remedies?

Store your kit and any leftover solution in a cool dry place out of direct sunlight. The solution sealed can be used for up to five days. Shake the solution between each use before applying.

How do you know if your homeopathic remedies are helping your trees and plants?

The correct remedy will often have a positive impact within 24 to 72 hours, if not sooner! It depends on the plant and the condition. Deep-rooted conditions may take longer, and weather also impacts your plant's recovery process. In rainy/wet situations you may need to reapply with more frequency.

How do you know when to repeat or change a remedy?

As a general rule, observe and evaluate! Wait 72 hours, and look back at your original profile to see what has changed. Do not expect everything to be resolved. If you see some improvement, you are doing well! DO NOT REPEAT the remedy. The guideline in homeopathy is: if you see improvement, you allow the remedy to continue its work. There is no need to repeat unless you see the improving plant begin to decline again.

Here's a quick reference guide:

- If the plant, tree, or soil looks better, WAIT!

- If not responding, repeat the remedy if you feel it is the correct remedy up to 3 times at 72-hour intervals. STOP if you see an improvement.

- If nothing has shifted, move to another remedy.

Remedies for General Plant Maintenance and Care

Arnica: apply to any new plant introduced into the garden. Use after any pruning, damage, dividing, and transplanting. It will promote root growth, healing, and overall vascular circulation of the plant.

Calendula: it will promote root regrowth, and healing. Provide it to any plant that looks weak after **Arnica** has been applied. It's helpful for trees or bushes that have cuts or bark removal from damage or poor pruning.

*Graphites: for neglected, dry, and limp plants where **Silicea** does not work!

*Petroleum: great for indoor or greenhouse plants that look dry, cracked, or have been overwintered in cold temperatures or lack of sunlight.

Silicea: for weak, neglected, dry plants. Plants will look limp and dry even shortly after water or always appear to be droopy.

Natural Pesticide Options for Leaf, Fruit Damage, Rot, and for Bacterial, and Fungal Conditions

*Natrum sulph: blight, leaf curl, brown rot, powdery or downy mildew from very damp warm weather, lengthy periods of humidity, or warm rain. May also see leaves frequently turning yellow.

*Thuja: leaf curl, leaf spot, brown rot, viruses that cause fruit and leaf deformities and growths. Powdery or downy mildew from very damp warm weather, lengthy periods of warm rain.

Natural Pesticide Options for Plant and Garden Insects and Wildlife

*Bombyx: deters the tomato hornworm, loopers, sawfly, moths, armyworms.

*Camphora: pest control inside and outside of the home; ants, stink bugs, mice, as a preventative and for maintenance. Great to apply to new plants before introducing the plant(s) into the garden. Deters animals such as deer and pests from nesting and nibbling on plants and flowers. Multiple applications may be needed due to weather, such as rain.

*Helix: deters slugs.

*Natrum sulph: deters gnats and other flying insects that occur or escalate during humid, damp summer weather. This remedy is very helpful in greenhouse environments.

*Petroleum: deters scale insects, mealy bugs.

Sulphur: great for insect infestations of moths, aphids, ants, or beetles. Great pesticide for the maintenance of cabbage, eggplant, squashes, cucumber, cantaloupe, and potato. This remedy is very helpful in a greenhouse environment.

Natural Options for Weather Damage

Aconite: damage from cold dry winds, and sudden snowstorm, or the plant is unprotected during transportation. Plants shocked by the cold.

Arnica: damage after hail, storm, or wind. Signs of breakage, broken stalks, limbs, etc. Promotes healing.

Belladonna: when the plant wilts quickly and leaves turn reddish brown or red spots—from long cold wet summers. Symptoms are sudden. The remedy acts as a source of heat and will warm the plant. The remedy may also be helpful for viral and bacterial symptoms when you see red spots on leaves.

*Natrum sulph: for damage from very damp warm weather, weather changes from cold to warm, lengthy periods of warm rain. Especially helpful for tomato plants.

*Petroleum: for damage from severe cold and frost. Look for cracking caused by the cold. Houseplants that receive too little sunlight and drafts from windows during cold periods.

Natural Germination, Fertilizer and Flowering

Calcarea carb: an important fertilizer remedy made from the calcium of oyster shells. Apply one dose of **6X** to new plants or after your seeds have germinated. **Calc carb** follows **Silicea** well. The remedy is also helpful in promoting flowering, fruit, and vegetable production throughout the blooming season.

Magnesium phosphoricum 6X: great for plants that fail after a cold or period or transport from nursery.

Leaves will slowly wilt and turn pale yellow. The remedy is especially helpful for tomato and pepper plants.

Silicea: great to assist with seed germination. Apply one dose of **30C** at the time of seeding. **Silicea** should only be applied once or twice per season to avoid stunting plant growth.

Summary of Homeopathy for Your Pets and Plants

There are many additional occurrences for both pets and plants that homeopathy can step in and support in powerful gentle ways. Observe your animals and plants and you will begin to see the common thread of symptoms between all beings and the homeopathic remedies that support these symptoms. Homeopathy for your plants and animals is a wonderful solution to study and implement in your homes and gardens to strengthen not only your vitality but the overall vitality of your environment and our planet.

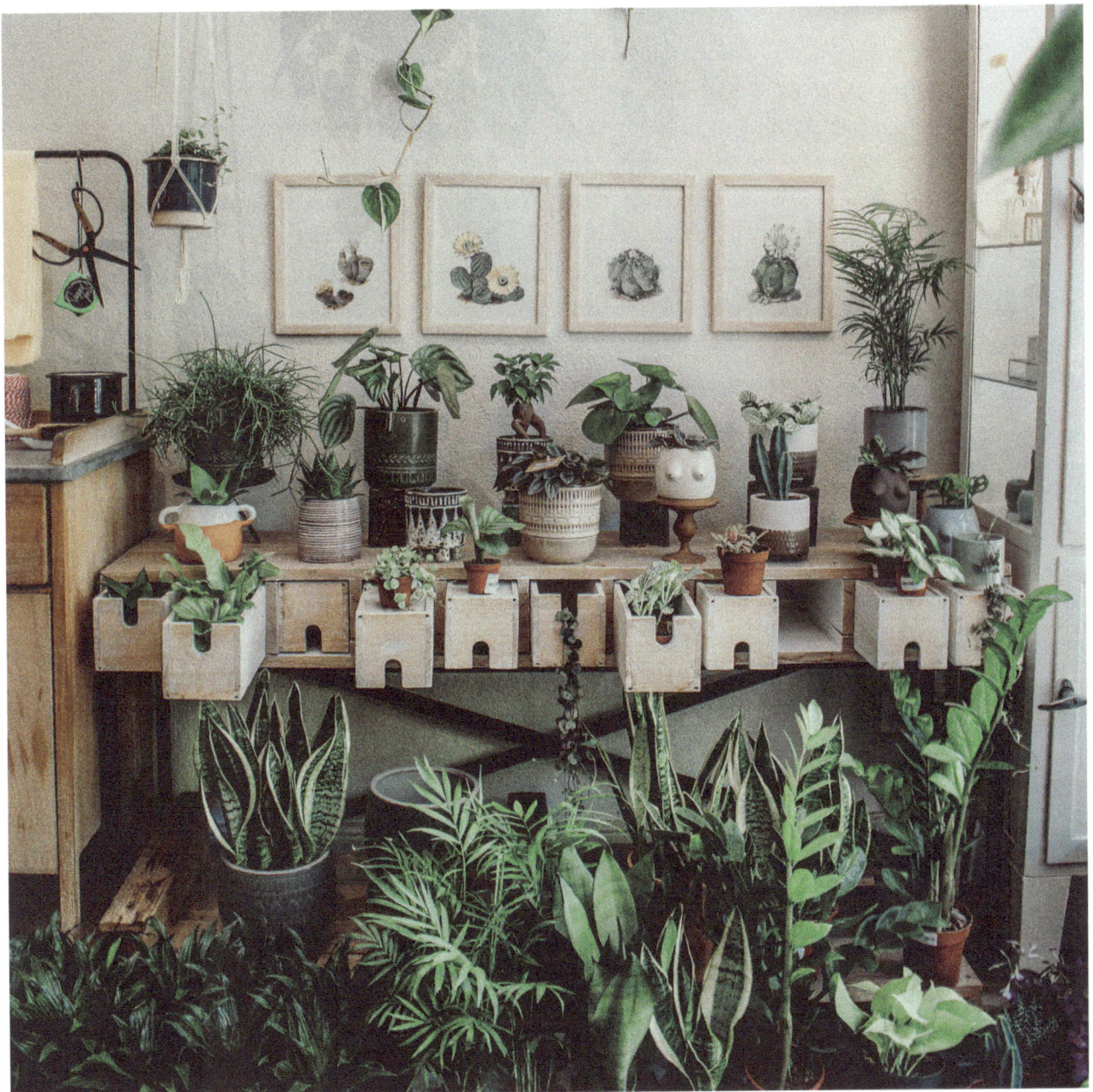

? WHAT'S THE FIRST REMEDY YOU THINK OF WHEN...

1. Your pet's injury has been cleaned well and you want to support the wound's closure.

2. Your dog has an abscess on their foot and you need something to help with possible infection and to promote discharge.

3. After finding your dog has raided the trash can, they are now throwing up and experiencing diarrhea.

4. You have been noticing your pet has been self-grooming more frequently and showing signs of hair loss.

5. You notice your animal has issues getting up and moving after resting, but is better after they are up and moving for awhile.

6. It is springtime, and your pet is experiencing profuse watering eyes, clear nasal discharge and a cough.

7. There is supposed to be a sudden extreme temperature drop and you want to help prepare your outside animals.

8. Your pet has had surgery and is still feeling the effects of anesthesia.

9. Your animal suddenly appears anxious, fearful and hurried and it is not typical of their behavior.

10. Your cat has just lost its bonded partner and is displaying its grief by constantly moving around and seemingly can't find a comfortable place to rest.

11. The temperature unusually dropped down close to frost levels last night and you want to support your plants.

12. Your bell pepper plant is growing but the pepper's are turning brown and are rotting after a rainy period.

13. Your tomato plants are being attacked by the dreaded tomato hornworm or other worm and you want to deter them.

14. Your vegetables, plants and bushes are being eaten by your friendly deer and you want to deter them.

15. Your strawberry plants are wilting quickly and the leaves have a reddish brown or have red spots. They were flourishing prior to a cold spell. You want to warm them and the soil.

16. Your rosemary plant has a scale like insect on it and it looks dry and cracked.

17. There has been a great deal of constant warm rain and humidity and many of your plants show signs of powdery mildew.

18. The winter weather damaged many of your trees and you have many broken limbs to address. You want to provide the tree aid in healing.

19. You have divided and transplanted a plant and you want to make sure the roots take hold.

20. A house plant seems to always need water and is very limp, very quickly after watering.

Answer key on page 325.

Appendix 1
What's the First Remedy? Quiz Answer Key

Chapter 3: Cell Salts	Chapter 4: First Aid	Chapter 5: Head	Chapter 6: Eyes
1. Ferr phos 2. Kali phos 3. Nat mur 4. Kali sulph 5. Kali phos 6. Calc fluor 7. Calc fluor 8. Mag phos 9. Kali mur 10. Nat mur 11. Silicea (Silica) 12. Ferr phos 13. Nat phos 14. Nat sulph 15. Nat phos 16. Ferr phos 17. Kali sulph 18. Calc sulph 19. Nat sulph 20. Kali phos	1. Arnica 2. Hypericum 3. Cantharis 4. Cantharis 5. Apis 6. Bryonia 7. Belladonna 8. Natrum mur 9. Carbo veg 10. Apis 11. Carbo veg 12. Cantharis 13. Nux vomica 14. *Glonoinum and Belladonna	1. Belladonna 2. China 3. Arnica 4. Arnica 5. *Natrum sulph 6. Arsenicum 7. Hepar sulph 8. Lycopodium 9. Ignatia 10. Ruta	1. Pulsatilla 2. *Symphytum 3. Pulsatilla 4. Silicea 5. *Phosphoric acid 6. Hypericum 7. Aconite 8. Arnica 9. Belladonna 10. *Euphrasia

Chapter 7: Ears	Chapter 8: Nose	Chapter 9: Mouth and Teeth	Chapter 10: Throat and Chest
1. Chamomilla 2. Mercurius 3. Mercurius 4. Aconite 5. Silicea 6. Chamomilla 7. Pulsatilla 8. Hepar sulph 9. Belladonna 10. Aconite	1. Aconite 2. *Allium cepa 3. *Euphrasia 4. Natrum mur 5. Arsenicum 6. Phosphorus 7. Ledum 8. Arnica 9. Arnica 10. Mercurius 11. Belladonna 12. Aconite 13. Phosphorus 14. Rhus tox	1. Arsenicum 2. Chamomilla 3. Hypericum 4. Arnica 5. *Calcarea fluor 6. Mercurius 7. Mercurius 8. Arnica 9. *Calc fluor 6X, *Calc phos 6X, and *Silicea 6X 10. Aconite 11. Belladonna 12. Rhus tox 13. Arnica with Hypericum 14. Hypericum 15. Hepar sulph	1. Bryonia 2. Lachesis 3. Phosphorus 4. Phosphorus 5. Belladonna 6. Hepar sulph 7. Mercurius 8. Aconite, first, then *Spongia 9. Ipecac 10. Ignatia

Chapter 11: Stomach and Abdomen	Chapter 12: Stool Issues	Chapter 13: Urinary Issues	Chapter 14: Male Issues
1. Nux vomica	1. Arsenicum	1. Apis	1. Sulphur
2. *Veratrum album	2. *Podophyllum	2. Staphysagria	2. Nux vomica
3. Bryonia	3. *Veratrum album	3. Arsenicum	3. *Baryta carb
4. Arsenicum	4. Bryonia	4. Lycopodium	4. Cantharis
5. Nux vomica	5. Nux vomica	5. Arsenicum	5. *Aesculus
6. Lycopodium	6. Silicea	6. Pulsatilla	6. *Graphites
7. Phosphorus	7. *Aesculus	7. Cantharis	7. Silicea
8. Arsenicum	8. Lycopodium	8. Pulsatilla	8. Lycopodium
9. Ipecac	9. Sulphur	9. *Causticum	9. Rhus tox
10. Carbo veg	10. Arsenicum	10. *Sarsaparilla	10. Staphysagria
			11. Phosphorus
			12. Nux vomica

Chapter 15: Female Issues	Chapter 16: Back and Neck	Chapter 17: Muscle, Joints and Bones	Chapter 18: Skin
1. Lachesis	1. Hypericum	1. Arnica	1. Nux vomica
2. *Magnesium phos	2. Arnica	2. *Eupatorium perf	2. Calendula
3. Nux vomica	3. Arnica on way to the Emergency Room (ER)	3. Sepia	3. Silicea
4. Bryonia	4. *Bellis per	4. Rhus tox	4. Silicea
5. Staphysagria	5. Sepia	5. *Calc phos	5. Ledum
6. Pulsatilla	6. Gelsemium	6. Bryonia	6. Calendula
7. *Bellis per	7. Arnica AND (this could be a frac-ture-do not move person, call for an ambulance)	7. Hypericum	7. Hypericum
8. Sepia	8. Rhus tox	8. *Symphytum and *Calc phos	8. Sulphur
9. *Sarsaparilla	9. Bryonia	9. Ruta	9. Apis
10. Sulphur	10. Silicea	10. *Bellis per	10. Rhus tox
11. Cantharis	11. Belladonna	11. *Strontium carb	11. *Anacardium
12. Sepia		12. *Mag phos	12. *Thuja
13. Staphysagria		13. *Bellis per	13. Hepar sulph
14. Staphysagria		14. Mercurius	14. Sulphur

Chapter 19: Mind and Emotions	Chapter 20: First three Years	Chapter 21: Childhood	Chapter 22: Young Adult
1. Ignatia	1. Aconite	1. *Causticum	1. Pulsatilla
2. Arnica	2. Chamomilla	2. Sulphur	2. Mercurius
3. Staphysagria	3. Chamomilla	3. Chamomilla	3. Natrum mur
4. Aconite	4. Lycopodium	4. *Ferrum phos	4. *Calcarea phos
5. Calcarea carb or Arsenicum	5. Calcarea carb	5. Mercurius	5. Nux vomica
6. Gelsemium or *Argentum nit	6. Arsenicum	6. Bryonia	6. Nux vomica
7. *Coffea or *Kali phos	7. Ipecac	7. Mercurius	7. Argentum nit
8. *Kali phos	8. Pulsatilla	8. *Phytolacca	8. *Bach Flower Rescue Remedy®
9. Nux vomica	9. Sulphur	9. Belladonna	9. Ignatia
10. Staphysagria or Nux vomica	10. Mercurius	10. Rhus tox	10. Lycopodium

Chapter 23: Influenza	Chapter 24: Travel related	Chapter 25: Surgery Considerations	Chapter 26: Pets and Plants
1. Gelsemium 2. Gelsemium 3. Arsenicum 4. *Baptisia 5. *Eupatorium per 6. Rhus tox 7. Gelsemium 8. Phosphorus 9. Bryonia 10. Oscillococcinum®	1. Nux vomica 2. Carbo veg 3. Gelsemium 4. Argentum nit 5. Arsenicum 6. Silicea 7. *Tabacum 8. China 9. Aconite 10. Arnica	1. Arnica 2. Aconite 3. Phosphorus 4. Calendula 5. Arnica, then *Bellis per 6. *Symphytum 7. Arnica (200c if available) 8. *Bach Flower Rescue Remedy® 9. *Causticum 10. Staphysagria 11. Hepar sulph 12. Nux vomica	1. Calendula 2. Hepar sulph 3. Arsenicum 4. Arsenicum 5. Rhus tox 6. *Allium cepa 7. Aconite 8. Phosphorus 9. Argentum nit 10. Ignatia 11. Aconite 12. *Thuja 13. *Bombyx 14. *Camphora 15. Belladonna 16. *Petroleum 17. *Thuja 18. Arnica 19. Calendula 20. Silicea

Appendix 2
Homeopathic Remedies Referenced in this Manual

Blue Helios 36 Remedy Kit in 30c Potency:

Aconite	Calendula	Ignatia	Nux vomica
Antimonium tart	Cantharis	Ipecac	Phosphorus
Apis	Carbo veg	Kali bich	Pulsatilla
Argentum nit	Chamomilla	Lachesis	Rhus tox
Arnica	China	Ledum	Ruta
Arsenicum	Drosera	Lycopodium	Sepia
Belladonna	Gelsemium	Magnesium phos	Silica
Bryonia	Hepar sulph	Mercurius	Staphysagria
Calcarea carb	Hypericum	Natrum mur	Sulphur

Remedies with no asterisk are found in the **Helios 36 Remedy Kit.**

Remedies WITH an *asterisk are NOT found in the kit but can be purchased online.

*See **Appendix 4—Additional Resources** on **page 348** for where to purchase homeopathic remedies.*

NAME IN THIS GUIDE	REMEDY FULL NAME	OTHER COMMON NAMES AND ABBREVIATIONS	ORIGINAL SOURCE
Aconite	Aconitum napellus	Aconitum nap/Acon	Monkshood
*Aesculus	Aesculus hippocastanum	Aesc	Horse-chestnut
*Aethusa	Aethusa cynapium	Aeth	Fool's parsley
*Agaricus	Agaricus muscarius	Agaricus mus/Agar	Fly agaric
*Allium cepa	Allium cepa	All-c	Red onion
*Aloe	Aloe socotrina	Aloe	Aloe succotrina
*Alumina	Alumina	Alum	Oxide of aluminum
Ammonium carb	Ammonium carbonicum	Am-c	Carbonate of ammonia
*Anacardium	Anacardium orientale	Anac	Marking nut
Antimonium tart	Antimonium tartaricum	Ant-t	Tartar emetic
*Antimonium crudum	Antimonium crudum	Ant-c	Sulphide of antimony
Apis	Apis mellifica	Apis mel/Apis	Honey bee
Argentum nit	Argentum nitricum	Arg-nit/Arg-n	Nitrate of silver
Arnica	Arnica montana	Arnica mon/Arn	Leopard's bane
Arsenicum	Arsenicum album	Arsenicum alb/Ars	Arsenic trioxide
*Arum triphyllum	Arum triphyllum	Arum-t	Jack-in-the-pulpit
*Aurum met	Aurum metallicum	Aur	Metallic gold

NAME IN THIS GUIDE	REMEDY FULL NAME	OTHER COMMON NAMES AND ABBREVIATIONS	ORIGINAL SOURCE
*Baptisia	Baptisia tinctoria	Bapt	Wild indigo
*Baryta carb	Baryta carbonica	Bar-carb/Bar-c	Carbonate of baryta
Belladonna	Belladonna	Bell	Deadly nightshade
*Bellis per	Bellis perennis	Bell-p	Common daisy
*Berberis	Berberis vulgaris	Berb	Barberry
*Bismuth	Bismuthum subnitricum	Bism	Nitrate of bismuth
*Bombyx	Bombyx processionea	Bomb-pr	Procession caterpillar
*Borax	Borax veneta	Bor	Anhydrous borate of sodium
Bryonia	Bryonia alba	Bry	Wild hops
Calcarea carb	Calcarea carbonica	Calc carb/ Calc-c	Cabonate of lime
*Calcarea fluor (and *cell salt)	Calcarea fluorata	Calc fluor/Calc-f	Calcium fluoride
*Calcarea phos (and *cell salt)	Calcarea phosphorica	Calc phos/Calc-p	Phosphate of lime
*Calcarea sulph (and *cell salt)	Calcarea sulphurica	Calc sulph/Calc-s	Calcium sulphate
Calendula	Calendula officinalis	Calendula off/Calen	Marigold
*Camphora	Camphora	Camph	Camphor
Cantharis	Cantharis	Canth	Spanish fly
*Capsicum	Capsicum aanuum	Caps	Cayenne pepper
Carbo veg	Carbo vegetabilis	Carb-v	Vegetable charcoal
*Carbolic acid	Carbolicum acidum	Carb-ac	Carbolic acid
*Causticum	Causticum	Caust	Tinctura acris sine kali
Chamomilla	Chamomilla	Cham	German chamomile
China	Cinchona officinalis	Chin/Cinchona off	Peruvian bark (quinine)
*Coca	Coca	Coca	Erythroxylon coca
*Cocculus	Cocculus indicus	Cocc	Indian cockle
*Coccus cacti	Coccus cacti	Cocc-c	Cocchineal
*Coffea	Coffea cruda	Coff	Unroasted coffee
*Colchicum	Colchicum autumnale	Colch	Meadow saffron
*Collinsonia canandensis	Collinsonia canandensis	Coll	Stone-root
*Colocynthis	Colocynthis	Coloc	Bitter cucumber
*Conium	Conium maculatum	Con	Poison hemlock
*Corallium rubrum	Corallium rubrum	Cor-r	Red coral
*Crotalus	Crotalus horridus	Crot-h	Rattlesnake
*Croton Tiglium	Croton tiglium	Croto-t	Croton oil seeds
*Cuprum	Cuprum metallicum	Cuprum met/Cupr	Copper
Drosera	Drosera rotundifolia	Drosera rotun/Dros	Sundew
*Dulcamara	Dulcamara	Dulc	Bittersweet
*Eupatorium perf	Eupatorium perfoliatum	Eup-per	Thoroughwort
*Euphrasia	Euphrasia officinalis	Euphr	Eyebright
*Ferrum phos (and *cell salt)	Ferrum phosphoricum	Ferr phos/Ferr-p	Phosphate of iron
*Fluoricum acidum	Fluoricum acidum	Fl-ac	Hydrofluoric acid

NAME IN THIS GUIDE	REMEDY FULL NAME	OTHER COMMON NAMES AND ABBREVIATIONS	ORIGINAL SOURCE
Gelsemium	Gelsemium sempervirens	Gelsemium semp/Gels	Yellow jasmine
*Glonoinum	Glonoinum	Glonoine/Glon	Nitro-glycerine
*Graphites	Graphites naturalis	Graph	Black lead
*Guaiacum	Guaiacum officinale	Guia	Gum guaiacum
*Hamamelis	Hamamelis virginica	Ham	Witch-hazel
*Helix	Helix tosta	Helix	Toasted snail
Hepar sulph	Hepar sulphuris calcareum	Hep/Hep-s	Calcium sulphide
Histaminum	Histaminum hydrochloricum	Hist	Histamine
Hypericum	Hypericum perforatum	Hyper/Hyp-p	St. John's-wort
Ignatia	Ignatia amara	Ign/Ign-a	St. Ignatius bean
*Iodum purum	Iodum purum	Iod	Iodine
Ipecac	Ipecacuanha	Ipecac/Ipec/Ip	Ipecac root
*Jaborandi	Jaborandi	Jab	Pilocarpus jaborandi
Kali bich	Kalium bichromicum	Kali-bic/Kali-bi/Kali-b	Bichromate of potash
*Kali carb	Kalium carbonicum	Kali-carb/Kali-c	Potassium carbonate
*Kali mur cell salt	Kalium muriaticum	Kali-mur/Kali-m	Potassium chloride
*Kali phos (and *cell salt)	Kalium phosphoricum	Kali-phos/Kali-p	Potassium phosphate
*Kali sulph (and *cell salt)	Kalium sulphuricum	Kali sulph/Kali-s	Potassium sulphate
*Kreosotum	Kreosotum	Kreos	Creosote (distillation of wood tar)
Lachesis	Lachesis muta	Lach	Bushmaster snake or surucucu
Ledum	Ledum palustre	Ledum pal/Led	Marsh tea
*Lobelia	Lobelia inflata	Lob	Indian tobacco
Lycopodium	Lycopodium clavatum	Lyc	Club moss
Magnesium phos (and *cell salt)	Magnesia phosphorica	Mag phos/Mag-p	Phosphate of magnesia
*Manganum	Manganum aceticum	Mang	Acetate of manganese
Mercurius	Mercurius vivus or Mercurius solubilis	Merc viv/Merc sol/Merc	Quicksilver or mercury
*Mezereum	Daphne mezereum	Mez	Spurge olive
*Millefolium	Millefolium achillea	Mill	Yarrow
*Natrum carb	Natrum carbonicum	Nat-carb/Nat-c	Sodium carbonate
Natrum mur (and *cell salt)	Natrum muriaticum	Natrum mur/Nat mur/Nat-m	Chloride of sodium
*Natrum phos cell salt	Natrum phosphoricum	Natrum phos/Nat phos/Nat-m	Phosphate of sodium
*Natrum sulph (and *cell salt)	Natrum sulphuricum	Natrum sulph/Nat sulph/Nat-s	Sulphate of sodium
*Nitricum acidum	Nitricum acidum	Nit-ac	Nitric acid
*Nux mochata	Nux mochata	Nux-m	Nutmeg
Nux vomica	Nux vomica	Nux-v	Poison nut
*Petroleum	Petroleum	Petr	Crude rock oil (kerosene)
Phosphorus	Phosphorus	Phos	Phosphorus
*Phosphoricum acidum	Phosphoricum acidum	Acidum phosphoricum/Phos acid/Ph-ac	Phosphoric acid

NAME IN THIS GUIDE	REMEDY FULL NAME	OTHER COMMON NAMES AND ABBREVIATIONS	ORIGINAL SOURCE
*Phytolacca	Phytolacca decandra	Phytolacca dec/Phyt	Poke root
*Picricum acidum	Picricum acidum	Pic-ac	Picric acid
*Podophyllum	Podophyllum peltatum	Podophyllum pel/Podo	May apple
Pulsatilla	Pulsatilla nigrans	Pulsatilla nig/Puls	Wind flower
*Pyrogenium	Pyrogenium	Pyrog	Putrescent meat
*Raphanus	Raphanus sativus	Raph	Black garden radish
Rhus tox	Rhus toxicodendron	Rhus-t	Poison ivy
*Rosa damascena	Rosa damascena	Ros-d	Damascus Rose
*Rumex crispus	Rumex crispus	Rumx	Yellow dock
Ruta	Ruta graveolens	Ruta grav/Ruta	Rue or bittersweet
*Sabadilla	Sabadilla officinalis	Sabad	Sabadilla officinalis
*Sanguinaria	Sanguinaria canadensis	Sang	Blood-root
*Sarsaparilla	Sarsaparilla	Sars	Smilax
*Secale	Secale cornutum	Sec	Ergot of rye
Sepia	Sepia officinalis	Sep	Cuttlefish ink
Silicea (and *cell salt)	Silicea terra	Silica/Sil	Silica or flint
*Spongia	Sponga tosta	Spong	Roasted sea sponge
Staphysagria	Staphysagria	Staphisagria/Staph	Stavesacre
*Sticta pulmonaria	Sticta pulmonaria	Stict	Lung-wort
*Stramonium	Stramonium	Stram	Jimson weed/Thornapple
*Strontium carb	Strontium carbonicum	Stront-c	Carbonate of strontium
Sulphur	Sulphur	Sulph	Sublimated sulphur
*Sulphuricum acidum	Sulphuricum acidum	Sulph-ac	Sulphur dioxide
*Symphytum	Symphytum officinale	Symphytum off/Symph	Comfrey or knitbone
*Tabacum	Tabacum	Tab	Tobacco
*Thiosinaminum	Thiosinaminum	Thiosin	Mustard seed oil
*Thuja	Thuja occidentalis	Thuja occ/Thuj	Arbor vitae
*Urtica	Urtica urens	Urtica-u	Stinging nettle
*Veratrum	Vertrum album	Veratrum alb/Verat	White hellebore
*Wyethia	Wyethia helenoides	Wye	Poison weed
*Zincum metallicum	Zincum metallicum	Zinc	Zinc
*Zingiber	Zingiber Officianale	Zing	Ginger

Appendix 3
Glossary of Homeopathic and Clinical Terminology

> *Quote from The Organon:*
>
> **"Among those medicines whose human condition-altering power has been investigated, the medicine whose observed symptoms are most similar to the totality of symptoms of a given natural disease will and must be the most fitting, the most certain homeopathic remedy. In this medicine is found the specificum for this case of disease."**
>
> *– Aphorism 147, by Samuel Hahnemann, Founder of Homeopathy*

This is a glossary of terms you will want to become familiar with as you study homeopathy. Also included are medical and physiological terms to aid in your general health knowledge and will assist in your understanding of homeopathy as well. Refer to this often as it will help your homeopathic understanding and use of homeopathic language.

ACRID

An unusually pungent, bitter or sharp taste or smell that is generally unpleasant.

ACUTE VERSUS CHRONIC* AILMENTS

An acute illness is one that has a gradual or abrupt onset, is self-limiting, and lasts for a short time—like a flu or stomach ache. A person with an acute illness will either recover and regain health or will die. A chronic illness is a set of symptoms that have not gone away after many months and limits the function of an individual. A common cold is considered an acute illness while recurrent seasonal allergies are considered a chronic condition. An ankle sprain is considered an acute problem while arthritis is considered chronic.

The body innately wants to heal. In chronic illness, the body tries to restore itself to health, but seems to get stuck along the way. Chronic symptoms may accumulate and change but don't go away.

Using homeopathy for treating a chronic disease can be very complicated and requires a high level of competence in homeopathy, as well as some medical education. This manual is designed to teach the use of homeopathy for home care in acute illnesses and injuries only. To this end, we have included some guidelines to help you decide when the condition you are addressing is or may be beyond the reasonable scope of home care, or when you may need the assistance of a skilled homeopath or other health care professional.

- Acute Illness produces symptoms that appear very quickly, are relatively short in duration, and go through a typical progression of changes. This covers injuries, fevers, flus, colds, cuts, bruising, teething, stomach upsets, etc. Ordinarily the vital force has its own self-healing resources and can find its own resolution. When the vital force isn't accomplishing this on its own, homeopathy can assist in encouraging the body to heal itself. Given the correct remedy, there will be less suffering and generally no suppression of symptoms.

- Chronic Illness is a long-term condition for which the body has no immediate internal solution. A chronic condition tends to get progressively worse over many months or years and remains as an ongoing health issue. In this case the self-healing mechanism has somehow been compromised. Repetition of acute illness is not referred to as acute anymore. If someone suffers repeated colds over a long period of time, the real problem lies in the dysfunction of the immune system, nutritional deficiencies, and/or environmental toxins. These conditions require constitutional homeopathic treatment which assesses every system of the body, including current symptoms, psychological make-up, family history, history since birth, and more. Through this treatment, lifestyle improvements are frequently identified and recommended.

*Important note: Chronic conditions should be treated by a clinically trained, experienced, and professional homeopath.

ALCOHOL POISONING

Alcohol poisoning happens when there is too much alcohol in the bloodstream and areas of the brain that control basic life support functions—such as breathing, heart rate, and temperature control—begin to shut down. Symptoms of alcohol poisoning: confusion. difficulty remaining conscious.

ALLOPATHY

Conventional medicine is referred to as allopathy. The word allopathy comes from the Greek words *állos* and *patheia* which translates into "other/different suffering." Allopathy is based on the principle of opposites (contraria contrariis). rather than the principle of "like cures like" (similia similibus curentur) that homeopathy is based on (see "Homeopathy"). The symptoms a person experiences are evaluated and a name, or diagnosis, is given to the condition. The person is then prescribed a chemical drug which is meant to stop the symptoms. For example, when an ear infection is treated with antibiotics, it may go away, but it often returns necessitating repeated doses of antibiotics. Frequent antibiotic use can result in a secondary reaction, such as stomach pain or heartburn, necessitating another drug.

AMELIORATION

When the condition of a person improves or shows a decrease in symptoms.

ANAPHYLACTIC SHOCK/ ANAPHYLAXIS

A severe allergic reaction to a substance that can be life threatening. See full description of **First-Aid for Injuries** in **Chapter 4** on **page 52**.

ANGINA PECTORIS

This is a medical condition due to coronary heart disease and it occurs when the heart muscle doesn't get enough oxygen and blood due to narrowed arteries. The pain that is experienced causes a sense of suffocation, oppression and constriction around the chest. The pain can also be experienced in the neck, jaw, shoulder and back of the arm.

ANTIDOTE

A homeopathic remedy can be antidoted meaning modified. The effects of a homeopathic remedy can be limited, partially neutralized or completely neutralized by certain specific homeopathic remedies. Additionally, certain substances such as coffee, strong odors; menthol, peppermint or eucalyptus (to name a few) and other agents such as cannabis can alter the effectiveness of a homeopathic remedy.

BILIOUS

In the case of vomiting, the expelled fluid is yellowish or greenish due to having bile in it. Throwing up bile is often a sign that the liver is producing an excess of bile from the liver.

BIOAVAILABLE

The ability of a substance to be absorbed by a living organism. It also refers to an amount of a nutrient that is available for absorption. Simply because there is an amount of a substance ingested, doesn't necessarily mean all of that substance will be fully absorbed and utilized by the body.

BLANCH

The process by which something is whitened. In terms of a health condition, it means to suddenly to turn white or become very pale.

BURSA

A fluid-filled sac located next to the tendons near the large joints in the shoulders, elbows, hips and knees that serve as a cushion and gliding surface to reduce friction between the tissues of the body. When the bursa gets inflamed, it is called bursitis.

CANDIDA (also known as Candida Albicans)

A yeastlike parasitic fungus that can sometimes cause thrush or other yeast-type infections.

CARPAL TUNNEL

There is an opening in the wrist on the bottom that is formed by the carpal bones and on the top where the transverse carpal ligament crosses the top of the wrist. Additionally there is a median nerve that can get inflamed that then causes what is called, carpal tunnel syndrome which can cause numbness, pain, weakness and tingling in the hand and wrist.

CATARRH

Excess mucus in the nose or throat.

CELL SALTS (A.K.A TISSUE SALTS)

Cell Salts are a biochemical system of medicine developed by a German physician, W.H. Schüssler. He developed an idea that tissues and cells of the human body can be broken down into twelve main inorganic mineral salts identified as calcium fluoride, calcium phosphate, calcium sulphate, phosphate of iron, potassium chloride, potassium phosphate, potassium sulphate, magnesium phosphate, sodium chloride, sodium phosphate, sodium sulphate, and silica. He further determined that when there was a disruption in the health of an individual, it was because of a disturbance in the levels of these salts in the body. He finally concluded that health could be restored by administering minute doses of these minerals prepared according to homeopathic preparation principles (6x and 12x potencies). Even though they are made by homeopathic principles, they are not considered homeopathic, but biochemic, as the salts still have a trace of the mineral in their content. Read more about **Cell Salts** in **Chapter 3**.

CERVICAL SPINE

The part of the spinal column that is the neck from the base of the skull to the top of the shoulders.

CHRONIC

See "Acute".

CLASSICAL HOMEOPATHY

The term classical homeopathy simply means individualizing homeopathic treatment and using a single remedy. This is a different philosophy than combination remedies. In classical homeopathic prescribing, the individual is considered as a whole (not just their allergies, headaches, etc.) for symptoms from the body, mind, and spirit are all taken into consideration when choosing an appropriate homeopathic remedy. Classical homeopathy best matches the totality of the individual's symptoms and personality with the homeopathic remedy in order to stimulate the body's own natural healing response.

COLITIS

Inflammation of the large intestine/colon.

COITION

The act of engaging in sexual intercourse.

COMBINATION REMEDIES

Some homeopathic products combine several different homeopathic remedies, each of which is known to be helpful for a certain common symptom associated with the condition listed on the packaging or label. The premise is that the combination will address that condition for the majority of individuals. For example, a combination product for allergies might contain the five most frequently prescribed homeopathic remedies for allergies. These combination remedies are often safely and effectively used for simple acute conditions; however, they do not constitute classical homeopathy. Combination products can be a wonderful way for a newcomer to begin her/his homeopathic journey.

CONCOMITANTS

A concomitant literally means "naturally accompanying or associated". In a homeopathic context, it is referring to symptoms that occur at the same time as part of the main complaint of a person's condition. They are not necessarily directly connected to the main complaint. For example, every time I get this headache, I also have diarrhea.

CONJUNCTIVITIS

Commonly known as "pink eye," is an infection of the outermost layer of the white part of the eye (that gets very red) and the innermost layer of the eyelid.

CONSTITUTION/CONSTITUTIONAL TREATMENT

Overall health is determined by a person's heredity, life history, lifestyle, environment, and past treatments and is considered his/her constitution. Homeopathic constitutional treatment involves a careful assessment of a person's constitution and current total symptomatology. After the analysis of this information; a remedy is selected that best matches the totality of the symptoms in order to stimulate the person's inner healing at the deepest level. Since constitutional treatment requires an in-depth and objective view of the individual from a broad perspective, this is best achieved under the care of a professional homeopath.

CORNEA

The transparent surface of the eye that lies in front of the iris and pupil. The cornea is what allows light to enter the eye.

CORYZA

Inflammation of the nasal cavity that generally causes a runny nose, possible congestion and loss of smell.

COCCYX

The small curved bone at the end of the spine that is commonly called the "tailbone."

DEBRIDEMENT

The medical process of removing dead tissue (a procedure done for the removal of serious burn tissue and dead skin from bedsores).

DEEP VEIN THROMBOSIS (DVT)

A blood clot that forms in a deep vein, usually in the upper leg or calf, typically while flying or remaining seated for long periods of time.

DERMIS

This is skin that lies under the epidermis (see explanation below). It comprises the middle layer of skin and is a dense layer composed of connective tissue, blood and lymph vessels, sweat glands, hair follicles and a sensory nerve network.

DECUBITUS ULCERS

These ulcers are commonly called bedsores or pressure sores. These sores develop from someone being bedridden or wheelchair bound from prolonged pressure on the skin, especially over bony protuberances.

DISEASE

In homeopathy, dis-ease (lack of ease), is simply an illness or sickness. It is a disturbance or a derangement in the vital force as a consequence of infection, stress, a weakness in the system or from environmental contaminants that affect the proper functioning of the organism.

DOSE/DOSING

A dose is the unit of measurement in Homeopathy that refers to the particular means by which a remedy is prepared and the resultant amount. Dosing refers to the instructions as to what remedy and how the remedy is taken (liquid, pillules or lactose tablets) in what potency and in what frequency.

EDEMA

An accumulation of excess serous (pale yellow or

transparent) fluid that builds up in cells, tissues and body cavities. It can be benign and mild or a serious sign of heart, liver, kidney failure and other diseases.

ENURESIS

Nighttime bedwetting.

EPIDERMIS

The outer layer of skin that tends to be nonvascular and nonsensitive that covers the corium (the "true" skin).

EPISIOTOMY

An incision that is made between the vagina and anus during childbirth. Prevents the perineal tissue from tearing.

ERUCTATIONS

An homeopathic word for belching (burping). It is the raising of gas or acidic fluid from the stomach resulting in a burp.

EUSTACHIAN TUBE

It's a tube that provides a passageway from the throat to the middle ear. Sneezing, swallowing and yawning, help to keep your eustachian tubes open that in turn keeps air pressure and fluid from building up in the ear. The eustachian tube can get plugged. The main function of the eustachian tubes is to keep the middle ear healthy by draining fluids, equalizing pressure and protecting the middle ear from pathogens that can cause an infection.

EXCORIATE

Superficial abrasions caused by scratching or scraping resulting in chapped, chafed. worn off or raw skin.

FLATUS/FLATULENCE

It is when there is wind present in the intestine or stomach and produces eructations (gas) that remains trapped or gets expelled from the rectum. It is generally a result of bacterial action on waste matter and is composed primarily of hydrogen sulfide and varying amounts of methane.

GANGRENE/GANGRENOUS

A type of death to the tissue that is caused by lack of blood supply. There can be a change in skin color, generally red or black. There can be pain, swelling, numbness, evidence of the skin breaking down or coolness of the skin to the touch. It can also be caused by an infectious agent such as bacteria.

GASTRIC DISTENSION

When there is a gas buildup (wind) in the lower belly, it can become bloated resulting in a rounded belly and sometimes with the sensation of pressure and fullness.

GASTRITIS

Inflammation of the stomach.

GASTROENTERITIS

Inflammation of the stomach or intestines or both.

HEALTH

"Homeopaths define health as a state of freedom existing on three interrelated levels. The physical, the emotional, and the mental. A healthy person experiences physical vitality and freedom from physiological malfunction, emotional peace and freedom of expression, and mental clarity with creativity. The most serious symptoms affect the deeper, more vital parts of the person. Evaluation of our overall state of health, according to the homeopath, depends on the mental state, next our emotional state, and then on our physical state."[1]

HEMATOMA

It can simply be referred to as a "black and blue mark." However, it is actually a swelling filled with blood resulting from a break in a blood vessel.

HERING'S LAW OF CURE

Constantine Hering, a German homeopath who emigrated to the U.S. in the 1830's, observed that healing occurs in a consistent pattern. He described this pattern in the form of three basic laws which homeopaths can use to evaluate and recognize that healing is occurring. "The main use of Hering's laws

---

1   *Everybody's Guide to Homeopathic Medicines* by Cummings and Ullman, page 12.

for you will be in home-treatment situations. You'll want to know whether the medicine you have given is helping... In acute situations, the homeopathic healing response is usually rapid and complete, and the progress of symptoms as it follows the laws often will be too rapid to notice. Whenever you are in doubt about a person's response, however, consider the changes in symptoms in light of Hering's laws."[2]

For more details, see **Chapter 1—Hering's Law of Cure** *on* **page 18**.

HFM

Hand, foot and mouth disease caused by the coxsackie A16 virus that produces a rash.

HISTAMINE

In the human body, histamine is a chemical found in many of the cells and is considered part of the immune systems to protect the body from foreign invaders. In the case of allergies, the body perceives certain substances (ordinarily not harmful to the body) as being harmful and produces what is known as an allergic reaction. This prompts the body's cells to act on a person's head, eyes, ears, nose, throat, lungs and gastrointestinal tract causing symptoms.

HOMEOPATH

A homeopath is someone who practices the healing art of homeopathy. Historically, homeopaths in the United States have been primarily licensed medical doctors, naturopaths, and osteopaths who were interested in and added homeopathy to their practice. As of this printing, there are around 100 homeopathic medical practitioners listed through their association – The American Institute of Homeopathy. In the last century, there has been another surge of lay people in the US (not otherwise licensed in any medical profession) who are being trained as professional homeopaths and have become certified classical homeopaths through the stringent requirements of The Council for Homeopathic Certification. As of this printing, there are over 1,000 nationally certified classical homeopaths listed. Additionally, though not listed anywhere, there are many other private individuals who are studying homeopathy through study groups, online programs, webinars, and other learning opportunities so they can use homeopathy for themselves and their families.

HOMEOPATHY

See description in **Chapter 1** *on* **page 17**.

HOMEOPROPHYLAXIS

Homeoprophylaxis is the preventative use of specific homeopathic nosode remedies to help educate one's immune system to infectious diseases prior to encountering them.

HOMEOSTASIS

Every living being is always in a fluctuating state of homeostasis. It's a state of equilibrium, the condition of optimal functioning for an organism. An example of homeostasis is the human body keeping an average temperature of 98.6 degrees. When a fever presents, it's the body's best response to an invading organism in an attempt to destroy the bacteria or virus with heat to assist the body in regaining homeostasis.

HYPOTENSION

In layman's terms this is low blood pressure. What is happening is that the parameters of healthy blood pressure are below normal levels. Both systolic (contracting) pressure (the top number on your blood pressure reading) and diastolic (expanding) pressure (the bottom number on your blood pressure reading.)

INCARCERATED GAS

An accumulation of gas in the intestines that gets stuck.

INTERMITTENT

Intermittent means the symptoms occur at irregular intervals, not continuous or steady. Compare with Persistent.

IRRITABLE

Irritable means the person is easily annoyed or bothered, usually causing a foul mood and touchiness.

---

2   Ibid., page 14.

KEYNOTES

Keynotes are frequently seen common symptoms that appear in many different individuals who need the same homeopathic remedy. Such a symptom then becomes associated with that remedy. When it appears more intensely in an individual case, that remedy would be more strongly considered. An example is "desire for lemonade", a keynote of Belladonna, or "stinging pain", a keynote of Apis (bee venom).

KOPLIK'S SPOTS

Tiny spots, like grains of sand, that precede the actual rash that is characteristic of measles.

LAW OF DEFICIENCY

Whereas Homeopathy is based on the Law of Similars (see below), Cell/Tissue Salt usage relies on the Law of deficiency. That is when the conditions of the body, when out of balance, will point to one or several mineral deficiencies. The theory being that if the deficiency via the use of cell salt is corrected, the symptoms and body signs will improve or resolve.

LAW OF SIMILARS/ LIKE CURES LIKE

Homeopathy is based on the principle of "like cures like" or the Law of Similars. This means that a material substance that is capable of producing certain symptoms in a healthy person can also remove, address or alleviate these symptoms in an ill person when the same substance is given as a homeopathic remedy.

For more details review **Chapter 1—Like Cures Like** *starting on* **page 19**.

LOCATION

Location is where in the body a symptom is experienced. It's one of the main underpinnings of identifying a complete description of a symptom. For example, I have a headache. But, where is it? The options are many such as forehead, temples, top of the head (or vertex), back of the head (or occipital region), etc. or a combination of these. Since remedies have affinities for different locations of the body, knowing the exact location is important.

LYMPHOCYTES

Immune cells that produce antibodies.

MATERIA MEDICA

A materia medica is a book that lists the substances used to make homeopathic remedies along with detailed indications for their application. The information in a materia medica is compiled from provings and clinical observations. The Latin words "materia medica" mean "materials of medicines".

See the list of remedies and the substances from which they are made in **Appendix 2—Remedy Name Chart** *starting on* **page 327.**

MENSES

Literally means the menstrual flow that is associated with normal vaginal bleeding that occurs as part of a woman's monthly cycle.

MICROBIOME

Your microbiome is the collection of all microbes, such as bacteria, fungi, viruses, and their genes, that naturally live in and on our bodies. More commonly the microbiome refers to your gut health. The best way to maintain a healthy microbiome is to eat a range of fresh, whole foods, mainly from plant sources like fruits, vegetables, legumes, beans, nuts and whole grains.

MODALITIES

A modality is an action or circumstance that makes a person or their symptom better or worse. For example, joint pain that feels better with hot applications, or back pain that feels better when sitting, or head pain that is worse in the sun, etc. Modalities are an important part of a complete homeopathic analysis.

MOLECULAR STRUCTURE OF REMEDIES

After a homeopathic remedy is potentized to the stage of 12c or 24X (which is the same potency), it is impossible to detect any molecules of the original substance. At this stage, the remedy becomes "sub-molecular" and free of chemical side effects. The surprising fact is that homeopathic remedies are often potentized thousands of times higher than these "low potency" levels, yet when prescribed according to the Law of Similars, they still retain their ability to trigger healing responses in the unwell.

Generally, higher potency remedies act more deeply

and trigger longer lasting reactions than their low potency counterparts. However, recently, with nanotechnology, the latest research shows the very highest homeopathic dilutions contain "nanoparticles" of the original substance that has been potentized. Nanoparticles are between 1 and 100 nanometers in size. A nanometer is 1 billionth of a meter. A single atom is one-tenth of a nanometer, and subatomic particles are even smaller. Quantum mechanics confirms these tiny particles impact our macro world and can be useful in such things as medicine, electronics, and the environment. Thus, after decades, we now have some reliable scientific verification of why a homeopathic remedy can produce a healing reaction in the body.

MOTHER TINCTURE

The mother tincture is the first stage in the preparation of a homeopathic remedy made by soaking a plant, animal, or mineral product in a solution of alcohol and water. It distills the raw material for the first dilution in the process of successive dilutions of an individual remedy.

NETTLE RASH

Nettle (urtica dioica) is a weed that when touched can cause a stinging sensation and produces a fluid-filled rash that can be itchy and certainly uncomfortable.

NOSODES

A nosode is a homeopathic remedy prepared from diseased tissue or the product of a disease. For example: Tuberculinum is prepared from the mucus or pus from a person who has tuberculosis. Nosodes are NOT found in a home remedy kit and should only be used by trained professional homeopaths.

OCCIPITAL/OCCIPUT

The back of the head.

THE ORGANON AND APHORISMS

During Samuel Hahnemann's career, he condensed his principles of the philosophy and practice of homeopathic medicine, including the tenets for maintaining health, into a book of aphorisms (insightful philosophical ideas) called *The Organon*. It was written in Hahnemann's native German and translated into many languages over the years. There are six different editions in existence with each edition building upon the previous one and adding more insights as a result of his experience. Anyone who is interested in learning more about his philosophies or planning to become a homeopath is strongly recommended to read and study *The Organon*.

PALLIATIVE

The process of lessening pain or reducing pain or sickness when a cure is no longer possible. In terms of homeopathy specifically it can mean that the chosen homeopathic remedy was helpful, but not one that could facilitate resolution of an ailment, if the presenting complaint can be resolved completely.

PAPULES

Pink and red spots typically seen in the early stages of chickenpox.

PARALYTIC

This refers to someone who is affected by paralysis as with a disease or is paralyzed.

PARAMYXOVIRUS

A group of viruses that are responsible for childhood illnesses such as mumps, measles, and parainfluenza among others.

PARAPLEGIA

A condition that comes from damage to the spinal cord that results in complete paralysis of the low half of the body including both legs.

PEEVISH

Easily irritated, especially by unimportant things.

PERIOSTEUM

The membrane that covers the outer surface of the bones.

PERISTALSIS

The wave-like muscle contractions that move food through the digestive tract starting at the esophagus.

PERSISTENT

When describing a symptom, persistent means a

stubbornly unyielding symptom that doesn't stop. Compare with Intermittent.

PHOBIA

A deep-seated, chronically ingrained fear.

PLEURISY

Pleurisy is an inflammation of the lining of the lungs and chest (the pleura) that leads to chest pain when you take a breath or cough.

PLUSSING

The way to make your remedy a little bit stronger. *For details, see **page 36**.*

POTENTIZATION AND POTENCY SCALES

To minimize side effects and create gentler medicines, Samuel Hahnemann developed a simple and easily reproducible process known as potentization. This is the process by which all homeopathic remedies are made. It is a series of dilutions and **succussions** (vigorous shaking with pounding). All homeopathic remedies have numbers and/or letters that follow their names to indicate the potency of each remedy. Each homeopathic medicine is referenced by the name of the raw material or strain followed by the level of dilution and scale such as Arnica 6C (made from a mountain daisy) or Sepia 30X (made from cuttlefish ink). It is important to note that 6C or 30X are not quantities (as in Aspirin 100 mg), but levels of dilutions.

There are four scales of dilutions described in the homeopathic pharmacopeia of the United States (HPUS), which is the official compendium for homeopathic medicines.

THE CENTESIMAL SCALE (C Potencies)

The first scale that Hahnemann developed during the early years of homeopathy is the centesimal scale. As its name would suggest, it has a 1:100 dilution ratio. A 1C (C is 100 in Roman numerals) is 100 times more diluted than the raw material (plant, mineral, animal part); a 2C is 100 times more diluted than a 1C; a 3C is 100 times more diluted than a 2C, etc.

Each successive dilution is prepared by mixing 1% of the previous dilution with 99% of solvent, usually 70% alcohol, in a new vial. The vial is then vigorously shaken against a hard surface. This step, called succussion, is essential to obtain a homogenous and therapeutically active homeopathic dilution. The most common dilutions used in the US are 6C, 9C, 12C and 30C. 6C is a low dilution, 30C is a high dilution.

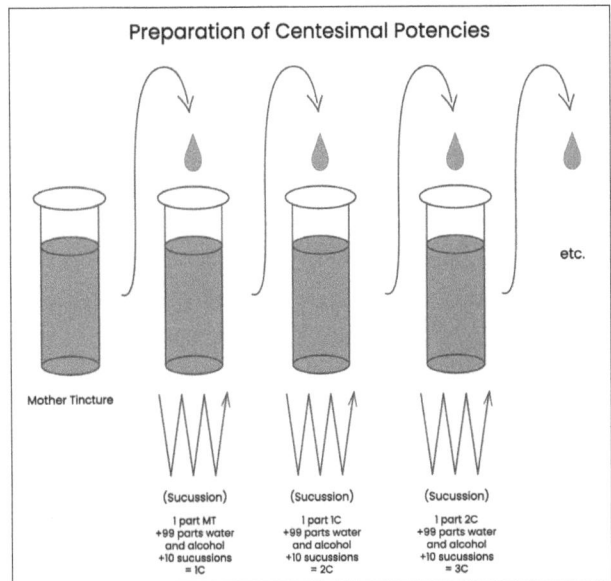

Preparation of Centesimal Potencies

Mother Tincture

(Succussion) — 1 part MT +99 parts water and alcohol +10 sucussions = 1C

(Succussion) — 1 part 1C +99 parts water and alcohol +10 sucussions = 2C

(Sucussion) — 1 part 2C +99 parts water and alcohol +10 sucussions = 3C

etc.

Diagram of How a C potency is Made. Graphic based on: homeopathy101.wordpress.com.

THE DECIMAL SCALE (X Potencies)

In this scale, the dilution factor is 10. A 1X is the raw material diluted 10 times (X is 10 in Roman numerals). A 2X is 10 times more diluted than a 1X, etc. Otherwise the process is identical to the C scale, including the succussion step. 1X to 6X are low dilutions, and 30X is a high dilution. A 30X is equivalent to a 15C. Some homeopathic practitioners, German especially, prefer the X scale, while others use the C scale. In some countries, the X scale is called the D scale (as in decimal).

THE CK SCALE (Korsakov Scale)

The CK scale was developed by Russian practitioner Simeon Korsakov. It is a centesimal scale of dilution (1% dilution) and succussion, with two differences from the C scale: each step of dilution is prepared in a single vial (versus a new vial per dilution), and the solvent is pure water (versus with 70% alcohol). Common CK dilutions are 6CK, 30CK, 200CK, 1,000CK (also named 1M for convenience),

10,000CK (or 10M), 50,000CK (or 50M) and 100,000 CK (or CM). These potencies are meant for the use of professional homeopaths only.

THE LM SCALE

This last scale of dilution was developed by Hahnemann at the end of his long life. Here, the dilution factor is 50,000 (LM in Latin numerals). They are also known as Q (quinquaginta millesimal) dilutions. A 2 LM is 50,000 times more diluted than a 1 LM. The series goes from 1 to 30LM. LM dilutions are traditionally sold as liquid drops or very small pellets (poppy seed sized) that are dissolved in water before use. LM potencies are administered very differently from the other potencies, in a process that is individualized to the particular case. Again, these potencies are meant for the use of professional homeopaths only.

For self-medication, it is best to use the C or X scale and start with low dilutions. Using LM or CK dilutions requires experience in homeopathy and should be reserved to skilled health professionals.

PROVINGS

A proving is the method used for understanding the effects of a potentized homeopathic substance. A sample of healthy people is given homeopathic doses of a substance with the objective of determining the symptoms the substance causes, and thus what symptoms it may have the capacity to alleviate when given in a homeopathic potentized dose. Participants in provings are monitored by master provers and are required to keep records of and report all their symptoms since taking of the remedy. The symptom picture of that remedy is compiled and then developed from these observations. Once the provers stop taking the remedy, the symptoms gradually go away. A materia medica is where you would find the symptom pictures of these homeopathic provings. Provings are only done on humans, not animals.

PUSTULAR

Yellow pus-filled eruption.

REMEDY

The term remedy is used to define a homeopathic medicine. A remedy is a highly diluted, potentized substance. Remedies start as a material substance, then triturated into a Mother Tincture, or ground to a fine substance, then added to water with some alcohol (as a preservative), then serially diluted and vigorously shaken (succussed). The resulting liquid is then dropped onto the outside of either sucrose or lactose sugar pellets. Remedies are most commonly administered as a liquid or taken as a dry pellet in a clean mouth and then dissolved under the tongue.

REPERTORY

The repertory is a reference book, which contains extensive lists of symptoms and the remedies that have been found helpful for that symptom through provings and clinical observations. The homeopath uses the repertory to determine which remedies may be helpful for the symptoms he or she is addressing. Repertories also provide information about the relative usefulness of a remedy for a particular symptom by using different typefaces for the remedies listed. These codes differ between repertories. The most commonly used repertory in the United States is Kent's Repertory. Repertorization, or the use of the repertory, is one facet of homeopathy that has been enhanced by the computer, and there are several computer repertories available.

RUBRIC

A rubric is a set of words used to denote a symptom found in a homeopathic repertory.

SACRUM

A large triangular bone that connects the lower part of the spine to the pelvis. It is also known as the sacral region.

SARCODES

Sarcode is a tissue or glandular extract created from healthy animal products that are made into a homeopathic remedy. For example, Thyroidinum is made from thyroid tissue. Sarcodes are NOT found in a home remedy kit and should only be used by trained professional homeopaths.

SCIATICA

The sciatic nerve is located in the lower part of the body and is formed by the union of five nerve roots in the lower spine. It is located deep within the buttocks and travels down the back of the thigh, all the way down to the heel and sole of the foot. Pressure on the sciatic nerve causes this condition called sciatica. Certain spinal conditions can put pressure on the nerve that causes inflammation and subsequent pain. The pain can be a mild ache or worsen into a sharp, burning pain that can feel like jolts or electric shock. Some people experience muscle weakness, tingling or numbness.

SENSATION

A sensation is the actual experience of what a symptom feels like for the person. For example, a headache could feel like stabbing, shooting, throbbing, pressure, sticking, etc.

SEPTUM

The bone and cartilage that divide the nasal cavity of the nose in half.

SIMILLIMUM

The simillimum is the most similar remedy corresponding to a set of symptoms expressed by the individual. It is this remedy that holds the greatest potential to relieve the person's symptomology.

SLOUGHING

The act or process of shedding skin, often the separation of dead tissue from healthy tissue.

SPHINCTER MUSCLES

Sphincters are circular muscles that open and close passages in the body to regulate the flow of substances.In the case of the anus, this is a group of muscles at the end of the rectum. The rectum is located at the last few inches of the large intestine (colon). These muscles surround the anus and control the release of stool. They can be found in other parts of the body, but mostly known for the ones regulating stool.

SUCCUSSION

Succussion is the act of vigorously shaking by banging the bottle or vial of a diluted preparation or substance on a book or other hard surface as it is being made into a remedy.
See **Potentization and Potency** *scales in this appendix for more information.*

SUPPURATE/SUPPURATION

The process of producing or discharging pus from an infected wound.

SUPPRESSION

Suppression is a term frequently associated with conventional or allopathic medicine. It's the result of giving a chemical medicine to prevent or relieve an unwanted symptom which can result in driving the disease deeper into the body. For example, people with itching skin affections may put a pharmaceutical cream on it to suppress the itch but this may drive the disease state deeper as evidenced by a new respiratory problem that surfaces like wheezing, asthma, or chronic cough.

SYMPTOMS

A homeopath sees that the body, through the activity of the vital force, is always working to keep itself well and in balance. When the body is threatened (by bacteria, viruses, trauma, stress, etc.), the vital force causes the body to produce symptoms such as pain, fatigue, mucus, and/or fever. These symptoms have a purpose: to ultimately restore well-being and balance. Here are some examples: Pain is a warning that something is not right; fever stimulates the immune system and deactivates many viruses and bacteria; mucus surrounds and carries off irritating material; fatigue causes a person to rest.

A homeopath considers symptoms to be the body's healthy and appropriate reaction to outside forces. Allopathy regards symptoms as manifestations of disease, which should be opposed or suppressed. For example, aspirin is given to lower fever and reduce pain, and antihistamines are given to dry up mucus. The homeopath seeks to support the individual's vital force to move toward health and balance, using the symptoms the individual produces as a guide to the selection of the correct remedy. Homeopaths treat the patient according to their own subjective description of their symptoms, not according to the disease.

"The homeopathic definition of the term 'symptoms' encompasses the physical and psychological, the obvious and subtle, the common and the unusual. Even if the person has a main symptom that is causing much discomfort, the homeopath must also assess all other physical and psychological symptoms. Characteristic emotional states, changes in the person's energy level, sensitivity to heat or cold, and numerous other factors must also be considered."[3]

"The assumption is that no matter what combination of conditions, complaints, and sufferings a patient experiences at any one time, all are the manifestation of a single 'disease,' an internal physiological disorder that is unique to the individual. The homeopath believes that no one organ of the body can be sick without affecting the person as a whole. Therefore, all symptoms must be taken into account; all are part of the body's effort to heal. It is crucial to understand that, in spite of the homeopath's desire to know all the minute details of the patient's symptoms, he or she does not treat symptoms. Instead the symptoms guide the homeopath to the medicine that can best stimulate the person's defenses."[4]

SYNCOPE

A brief loss of consciousness represented by fainting or passing out, caused by inadequate blood flow to the brain and generally is self-limiting and not connected to serious conditions

THROMBOSED

Affected with or obstructed by a clot of coagulated blood.

TRITURATION

The act of reducing a substance to a fine powder while incorporating it thoroughly with milk sugar by mixing with a mortar and pestle.

URTICARIA

A generic homeopathic term for hives and rashes.

UVULA

The cone-shaped piece of flesh at the back of the mouth at the entrance of the throat, and is an extension to the soft palace. It is composed of glands, small muscle fibers and connective tissue. It lubricates the throat by secreting large amounts of saliva and it helps to keep food or fluids from the space behind your nose when you swallow.

VARICELLA

Commonly called chickenpox.

VASOVAGAL (EPISODE/SYNCOPE)

This is the most common cause of fainting typically happening by a trigger such as the sight of blood or an intense emotion, usually fear or fright.

VERTEX

The top of the head, referred to as the crown.

VESICLES

Fluid-filled bumps that typically occur in the second stage of chickenpox.

VITAL FORCE

The vital force is the energy that enables all living things—human, plant or animal—to self-heal and/or to preserve life by adapting to environmental changes. It is the vital force that separates us from non-living matter. In the English-speaking world it has been called the life principle, life force, vitality, or dynamis. In other cultures, it has been known as qi, chi, or prana. Hahnemann called it the vital force. In the case of the human body, the vital force directs the different body systems to function as a harmonious whole, in much the same way a conductor directs the separate parts of an orchestra to produce a single, pleasing piece of music. When a plant or

---

3   Ibid., page 8.
4   Ibid., page 8.

animal is diseased, we look to the symptoms as clues for finding the correct remedy.

Symptoms are the secondary changes and are the products of a deeper disturbance. Apart from injury, the symptoms of disease and ill-health can only occur when there has been a disruption to the energetic vital force. This disruption can occur from mental shocks such as deep grief, prolonged anxiety, terror, disappointment, or even extreme joy. Physical shocks can come from infectious diseases, exposure to the elements, trauma, malnutrition, extreme exertion, and so on.

The vital force, when disrupted energetically by one of these shocks, enters a struggle to regain its balance and preserve life. During this struggle, the vital force produces signs and symptoms. These are not the disturbance but only the byproducts of the struggle. In the case of acute problems such as the flu, gastroenteritis, and headaches, the vital force is usually successful, and the person recovers. In other instances, an acute problem can gradually change into a chronic disease.

WATER BRASH

The production of an excess amount of saliva that mixes with stomach acid and has risen into the throat. This is usually a result for people with gastro-esophageal reflux disease. It can feel like heartburn and leaves a bad taste in the mouth.

Appendix 4
Additional Resources

Note: All the resources and the links that follow were verified at the time of this book's publication (July 2024). Including them here is solely for the reader's reference, not an endorsement by Homeopathy Educator LLC or Homeopathy Educator Press.

Suggested Readings

These three books are great starter books to add to your reading list:

Homeopathy: Start Here, Ann Jerome PhD, CCH, available through Amazon in both paperback and Kindle editions.

Homeopathy: Beyond Flat Earth Medicine, Dr. Timothy Dooley, MD, ND, available online at no cost or in bound form through online booksellers.

The Parent's Guide to Homeopathy, Shelley Keneipp, MH, DiHom(UK), available through the author's website www.LifelongHomeopathy.com.

Additionally, here are some practical reference books that can also be secured online to assist with your learning:

A Concise Repertory of Homoeopathic Medicines, Dr. S.R. Phatak.

Easy Homeopathy, Edward Shalts, MD.

Everybody's Guide to Homeopathic Medicines, Stephen Cummings and Dana Ullman.

Freedom from Infectious Diseases—The Homeopathic Solution, Manfred Mueller.

Homeopathic Medicine at Home, Maesimund B. Panos, MD and Jane Heimlich.

Homeopathic Medicine for Children and Infants, Dana Ullman.

Homeopathic Remedies, Asa Hershoff.

Homeopathy Basics, Priscilla Medders.

Homeopathy for Musculoskeletal Healing, Asa Hershoff.

Homeopathy for Pregnancy, Birth and Beyond, Miranda Castro, CCH, RSHom(NA), FSHom.

Impossible Cure, Amy Lansky.

Levels of Health, Professor George Vithoulkas.

Magic of the Minimum Dose, Dr. Dorothy Shepherd.

Materia Medica of Homoeopathic Medicines, Dr. S.R. Phatak.

More Magic of the Minimum Dose, Dr. Dorothy Shepherd.

Organon Reflections, Wendy Thacher Jensen.

Practical Homeopathy, Vinton McCabe.

Reach for a Remedy, Sheehy & Jones.

The Best Family Homeopathy Acute Care Manual, Kate Birch.

The Complete Homeopathy Handbook, Miranda Castro, CCH, RSHom(NA), FSHom

The Family Guide to Homeopathy: Symptoms and Natural Solutions, Andrew Lockie.

The Parent's Guide to Homeopathy, Shelley Keneipp, MH, DiHom(UK).
The Practical Handbook of Homeopathy, Colin Griffith, MCH, RSHom.
The Science of Homeopathy, Professor George Vithoulkas.
And for the very serious, we suggest *The Organon of the Medical Art (sixth edition)* by Dr. Samuel Hahnemann, the founder of homeopathy and edited by Wenda Brewster O'Reilly PhD. His entire book, originally written in German in 1842, is considered the homeopathic bible and a very interesting study in homeopathic and healing philosophy.

More Great Books

In addition to these specialty books, take a look at **Appendix 5: Bibliographic Resources** where you'll see the many sources used in this book. Many of them are books to consider adding to your bookshelf!

Cell Salt References

Homeopathic Cell Salt Remedies, Nigley Lennon and Lionel Rolfe.
Schussler's Biochemic Pocket Guide with Repertory.
The Biochemic System of Medicine, George Carey.
The Human Echo, Vinton McCabe.

Agriculture References

Narayana Verlag, Homeopathy, Natural Healing, Healthy Food, https://narayana-verlag.com.
Homeoplant—*Homeopathy for Farm and Garden*, Narayana Verlag, Homeopathy, Natural Healing, Healthy Food, https://narayana-verlag.com.
Homeopathy for Farm and Garden: The Homeopathic Treatment of Plants—6th revised edition, Vaikunthanath Das Kaviraj, https://narayana-verlag.com.
Homeopathy for Plants—5th revised edition, Christiane Maute®.

Animal References

Homeopathic Care for Cats and Dogs, Revised Edition: Small Doses for Small Animals, Don Hamilton D.V.M. (Author), Richard Pitcairn DVM (Foreword).
Homeopathy for Pets, George Macleod.
Natural Health for Dogs & Cats, Richard H. Pitcairn, DVM, PhD.
Practical Handbook of Veterinary Homeopathy, Wendy Thacher Jensen, DVM.

Basic Homeopathy and Related Podcasts

Homeopathy247 Podcast with Mary Greensmith, https://homeopathy247.com/podcast.
Homeopathy at Home with Melissa Crenshaw, https://melissacrenshaw.com/podcasts.
Homeopathy Hangout with Eugenie Krueger, https://homeopathyhangout.com.
Homeopathy for Mommies with Sue Meyer, https://ultimateradioshow.com/homeopathyformommies.
Homeopathyly for the People with Mette Mitchell, https://open.spotify.com/show/0UxwyKftU2Ov9o1BHw93pS.
Honest Homeopathy with Amelia Phipps, https://podcasters.spotify.com/pod/show/honest-homeopathy.
Intuitive Homeopathy Podcast with Angelica Lemke, Sarah Valentini, and Bridget Biscotti Bradley, https://www.homeopathyhive.com/podcast.
Practical Homeopathy with Joette Calabrese, https://joettecalabrese.com/podcast1.

Robert Scott Bell Show, https://podcasts.apple.com/us/podcast/robert-scott-bell-show-podcast/id392503709.
Strange Rare and Peculiar Podcast with Denise Straiges and Alistair Gray,
   https://academyofhomeopathyeducation.com/srp-podcast.
Wise Traditions - Weston A.Price Foundation, https://www.westonaprice.org/podcast.

Some Educational Films About Homeopathy

Just One Drop, https://justonedropfilm.com.
Magic Pills, https://magicpillsmovie.com.
Introducing Homeopathy, https://introducinghomeopathy.com.

How to find a qualified practitioner

To find an U.S. homeopathic provider, use the links below. Know that many homeopaths provide virtual consults so they don't necessarily need to be in your city or state.

- **The American Association of Naturopathic Physicians (AANP)**, www.naturopathic.org.
- **The American Institute of Homeopathy (AIH)**, https://homeopathyusa.org.
- **The Council for Homeopathic Certification (CHC)**, www.homeopathicdirectory.com.
- **The National Center for Homeopathy (NCH)**, www.homeopathycenter.org.
- **The North American Society of Homeopaths (NASH)**, www.homeopathy.org.

If you live in the UK, you can search at:
- **Homeopathy UK**, https://homeopathy-uk.org/find-a-homeopath-search.

If you live in Canada, you can search at:
- **The Canadians for Homeopathy**, https://canadiansforhomeopathy.com/find-a-homeopath.

If you live in Australia, you can search at:
- **The Australian Homeopathic Association**, https://www.homeopathyoz.org.

If you live in India, you can search on:
- **Bark**, https://www.bark.com/en/in/homeopathy.

In addition to these resources, there are other online registries so it would be wise to do a more thorough internet search for homeopathic practitioners specific to your country.

How to Gain More Experience and Knowledge

- **Start a study group** using this book to help guide you to choose appropriate remedies.
- **Connect with an experienced practitioner** to get homeopathic care for yourself and your family.
- **Search the internet** for where you can access homeopathy webinars, both free and fee-based.
- **Get a kit and try out** using your remedies for acute issues - it's the best way to learn!
- **Do some of Trinity Health Hub's "Health Self-Reliance" online, on-demand learning programs** for self care focusing on homeopathy. Also have more in depth training for all levels of homeopathic interest, https://trinityhealthhub.com/hsr.
- **Visit Dana Ullman's website** for books, blogs, remedies and interesting articles, https://homeopathic.com.

- **Investigate the Homeopathy Plus website**. Lots of remedy descriptions, informative free e-newsletter, https://homeopathyplus.com.
- **Join Mary Aspinwall's Homeopathy Study Group** on Facebook with over 40K members! Amazing networking and education while learning more with others online.
- **Check out Whole Health Now**. It offers a wide array of courses, from beginning to advanced continuing education. Their website has a lot of interesting reference information, including a timeline of homeopathy, and articles, well known homeopaths, https://www.wholehealthnow.com.
- **Click on Google "Free Homeopathy Webinars"** and you will see many topics, amazing presenters and organizations to learn from, all for free!
- **Set up an account for Joette Calabrese's free resource library,** https://joettecalabrese.com.
- **Utilize this free online remedy finder,** https://homeosource.org.
- **Learn about natural alternatives for various conditions,** www.alternativemedicine.com.
- **Educate yourself about diseases, diagnoses and medical terms,** www.webmd.com or www.medlineplus.gov.
- **Get acquainted with information about drug interactions and side effects,** www.rxlist.com.
- **Connect with the Holistic Moms network,** www.holisticmoms.org.

Homeopathic Research

To learn more about current research into homeopathy, go to **Homeopathy Research Institute** located at https://www.hri-research.org.

To read some research articles online, go to the **American Institute for Homeopathy** on their research page: https://homeopathyusa.org/aih-guide-to-homeopathic-research.

Phone or iPad Apps

Search your device's App Store for these starter apps. There are other more advanced ones but these are good to get started with:

- Mary Greensmith's app **Homeopathy@Home** for iPad and iPhone, $2.99.
- **Homeopathyly: Easy Home Prescriptions** for iPhone, $4.99.
- **Homeopathy for Everyone** for iPhone, FREE.
- **Homeopathy Medicine Finder** from Boiron for iPad and iPhone, FREE.
- **Helios Homeopathic Remedy Finder** for iPad and iPhone, FREE.

Where to Purchase Homeopathic Remedies

ABC Homeopathy, https://abchomeopathy.com/shop.php.
Ainsworth (UK based), https://www.ainsworths.com.
Amazon.com, https://www.amazon.com/Single-Homeopathic-Remedies/b?ie=UTF8&node=3767781.
Boiron, USA, https://boironusa.com.
Hahnemann Labs, https://www.hahnemannlabs.com.
Helios (UK based), https://www.helios.co.uk/. Best 36 remedy 30c kit available online.
Homeopathic Remedies Online, https://homeopathicremediesonline.com.
Homeopathy Store, https://www.homeopathystore.com.
Hyland's, https://hylands.com.
Ollois (lactose-free), http://ollois.com.
Thompson's Homeopathic Supplies LTD (Toronto, Ontario), https://www.thompsonshomeopathic.com.

Washington Homeopathics, https://www.homeopathyworks.com. At the time of publication, they were again offering 50 remedy 30c kits.

Where to Purchase Cell Salts

You can purchase cell salts individually or as a kit of 12 on the internet or in some health food stores. As of the time of the publication of this book, these were some options we found. Double-check the ingredients if concerned about a milk, dairy, or sugar allergen:

BeeHealthy Homeopathic, https://www.beehealthyhomeopathic.com/collections/tissue-salts.

Hylands, https://hylands.com/collections/cell-salts. Lactose tablets.

Jackson Naturals (Vegan Cell Salts), https://jacksonsnaturals.com. Sucrose tablets.

Miranda Castro's Shop, https://mirandacastro.com/shop. Lactose tablets.

Ollois, https://ollois.com/products/cell-salts-kit. Lactose Free, Vegan, Kosher.

The Homeopathy Store, https://www.homeopathystore.com/collections/schuessler-cell-salts. Liquid sprays.

Homeopathic Schools

ACHENA (Accreditation Commission for Homeopathic Education in North America) is an independent accreditation agency that assesses the educational standards of homeopathic schools and programs. Homeopathic schools and programs that receive ACHENA accreditation have met recognized standards of excellence aimed to protect the public and promote professionalism.

* = ACHENA approved at time of printing
** = Pending ACHENA at time of printing

- ***Academy of Homeopathy Education,** www.ahe.online.
- **Allen College of Homeopathy,** www.allencolleg.co.uk.
- ***American Medical College of Homeopathy at PIHMA,** www.AMCofH.org.
- ***British Institute of Homeopathy International,** www.bihint.com.
- **Caduceus Institute of Classical Homeopathy Training,** https://homeopathytraining.org.
- ***Canadian College of Homeopathic Medicine,** www.homeopathycanada.com.
- **Centre for Homeopathic Education (CHE)** (London), www.chehomeopathy.com.
- **College of Homeopaths of Ontario,** www.collegeofhomeopaths.com.
- **Homeopathy School International (HIS),** www.homeopathyschool.org.
- **International Academy of Classical Homeopathy (IACH),** George Vithoulkas, www.vithoulkas.com.
- **London College of Homeopathy,** UK, https://lchomeopathy.com.
- **Los Angeles School of Homeopathy,** www.Lahomeopathicschool.com.
- **Montreal Institute of Classical Homeopathy (MICH),** https://www.michmontreal.com.
- **New England School of Homeopathy (NESH),** https://nesh.com.
- **New York School of Homeopathy (NYSH),** https://nyhomeopathy.com.
- ***Northwestern Academy of Homeopathy,** www.homeopathictraining.org.
- **Ontario College of Homeopathic Medicine (OCHM),** https://ochm.ca.
- ****Prometheus Homeopathic Institute (PHI),** https://prometheushomeopathicinstitute.com.
- **Resonance School of Homeopathy,** https://www.resonanceschoolofhomeopathy.com.
- **The Homeopathic Academy of Southern California (HASC),** https://homeopathic-academy.net.
- ***The School of Homeopathy,** www.homeopathyschool.com.

Homeopathic Associations in the USA

Although Homeopathy Educator LLC is a for-profit entity, excess yearly revenues from the sale of this book, after reasonable expenses, will be donated equally among these 12 existing homeopathic associations in the United States.

1. **Academy of Veterinary Homeopathy (AVH)**, https://theavh.org.
2. **Accreditation Commission for Homeopathic Education in North America (ACHENA)**, https://achena.org.
3. **American Association of Homeopathic Pharmacists (AAHP)**, https://www.theaahp.org.
4. **American Institute of Homeopathy (AIH)**, https://homeopathyusa.org.
5. **Americans for Homeopathy Choice (AFC)**, https://homeopathychoice.org.
6. **Council for Homeopathic Certification (CHC)**, https://www.homeopathicdirectory.com.
7. **Free and Healthy Children International (FHCI)**, https://freeandhealthychildren.org.
8. **Homeopathic Academy of Naturopathic Physicians (HANP)**, https://hanp.net.
9. **Homeopathic Nurses Association (HNA)**, https://www.nursehomeopaths.org.
10. **Homeopaths Without Borders (HWB)**, https://www.hwbna.org.
11. **National Center for Homeopathy (NCH)**, https://homeopathycenter.org.
12. **North American Society of Homeopaths (NASH)**, https://homeopathy.org.

Local, State, Regional, National Membership Organizations for Homeopaths in North America

- **Arizona**: The Homeopathy Association of Arizona, https://homeopathyaz.com/about.
- **Arizona**: Arizona Homeopathic and Integrative Medical Association, https://arizonahomeopathic.org.
- **California**: Bay Area Homeopathy Association, https://www.bayareahomeopathyassociation.org.
- **California**: The California Homeopathic Medical Society, https://homeopathywest.org.
- **Canada**: Canadian Society of Homeopaths (CSOH), https://www.csoh.ca.
- **Canada**: West Coast Homeopathic Society (WCHS), https://www.wchs.info.
- **Florida**: Florida Homeopathic Society, https://floridahomeopathicsociety.org.
- **Maine**: Maine Association of Homeopaths, https://homeopathyinmaine.com.
- **Minnesota**: Minnesota Homeopathic Association (MHA), https://www.mnhomeopathicassociation.org.
- **Nevada**: Nevada State Board of Homeopathic Medical Examiners (NVBHME), https://nvbhme.org/licensees.html.
- **Oregon/Idaho**: Pacific Northwest Homeopathy Association (PNWHA), https://pnwha.org.
- **Texas**: Texas Society of Homeopathy, https://texassocietyofhomeopathy.com.

Consumer, Grassroots and Advocacy organizations for homeopathy

Americans for Homeopathy Choice, https://homeopathychoice.org.
HOHM Foundation, https://hohmfoundation.org.
Homeopaths Without Borders—NA (North America), https://www.hwbna.org.
Homeopathy Institute of the Pacific (HIP), https://www.homeopathyip.org.
Homeopathy for Health in Africa (HHA), https://homeopathyforhealthinafrica.org.
Homeopathy UK, https://homeopathy-uk.org.
National Center for Homeopathy, https://homeopathycenter.org.
The Traveling Homeopaths Collective, https://thc.org.uk.
The Society of Homeopaths (also known as 4Homeopathy), https://homeopathy-soh.org/about-us/4homeopathy.

Appendix 5
Bibliographic Resources

The following are resources our authors used when creating their content:

American Academy of Pediatrics, http://www.healthychildren.org.

A Synoptic Key to the Materia Medica, C.M. Boger.

British Homeopathic Association, http://britishhomeopathic.org.

Desktop Guide to Keynotes and Confirmatory Symptoms, Roger Morrison, MD.

Dr Homeo website—Dr Vikas Sharma, http://www.drhomeo.com.

Essentials of Human Anatomy and Physiology, Elaine Marieb, RN, PhD.

Everybody's Guide to Homeopathic Medicine, Stephen Cummings, MD and Dana Ullman, MPH.

Family Health Guide to Homeopathy, Dr. Barry Rose.

Gentle Little Souls: All about the Cell Salts, Miranda Castro, FSHom, *Homeopathy Today* magazine, July/August 2008.

Helios Homeopathy: A Brief Guide to 36 Remedies with Illustrations, http://materiamedica.uk.net.

Homeopathic Cell Salt Remedies, Nigey and Lionel Rolfe.

Homeopathic Clinical Repertory (Third Edition), Robin Murphy, ND.

Homeopathy for Musculoskeletal Healing, Asa Hershoff, ND, DC.

Homeopathic Medical Repertory (third revised edition), Robin Murphy, ND.

Homeopathic Medicine at Home, Maesimund Panos, MD and Jane Heimlich.

Homeopathic Medicine for Children and Infants, Dana Ullman, MPH.

Homeopathic Prescribing, S. Kayne and L. Kayne.

Homeopathic Remedies, Asa Hershoff, ND, DC.

Homeopathic Remedy Guide, Robin Murphy, ND.

Homeopathic Self-Care, Robert Ullman, ND and Judyth Reichenberg-Ullman, ND, MSW.

Homeopathy for Childhood Illnesses, Miranda Castro, FSHom, https://www.mirandacastro.com/homeopathy-for-childhood-illnesses.

Homeopathy for Everyone, http://hpathy.com.

Homeopathy for Pregnancy Birth and Your Baby's First Year, Miranda Castro, FSHom.

Homeopathy Papers, Robert Medhurst, https://hpathy.com/homeopathy-papers.

Lotus Materia Medica (third edition), Robin Murphy, ND.

Materia Medica of Homeopathic Medicines, S.T. Phatak.

Mayo Clinic, www.mayoclinic.com.

National Center for Homeopathy, www.homeopathycenter.org.

Nature's Materia Medica (fourth edition), Robin Murphy, ND.

New Manual of Homeopathic Materia Medica with Repertory, William Boericke.

Nurture Your Inner Athlete with Homeopathic Cell Salts, Tanya Renner, CCH, RSHom (NA), *Homeopathy Today* magazine, Summer 2015.

Pocket Manual of Homoeopathic Materia Medica with Repertory, William Boericke.

Prisma: The Arcana of Materia Medica Illuminated, Frans Vermeulen.

Radar Opus Software, Version 10.

The Biochemic System of Medicine, George W. Carey.

The Companion to Homeopathy, Colin Griffith MCH, RSHom.

The Complete Homeopathy Handbook, Miranda Castro, FSHom.

The Family Guide to Homeopathy, Dr. Andrew Lockie.

The MetaRepertory (fourth edition), Robin Murphy ,ND.

The Organon of the Medical Art (sixth edition), Samuel Hahnemann.

The Parent's Guide to Homeopathy, Shelley Keneipp, MH, DiHom (UK).

The Practical Handbook of Homeopathy, Colin Griffith, MCH, RSHom.

The Savvy Traveler's Guide to Homeopathy and Natural Medicine: Tips to Stay Healthy Wherever You Go, Judyth Reichenberg-Ullman, ND and Robert Ullman, ND.

Vacation Worry-Free with Homeopathic Cell Salts, Tanya Renner, CCH, RSHom (NA), **Homeopathy Today** magazine, Summer 2019.

Vaccine Free Prevention and Treatment of Infectious Contagious Disease with Homeopathy, Kate Birch.

WebMD First Aid, https://www.webmd.com/first-aid/first-aid-a-to-z.

Yasgur's Homeopathic Dictionary and Holistic Health Reference, Jay Yasgur, R.Ph., M.Sc.

Your Natural Medicine Cabinet, Burke Lennihan.

Index

Symbols

B

X

Y

Z